what people are saying...

This is it — this is the real answer to our eating woes! Our American diets are a mess. *If It's Not Food, Don't Eat It!* guides us back to the natural way we were intended to eat. This is not another "fad" diet. It is something every person can use. With this book, the road to better health has finally been clearly paved!
— *Tara Berro, M.S., Sports Physiologist & Trainer - Malibu, CA*

If It's Not Food, Don't Eat It! is a must for every chiropractor's waiting room!"
— *Amy Dusek*, Editor, *Today's Chiropractic* magazine

Kelly Hayford's book serves as the building block to good health by gently and clearly stating the importance of real foods in our fake-food society. It is a timeless recipe for healing and prevention. Everyone in America should read this book over and over again.
— *Dr. Vic Shayne, Clinical Nutritionist – Food Science Researcher*

My sister-in-law gave me a copy of *If It's Not Food, Don't Eat It!* and it has truly changed my life. I could write my own book about all the things I have tried to get rid of the persistent migraines I have experienced every day for nearly three years. This book put an end to all that pain and suffering! I also have so much more patience and I feel like a whole person for the first time in my life.
— *Patrice Jane Orr, Littleton, CO*

What an eye opener! *If It's Not Food, Don't Eat It!* contains great information, is easy to digest, and entertaining as well. I would suggest EVERYONE read this book, it can benefit us all!
— *Carole Handler, Tucson, AZ*

Well done! I am impressed by the comprehensive research contained in *If It's Not Food, Don't Eat It!*, as well as its overall message and timeliness. Most importantly, this book is easy to read and filled with inspiration and practical ways in which anyone, including the novice, can improve their overall health and wellbeing.
— *Dr. John F. Demartini*, Best-selling author of *Count Your Blessings*

My 11 year old son had headaches for most of his life. He would often have to come in from playing to lie down and cry from the pain. Then I started following Kelly's first guideline to *Eating for Health*, "if it's not food, don't eat it!" It was actually not that hard to do. He has not had a headache since. As for me, I feel better than I have felt in a very long time and am getting better every day.
— *Becky Gatlin, Spring, TX*

If It's Not Food ...Don't Eat It!

THE NO-NONSENSE GUIDE TO AN EATING-FOR-HEALTH LIFESTYLE

KELLY HAYFORD, M.A., C.N.C.

Nutrition & Health Coach

Delphic Corner Press
P.O. Box 17394
Boulder, CO 80308-0394
Order Fulfillment: 303.746.8970

To receive a free online newsletter on *Eating for Health* and other tips for maintaining a balanced state of well-being, register directly at website: www.FoodFitnessByPhone.com

Cover Design: Tracy Hayford, Designworks, 209.679.2006
Cover Photos: Don Murray Photography, www.donmurray.com
Graphic Assistance: Carolyn Tate, www.tatedesigngroup.com

Disclaimer: The information contained in this book is for educational purposes only and is not intended to replace or subvert the intervention or participation of a qualified medical professional for diagnosis or disease treatment.

ISBN: 0-9765668-0-x
Library of Congress Control Number: 2005901160

In Memoriam

to my mother

Leora Frances Kemble Hayford,
Thank you for stirring the wind beneath my wings. Fly free now.

Table of Contents

Foreword

At the heart and soul of natural healthcare, and missing from the practice of modern medicine, is nutrition — the foundation of healing, cellular energy, growth and disease prevention. Proper nutrition is a basic, biological need, which is why the title of this book speaks volumes: *If It's Not Food, Don't Eat It*. This is the most direct and life-saving advice of our modern era. But to the uninitiated, this proclamation might sound so simple as to be overlooked as trite advice. After all, why would anyone eat something that's not food? Well, if you're posing such a question, this book will serve and uplift you in unimaginable ways. I only wish such a book had existed when I was first starting out in this field many years ago.

What most people eat in our nation today cannot really be classified as food, or nutritious. Certainly, we have been misled — through persistent, clever and deceptive advertising — to believe that processed, chemical-laden, toxic and artificial substances qualify as food. Advertising has turned our collective cultural perception of food upside-down. In direct contradiction to our biological, cellular needs, we have become a nation fed on foul nutrition, with chemicals being insidiously substituted for nutritious foods. Our chemical, nutrient-deficient daily diets have caused the escalation of disease, suffering and death — even in the face of our so-called "advanced" medical system.

The truth is that modern medicine has lost a lot of its appeal and followers. Dissatisfied with its lack of health-promoting results, our civilization has reached back into the past and revived the philosophy of natural healthcare. Thousands of medical doctors have joined the cause as well, but at the leading edge are advocates like Kelly Hayford who have entered this revitalized industry because it is their passion. They learned, as I have — from personal experience conquering chronic illness — that natural healthcare works without side effects, and it carries the seeds for a happier, healthier, more fulfilling life.

Kelly Hayford, in this life-saving book, teaches us how to regain our health using the most natural, ancient cures known to humankind. Using food as the basis for healing is not only a primal solution to our maladies, it is actually the only avenue of healing recognized by our cells. Eating right heals, yet causes no side effects. This is never true about drugs, which the body considers foreign invaders.

As living, complex, dynamic (always changing) biological beings, real, whole, untainted foods are the only substances meant to be ingested into our delicate, complex bodies. Nature's unadulterated foods resonate within us as they nourish us. All other substances, including drugs, artificial ingredients, and processed (dead) pseudofoods, are injurious to our bodies.

Certainly, as we look around, we notice that our friends and relatives (if not we ourselves) are sick, overweight, dying of cancer, drugged, chronically fatigued or suffering from innumerable health problems. But without our national media recognizing and reporting our escalating national health crisis and the perpetrators of our demise, we fail to understand the enormity of our dilemma. Our national media — newspapers, radio and television networks, which once served to keep us informed of important events, is now used against us to promote that which sickens us instead of that which can rescue us. The media deceive us, motivate us to buy what is injurious to our health, and suppress the proponents of chemical-free solutions to our problems. Our media serves its advertisers, not us its readers, viewers and listeners. This might be good for business, but it's killing us, quite literally.

Fortunately, not all media has been usurped. We still have myriad avenues of life-saving sources. This book, in my opinion as a researcher, ranks among the best. The author shows us that the solution to most health problems is simpler than most people could imagine. Kelly Hayford has the ability and insight — borne of her own personal victory over ill-health — to reconnect us with our natural state. Her health advice is built upon common sense and the power of nature and real foods to heal, prevent illness and perpetuate vitality.

Kelly Hayford bestows upon us, in complete candor, the invaluable paradigm of the Natural Healthcare Revolution: *To overcome our health problems, we must embrace a lifestyle change, not a treatment method.* Natural healthcare resonates with our biological, emotional, mental and spiritual needs. For healing and prevention of disease, there is no substitute for the innate wisdom, power and potential of nature presented in this book.

— Dr. Vic Shayne, PhD - Clinical Nutritionist, Food Science Researcher

Author, *Man Cannot Live on Vitamins Alone, Whole Food Nutrition,* and *Illness Isn't Caused by a Drug Deficiency*

Acknowledgements

Appreciation must first go to my father who encouraged me to write a book since I could first hold a pen. Next, a special thank you to all my initial clients and program participants who encouraged me to write this book in particular. It is you who taught me what you wanted to know, and what I needed to put in this book. And it is for you and all others like you who thirst for a better way to live that this book is written.

Throughout this project I have been blessed with an incredible array of people willing to help. My gratitude goes to Mireya VanAmee, Tara Berro, Susann Shier, O. Frank Turner , Carole Handler, Don Murray, Jude Willhoff, Kirk Slowe, Mary Soliel and Albert Iggi for their help in the developmental and production stages of this book. Thanks for lending me your ears, your eyeballs, your opinions and your skills on so many occasions.

Tracy Hayford and Carolyn Tate cannot be thanked enough for their incredible graphics skills and all the long hours they applied to the creation of the cover for this book. Thank you also to John Martin for your keen editorial skills and enthusiastic support; and to Vic Shayne for writing the foreword, being a willing and knowledgeable resource, and your editorial contributions as well.

Much gratitude to Jackie Sach, Denise Miller, and Dave Monette for believing in this project, and all your support in moving it in the direction of getting it out into the world. A special heartfelt thank you to Gurucharan Singh Khalsa for envisioning the possibility for healing so many years ago, and to Dr. John Demartini for teaching me the value of my voids. To Paul Nordin, no words can adequately convey my appreciation.

And finally, my humbled gratitude goes to that all-powerful and pervasive force that guides us when we let it, to accomplish things and serve in ways we never knew possible.

Introduction

In the introduction to his classic book *Diet & Nutrition*, Dr. Rudolph Ballentine wrote, "Clive McCay, one of the outstanding nutritionists of this century, writing in the 1930's, estimated that in order to keep up with the published literature on nutrition, one would have had to read one article every three minutes during his entire working day of eight hours."

Today, he would probably estimate a tenfold increase given the vast array of information with which we have been inundated in the decades since. And the amount of information seems to just keep growing.

Most everyone would agree that what they eat has an effect on their body and their health. However, everyone seems to be at odds as to what to eat, when to eat it, and how much of it to eat. Although nutritionists and scientists are busy unraveling the mysteries of food and the role it plays in human health and *disease*, each new food substance introduced or theory offered as explanation only seems to add more controversy and more confusion.

No one knows this better than the people who seek out this information in an often desperate attempt to maintain or restore balance and health to their bodies. Despite the confusion (or as a result of it!), millions voraciously devour whatever they can on the topic of diet and nutrition in an effort to lose weight, get relief from symptoms, or cure what ails them.

I discovered long ago that everyone has a different definition of "balanced diet," "in moderation," and what's healthy and what's not when it comes to food. And that often, those definitions vary widely.

The guidelines presented here are the product of my own experiences that began as a search for symptomatic relief and later became a search for a way to elude potentially life-threatening illness. I, like many others, learned the hard way that eating for health is necessary to have a desired quality of life, and sometimes to have a life at all.

The Beginning

Yoga Retreat
Ram Das Puri, New Mexico - June, 1989

A ribbon of steam flavored with Indian spices drifted through the screen door from the large pots cooking in the community kitchen, carrying with it the promise of a savory dinner to come. People gathered under the sparse shade of a lone tree in the middle of an otherwise vast expanse of hot summer sun, slurping up pieces of freshly cut watermelon.

In between propelling watermelon seeds, my friend beckoned for me to have a piece. Both hands full, he pointed with his elbow to the large platter of brightly colored fruit as he nodded at me. "Come on, have some. It's really sweet," he encouraged.

When my telltale eyes met his, his expression shifted as he remembered my plight. My digestion and overall health had degenerated to such a degree that my symptoms and syndromes were too many to list, and there was very little food I could eat. Plain steamed zucchini and rice were my private sustenance. In social situations, I had learned to hold in my personal anguish and reply to such offers of culinary delight with a polite, "No, thank you. I don't care for any right now." It had served me well in many situations. No one even suspected the waves of despair that flowed through me in those moments.

But this moment was different. After so many years, each one progressively worse, my despair had reached an all time low. Attempts to eradicate my declining condition had been futile. Medical doctors had made things worse and natural healthcare practitioners, one after the other, all reached a point when they silently shrugged their shoulders and gave up, leaving me with a little less hope each time.

And now, there I stood. An inner desperation for understanding that bordered on hopelessness welled up inside of me. Over the previous few days, having stretched my weak, ailing body into yogic postures and meditated for hours on end, I spoke out at a new level of vulnerability. In a quiet voice heavy with despair I queried, as if to the Creator itself, "Will I ever be well again? I just want to know why this is happening to me."

At that moment a warm gust of wind blew up a swirl of dust, as happens at that magical mountain retreat. And my friend, who I had forgotten was standing there, replied in an all-knowing voice unlike his own, "Yes, you will be well again. You will learn. And then you will teach others and help them to be well, too."

Section One

the foundation

Building an Eating Lifestyle Based on Solid Ground

When Betty first came to me she was in constant pain. She was taking seven different medications, had severe osteoarthritis, could barely walk, and had to catheterize herself daily. She had heard that making certain dietary changes could be beneficial to her health, and that there were natural herbs and supplements that might be helpful as well. But she didn't know much about it and because her condition was so severe, she doubted that such an approach could actually do anything for *her*. In addition, her healthcare plan did not cover such expenses. Betty came to me only because the price of her medications was increasing to a level she could no longer afford, and her persistent friend had insisted.

Upon reviewing her food diary, a requirement for all incoming clients, I asked Betty if any of her doctors had ever inquired about her diet or given her any dietary guidelines. She told me that none had ever asked. Her food diary revealed a *Standard American Diet (SAD)*. It looked like something an average American might be eating, and that was the problem.

Betty was skeptical about my recommendations at first, but I kept encouraging her to give them a try. "Trust me," I would say, "the results will convince you." Out of desperation she reluctantly followed my advice, and was delighted, when in just a few short weeks, she was able to go off four of her medications, became virtually pain-free, could walk without using her walker, had lost a few pounds, and was generally beginning to feel much better. In addition, Betty's latest cholesterol test results were below what they had been when she was taking cholesterol-lowering medication.

What did Betty do to achieve such dramatic improvements in her health in such a short period of time? It might surprise you to know that Betty didn't cut or count calories or carbohydrates or fat, go on a special diet, deprive herself of favorite foods, take a special pill or herbal formula, undergo hypnosis, or start an intensive workout program. She simply made the switch from the low-quality, chemical-laden processed food brands she had been eating for years to higher quality, additive-free natural food brands of the same foods. She also began to include a small amount of whole, fresh, natural foods, primarily a couple of fresh fruits or vegetables, into her diet each day.

How can this be so? This is so because the most popular brands of processed, packaged chemical-laden foods (pseudofoods) so widely consumed today are injurious to the body. In fact, poor eating habits characterized by the regular consumption of these fake foods, saturated with refined sugar, sodium, unhealthy fats, and toxic chemicals, are the greatest weapon of mass destruction the world has ever known. Not a weapon in the usual sense, but a weapon nonetheless, as a result of the devastation it is causing, as Betty was experiencing. But Betty isn't the only one suffering.

As a result of the regular consumption of low-quality nutrient-deficient food, our nation has recently entered into the beginning stages of a major health crisis; a health crisis of such magnitude that it has the potential to change life in America as we know it. This poor eating syndrome is the most insidious kind of weapon of mass destruction because, aside from the obvious diet-related conditions such as heart disease, diabetes, and obesity, few people realize that it is the root cause of *all* chronic *dis*-ease. I use the term *dis*-ease as it encompasses not only established diseases, but any symptoms or conditions people experience that cause their bodies or minds to become ill at ease.

---

the standard american diet

In America between 1980-1997, the average per capita consumption of major food commodities per person, per year included:

- 111 lbs. red meat	- 580 lbs. dairy products
- 29 lbs. ice cream	- 53 gallons soft drinks
- 66 lbs. fats and oils	- 39 gallons alcohol
- 150 lbs. wheat	- 24 gallons coffee
- 154 lbs. sugar	

U.S. Census Bureau, *Statistical Abstract 1999*

Betty is just one of millions who are unaware of the chronic *dis*-ease her *Standard American Diet* was causing. Fortunately, by making a few small changes, she was able to begin to turn her health around. The way we eat in our modern post-industrialized society is so far out of balance from what nature intended that when people like Betty begin to restore that balance by even marginally eating in a way that nature *did* intend, dramatic results occur. Many, if not all, of the symptoms — which are merely warning signals from the body that we're doing something wrong — diminish significantly or completely go away. Although Betty might never be able to completely reverse some of her *dis*-eases as they have progressed too far, she has been able to get relief from many of them, more relief than what any drugs or medical procedures had provided in the past. As she continues to eat for health at higher and higher levels, she will bring her state of health and well-being to higher and higher levels as well.

why didn't anyone tell me?

"It's really amazing the results I'm getting and how easy it's been," Betty told me during a phone consultation we had a few weeks later. "I can't believe how much better I feel. I never would have imagined this was possible." Her voice became somber, as she further reflected, "Why didn't anyone tell me? Why didn't I know this before? Things just kept getting worse and worse. If only I had known that such simple changes in my diet could make such a big difference, I wouldn't have had to suffer so much, for so long."

Her words sounded all too familiar. They were almost the exact words that I had muttered to myself many times years ago, as I began to discover the relationship between the food I ate and my declining health. I just couldn't figure out why no one had told me and why those around me hadn't known either. Why was it such a mystery? The more I learned, the more it seemed that what I was learning should be common sense.

Others who have experienced dramatic results from *Eating for Health*, as I call it, have expressed these same sentiments, sentiments that arose from their firsthand discovery of the ravages our popular food culture was having on their health.

building a new foundation

Why have poor eating habits become the norm rather than the exception for the overwhelming majority of people in this country? Why have we as a society increasingly lost sight of the value of eating nutritious foods for the preservation of our health and well-being? That's what *Section One* is all about.

The first chapter unravels the origins of our current unhealthy food climate, including an exposé on the antics of the food industry in concert with the media, as well as a startling look at how poor quality, processed foods are robbing America of its health on a grand scale. Without this awareness and understanding, efforts to progress along healthier lines are frequently hindered. The remaining two chapters of *Section One* focus on building a new foundation for creating a healthier eating lifestyle based on the concepts of *Eating for Health;* the most important concept of which became the title of this book: *if it's not food don't eat it.*

At its very core, *Eating for Health* is about putting your health at the forefront of your mind when making food choices. It is not a fad or a special diet. It is a return to the natural way of eating that existed before our food culture became dominated by an urban landscape and the profit-minded mega-pseudofood industry, with a little refinement, a little personalization, and a little allowance for modern living.

When applied consistently over time, *Eating for Health* brings about what many refer to as amazing results. Although once you fully understand the relationship between diet and *dis*-ease, these amazing results will seem more like common sense. Quite often people experience immediate results as well. It is miraculous what the body can do when it is given the right fuel — energy is restored, excess weight is shed, body systems are regenerated, *dis*-ease is reversed, and nagging symptoms disappear. Of course everyone is different and will therefore experience different results depending on a variety of factors, such as present and past health conditions, age, weight, current diet and levels of exercise. However, given time, those who consistently follow the concepts put forth in this book will reap beneficial results, no matter what condition they were in when they began.

As with anything, what you put into it will determine what you get out of it. And therein lies the challenge. After a lifetime of eating in a habitual manner, it is difficult to break free and begin anew. Many people don't know where or how to begin. Because this task might seem daunting, many people keep putting it off or flip-flopping back and forth and end up feeling defeated.

The pages ahead will help you enormously in simplifying this task of eating healthier and actually enjoy doing it. In this section you will learn five simple guidelines and four levels of *Eating for Health* designed to make it easy for you to choose foods that are supportive and nourishing for the human body in general, and for your individual body specifically. Subsequent sections offer practical tools, recipes, and most importantly, strategies for dealing with the social and mental gymnastics that do so much to undermine our food choices and behavior. The next chapter, in particular, will generate powerful motivation for you to start *Eating for Health* now, and make it a lifetime habit.

Chapter One 🍎

why me, why now?

Our Popular Food Culture & The Toll It's Taking on Our Health

Most people first become interested in improving their diet because they want to lose weight. I first became interested for other reasons. After college I served as a Peace Corps volunteer in Morocco and became a host to a variety of microbial critters that left me with chronic dysentery for most of my service. A couple of years later, I was still having digestive and eliminative disturbances that included bouts of diarrhea that alternated with constipation. Although a nuisance, these were private matters I could deal with. An associated problem of a gaseous nature, however, became increasingly hard to keep to myself. It was this problem, and the fact that no antacid, no herbal formula, no charcoal tablet, not even Beano provided any relief, that launched my strongest desire to learn more about food and its effect on bodily functions. Especially after the frequency and severity of this problem pinnacled into one of the most embarrassing moments of my life.

There is only one corner of the universe that you can be certain of improving and that's your own self.

Aldous Huxley

It happened one afternoon while teaching math to fourth graders at a Catholic elementary school. Up until that day, I had managed to keep this problem under wraps by discretely slipping out into the empty hallway for a moment of relief. However, on this particular day I was caught off guard.

As the familiar feeling of growing pressure arose, panic ensued as I realized I was standing at the back of the room between two rows of desks, farthest from the door and closest to the children. My first inclination was to try to make it to the door, but one step forward warned me that this would only increase the estimated time of arrival. So I did the only thing I could. I stood as still as possible, clenched every muscle possible, and silently prayed to every Saint possible, all the while continuing my geometric discourse on right angles and the hypotenuse as nonchalantly as possible, so as not to draw attention to what was preparing to make itself known. But try as I might to stop it, a silent but deadly one, as the children would say, won out.

What now? I thought to myself. It would surely not go unnoticed. This growing little problem was actually bigger than average. So big, that nobody in their right mind would have wanted to stake a claim to it, especially not the teacher. So, that's exactly what I decided to do, maintain my dignity through silent denial and let the blame fall where it may.

I put this desperate plan into action by casually strolling down the aisle distancing myself from the scene of the crime, leaving behind a chorus of accusations and pointing fingers.

"*Eeew*, gross, you farted!"

"I did not, you did!"

"It wasn't me, it was *him*!"

This childish chorus convinced me that my cowardly maneuver had been a success. Then all of a sudden I heard a little boy exclaim in what was intended to be a whisper, "It was Ms. Hayford!" — which set off a chatter of disbelief that soon turned into a confirmation of uncontrollable giggles.

I was mortified.

After this incident I became desperate to resolve this annoying problem that was not only causing me great internal discomfort, but was also beginning to cost me the respect of those around me. Because I had tried every generally recommended protocol, I was forced to explore other alternatives, the most obvious of which involved my diet. But I didn't know this at first. Because my problems started, for the most part, during and after my stint in Morocco and because no doctor had ever indicated diet as a solution, I didn't think that what I was eating was the

> You grow up the day you have the first real laugh –
> at yourself.
>
> Ethel Barrymore

issue or that making changes would make any sizeable difference. That's where I was wrong.

food matters

In fact, that's where most people faced with nagging symptoms and *dis*-eases go wrong. They mistakenly believe, as Betty and I had initially, that their particular symptoms or *dis*-eases are not related to the food they eat, but rather are hereditary or the result of some kind of virus, bacteria, or mysterious disease. As you will soon learn, your health is *always* related to and affected by the food you eat. For example, science is now discovering that much of what was once considered hereditary is actually a result of the perpetuation of poor eating and lifestyle habits. Much of what has become *culturally* acceptable to eat is *not* acceptable to the human body. That's why these symptoms and *dis*-eases of the body develop in the first place. They are our bodies' way of telling us that what we're eating or doing in our lives is not working.

Inspired by the success stories of others, new health-related information being released, and the failure of medical and similar approaches aimed at treating the symptoms rather than eliminating the causes, an increasing number of people are becoming aware of this relationship between diet and *dis*-ease and taking measures to revamp their diets. For those of you who are overweight or are experiencing other health challenges and can relate to Betty's or my story, the answer to the question of *Why Me, Why Now?* when it comes to *Eating for Health*, is probably becoming clear, if it wasn't already. To others, it may not be clear —yet.

Many people may not currently be having symptoms and might be feeling pretty good, believing that they are either doing the right thing, or believing that what they are doing is not affecting their health. For those of you who fit this description, you may not feel compelled to eat for health at this stage, but that does not mean there is any less *reason* for you to do so.

Symptoms are the last thing to show up and the first thing to disappear. Just because someone is not currently experiencing any adverse symptoms or *dis*-eases, it doesn't mean that there may not be some in the works, no matter what their age. Many people knowingly continue unhealthy eating habits because they *feel* O.K., not realizing that diseases can simmer in the body long

> Nutrition directly affects growth, development, reproduction, well-being and an individual's physical and mental condition.
>
> Health depends upon nutrition more than on any other single factor.
>
> Dr. William Sebrell

before any symptoms appear. Think of people who are habitual smokers. They are running toxic *dis*-ease-causing agents through their bodies multiple times a day, every day. Even though they may not currently have smoker's cough or have been diagnosed with emphysema or lung cancer, they are still consistently causing a great deal of damage to their bodies. Eventually it will catch up with them in one form or another.

The same is true of habitually poor eaters. Besides missing out on the vital nutrients that quality foods provide, they are running toxic *dis*-ease-causing foods through their bodies every day, often multiple times a day. Although they may not currently have heart disease, diabetes, or cancer (or at least have not yet been diagnosed with anything), they are still consistently causing a great deal of damage to their bodies. This will eventually catch up to them in one form or another, if not in the form of a catastrophic disease, most certainly in the form of a compromised quality of life.

Which leads us to another set of people who may believe that they *are* eating healthfully, but who may be surprised to learn that, in fact, they are not. One of the biggest challenges facing America today is that many, many people do not *realize* that they are eating poorly. After all, they're eating what everyone else is eating, and there's a big clue right there. If someone is eating what has come to be known as the *Standard American Diet* — basically, what everyone else is eating these days — just like the habitual smoker, they are headed for trouble.

Much of what I learned over the course of my own healing journey helps answer the question, "Why didn't anyone tell me?" The rest is information I discovered when I first began doing public speaking and teaching a program called *Eating for Health*.

Having been involved in natural health care for many years, I was aware that conditions in America were somewhat bleak when it came to health. However, I never imagined that the state of health in this country was as bad as it is until I started collecting statistics and putting them together. Quite frankly, I find dietary and health-related statistics in America today to be alarming and disturbing. Ever since, I have felt a moral obligation to make other people aware of what's going on. My guess is that because I was not aware of the gravity of the situation, most other people probably are not aware as well. And if they were, they

The laws of health are inexorable; we see people going down and out in their prime of life because no attention is paid to them.

Paul C. Bragg

might be more motivated to make changes in their current eating and lifestyle habits.

if only I had known...

I remember my mother telling me that back in the early fifties when she started smoking as a teen, it was the popular thing to do and they were completely unaware of the tremendous health risks involved. It wasn't until years later that the Surgeon General stamped his warning on the side of every tobacco pack — after she was already hooked on cigarettes, a habit that would eventually cost her a lung. Throughout my childhood, as my mother struggled to free herself of this insidious habit, she frequently expressed how much she wished she had known from the outset the stranglehold and potentially devastating health consequences of smoking. If she had, she never would have started in the first place. Reminiscent of the sentiments expressed by Betty, myself and countless others with regard to the potentially devastating health consequences of eating the *Standard American Diet*, she repeatedly lamented, "If only I had known..."

> Knowledge is not an endless cycle, but an upward reaching spiral.
>
> Emmet Fox

These words, ringing in my ears from so many different voices, are what prompted me to compile a set of what I call *Scary Statistics* to inform people about the tremendous decline in health standards that has emerged as a result of the prolonged poor eating habits of the majority of people in America. I shared it for the first time by reading it aloud at an *Eating-for-Health* program. A few weeks later, one of the participants, named Joanie, sent me a beautiful note.

Joanie was less than enthusiastic about attending the class initially (more accurately, she was dragged there by a health-conscious friend who was increasingly concerned about the way she ate). She was a young woman in her late twenties who confessed to the group that she ate fast-food meals daily, sometimes twice a day, and the rest of the time indulged in frozen entrees and junk foods, including two to three caffeine- and sugar-packed soft drinks a day. She had never cooked a regular meal, even though she had been on her own for several years now with a husband and a small child. She admitted that she was probably one of the worst eaters she knew, but really didn't see any reason to make any changes because, except for an extra ten pounds she wouldn't mind losing, she didn't see any problem with what she was doing. That was, up until she became aware of the *Scary Statistics* and other information I presented in the program, which later inspired her to write me the thank you note.

In the note, she told me that she'd had no idea of the potential harm she was causing herself, and that no one else had ever been successful in motivating her to make dietary changes until this program. She wanted to thank me for sharing this information and *scaring* her into making healthful changes in the way she ate. I was grateful to have reduced by at least one, the number of people who might one day have come to lament, if only I had known. But I also felt awkward about her use of the phrase *"scared* me into making changes" and reflected on using this as an approach.

My reflection confirmed that I was doing the right thing. It made me realize that making people aware of *Scary Statistics* in an effort to inspire them to make changes in their diet and lifestyle, is no different from a mother slapping the hand of her child aiming to stick its finger in a light socket. Tough love is sometimes in order, especially when complacency has taken over. Like the mother doing the hand slapping, it is not popular to tell people things they don't want to hear. However unpleasant it might be, sharing the *Scary Statistics* can be very useful.

Once made aware of what is going on in our country today and how we got here, and the unconscious influence it has had on them as individuals, I have watched people make lasting changes in their diet and lifestyle habits that they had struggled with for years or had never had the courage or impetus to do before. Without fail, these same people express that they wish they had started *Eating for Health* long before, because since they have, they have either lost weight, increased their energy, or alleviated symptoms. In general they feel so much better. They also express that the overall quality of *every* area of their lives has improved and making changes was much easier than they had imagined.

Before reading through the *Scary Statistics*, it is important to realize that although some might disagree as to the exact numbers, everyone does agree that diet plays a significant role in preventing disease, as well as in assisting with any current conditions. Please keep this *Encouraging Statistic* in mind as you read through the *Scary Statistics* that follow:

Do not waste worry. If you're going to worry, worry well.

Put that energy to good use, aim it at an answer.

Don't forget: nothing diminishes anxiety faster than action.

Walter Anderson

encouraging statistic

- *60-90% of chronic, degenerative disease can be prevented by diet and lifestyle.*

Remembering this *Encouraging Statistic* will help you maintain a sense of hope and perspective as you read through the following *Scary Statistics*, which, unless otherwise indicated, have been taken from recent reports by the *Centers for Disease Control, The American Heart Association* and *The American Cancer Society.*

I titled them *Scary Statistics* for a reason. If, while reading through them, you find yourself feeling a little uncomfortable, don't be surprised. Resist the human tendency to go into denial when hit with unpleasant news, however, because denial about the current state of things is a big part of the problem. In other words, don't get depressed and immerse yourself in a gallon of double-fudge ice cream figuring *what's the use?* Just take a few deep breaths and keep reading. Remember the *Encouraging Statistic* above, and that the rest of this book is filled with practical information to help you and your loved ones significantly reduce the risks of chronic *dis*-ease and reverse those already acquired by making *Eating for Health* a daily reality. Based on consistent feedback I receive, I promise you that armed with this valuable know-how, which many of you may not have had during unsuccessful attempts in the past, *Eating for Health* will be much easier and more pleasant than you may think.

The following *Scary Statistics* are a representative sample of some of the most frequently occurring and debilitating conditions and chronic diseases plaguing America today that are inextricably linked to diet and lifestyle. They do not include the many other ailments, such as arthritis, sinusitis, depression, digestive disorders, osteoporosis, Alzheimer's, ADD and ADHD that also plague the population of this country, and that also have undeniable links to nutrition. In fact, it is rare to have a *dis*-ease of the human body or mind that is *not* somehow linked to nutrition. So, with the intention of further reducing the number of people who might otherwise have someday lamented, "If only I had known…" and to motivate those who already do know, here is a selection of…

> Remember always, you are punished by your bad habits of living, not for them, but by them!
>
> Paul C. Bragg

scary statistics

weight:

- 64% of the people in America are overweight — the highest percentage of any country in the world.
- Of those, 30% are classified as obese.
- The rate of obesity has doubled for children and tripled for teenagers in the last 20 years.
- In addition to a significantly higher risk for many health problems and chronic diseases, overweight people have a 45% higher risk of developing many cancers.

We are very conservative when it comes to health and very liberal when it comes to disease.

Gary Null

specific chronic diseases

Chronic diseases are defined as illnesses that are prolonged, do not resolve spontaneously, are rarely cured completely and *are preventable.*

heart disease

- Heart disease is the number one cause of death in America.
- Cardiovascular diseases account for more than 40% of all deaths in the United States.
- Women comprise more than half of the people who die each year of cardiovascular disease.
- At least 58 million Americans have some form of cardiovascular disease, including high blood pressure.

diabetes

- 18 million people in America have diabetes — 6 million don't know they have it. Another 41 million have pre-diabetes, and most of them don't know they have it.
- Type 2, or adult diabetes, which has been considered until recently a disease of aging normally striking adults over 50, is now afflicting pre-teens and teens in alarming numbers.

- There was a 70% increase in adult diabetes for people between the ages of 30-39 from 1990-1998.

- The overall increase in adult diabetes was 33% between 1990-1998.

- Diabetes is the #1 cause of blindness, kidney failure and amputations. Each year, among people with diabetes:

    ~ *12,000-24,000 become blind due to diabetic eye disease*

    ~ *more than 100,000 experience kidney failure*

    ~ *86,000 undergo lower-extremity amputations*

cancer

- One out of every 2.5 people will develop some form of cancer in their lifetime — that's almost half the population.

- Over the next 5 years, cancer is predicted to surpass heart disease as the number one cause of death.

- 53% of Americans believe that most cancers are the result of genetic factors, while in reality only 5-10% of most types of cancer result from genetic factors.

- Since 1973, the overall cancer rate has increased by 40%.

note: A very recent study indicates that overall cancer rates have declined by 0.8% between 1990-1997. This is miniscule compared to the enormous increase over the last 30 years and says nothing about the many individual cancer rates that have skyrocketed.

chronic disease in general

- More than 90 million Americans live with chronic illnesses.

- Chronic diseases account for one-third of the years of potential life lost before age 65.

- Poor nutrition and lack of physical exercise are associated with 300,000 deaths each year, factors that

nutrition & cancer

According to Sir Richard Doll, M.D. a leading cancer researcher at Oxford University in England, upwards of 70% of all cancer cases are probably related to diet. (Harvard estimates it to be 50%.)

American Cancer Society

The National Cancer Institute recommends 5 servings per day of fruits and vegetables, but only 9% of the population, and only 20% of "gatekeeper" family physicians say they consume the daily 5 servings.

Nutrition Action Healthletter

84% of cancer patients do not eat cruciferous vegetables, the most recommended food for preventing and fighting cancer. 82% do not get adequate amounts of fiber for disease prevention.

Patrick Quillin,
Beating Cancer with Nutrition

may soon overtake tobacco use as the leading cause of death.

• Chronic diseases account for 70% of all deaths in the United States.

It is important to remember that the diseases mentioned above are chronic *degenerative* diseases. People don't just suddenly have a heart attack or suddenly "get" cancer or Type 2 diabetes. These are diseases that develop in the body over a number of years. Tragically, they are not due to circumstances beyond someone's control. They are self-inflicted conditions. Given the high percentage of deaths attributed to chronic diseases caused by diet and lifestyle, we are in an era where the majority of people in this country are literally, and frequently unknowingly, committing a prolonged rendition of socially-sanctioned suicide.

If 70% of deaths in America were the result of accidents, terrorist activity, or infectious diseases, people would be storming government offices demanding that action be taken at a government level to eradicate the problem. Instead, a tremendous number of individuals and families are playing out what has become a culturally accepted epidemic of *preventable* chronic disease in the privacy of their own homes, living quiet lives of desperation tending to *dis*-eases. These statistics aren't just numbers on a page, these are people we see every day — they are our aunts and uncles, our parents and grandparents, our children, our friends, ourselves.

The preceding statistics only provide a profile for those who already *have* the above-mentioned chronic diseases. The overall picture of things is actually much worse when you consider the many other chronic diseases not listed, not to mention the perils associated with the degenerative process. Plagued with a multitude of symptoms, syndromes, and discomforts, as their bodies progressively deteriorate, most people live a sub-standard quality of life during the years leading up to an established chronic disease. They suffer from sinus troubles, allergies, arthritis, chronic fatigue, lowered immune function, headaches, indigestion, constipation, high blood pressure and the list goes on.

Just look at all the people around you who are either sick, fat, tired, or all of the above. And this is increasing dramatically

As for me, except for an occasional heart attack, I feel as young as I ever did.

Robert Benchley

among people at progressively younger ages. *A 70% increase in Type 2 diabetes over an 8 year period among those between the ages of 30-39* — now, that's truly a scary statistic. Especially when you consider that Type 2 diabetes has always been classified, up until very recently, as a disease of aging. Most people in our country today are rapidly aging and degenerating well before their time. While the average lifespan in the industrialized world has steadily increased, the quality of life has simultaneously declined.

In light of the *Encouraging Statistic* above, that an estimated 60-90% of chronic disease is preventable, and the fact that in a recent study, 97% of the adults polled listed maintaining good physical health as the number one most important thing in their lives, it may seem a bit puzzling why this epidemic of preventable *dis*-ease is occurring in this country, and spreading throughout the world. There are multiple factors to consider when unraveling this puzzling phenomenon. Environmental factors, smoking and lack of physical exercise, all play a role in the declining state of health. However, poor nutrition is *the* most significant factor contributing to poor health for the vast majority of people in America today, and a growing number of other countries.

It is mind boggling to think that enormous amounts of time and money are being dedicated to finding *cures* for chronic, degenerative *dis*-eases, when the very *causes* are in our kitchens and restaurants. As a society, we are literally digging our graves with our forks. The primary reasons for this have to do with the current cultural belief systems that have developed over the last couple of generations; cultural belief systems that have become ingrained in each of us and greatly influence the food and lifestyle choices the majority of us make, usually without consciously thinking about or being aware of the short and long term ramifications. Those who are aware of their poor nutritional habits and continue them anyway, often do so because they feel powerless to do anything about them.

The first step toward becoming empowered to make changes in this arena of perpetual poor eating and subsequent epidemic of chronic *dis*-ease, is to have a greater understanding of our current popular food culture and how it all came to be.

It's no longer a question of staying healthy.

It's a question of finding a sickness you like.

Jackie Mason

diet, *dis*-ease & denial

Our modern culture has lost sight of the wisdom of the ages and Mother Nature when it comes to what we feed our bodies, and has also come to greatly diminish the impact of diet on our health. The resulting cultural moré is to throw caution to the wind when it comes to what we eat, while upholding physicians and the medical field as the first line of defense when it comes to eradicating any mental or physical *dis*-ease. It is undeniable that *preventing dis*-eases is always much better and much less expensive than treating them, but we have lost sight of this wisdom as well.

One of the best analogies I know to illustrate how we as a culture have come to think about health and the food we eat uses the automobile as a metaphor for the human body, which is very poignant, given that our body is the vehicle in which we go through life. It goes something like this:

Imagine that Mr. Whitless has just bought a new car. He's been filling it up with a new kind of fuel. Unlike gas originally used to fuel cars, this fuel has gone through so many different processes that it no longer even resembles the original gas. In addition, it is filled with toxic chemical preservatives, artificial colorings, flavor enhancers, artificial sweeteners, and the like -- none of which were ever meant to go in a car, and in fact, have been proven to be detrimental to its function.

At first, Mr. Whitless' new auto begins to cough, spit and sputter. Then it becomes difficult to start and keep going. After a short time various parts start to break down. So, Mr. Whitless starts taking the car to the mechanic. Each time the mechanic asks what the symptoms are, and then with his mechanical expertise, he goes about identifying the dysfunctional or degenerated parts and repairs or replaces them. He then sends Mr. Whitless on his way; never checking to see what Mr. Whitless is filling his tank with or merely giving the matter lip service with passing comments, such as, "Now be sure you're fillin' 'er up with good gas and oil." To which Mr. Whitless nods in agreement, believing that this is what he's doing. After all, the gas he's using is the latest thing and everyone he knows is using it as well.

As a third party observer to this scenario, any average person who knew anything about cars would think this was absurd and that Mr. Whitless had a most suitable name. They

It's strange that some men will drink and eat anything put before them, but check very carefully the oil put in their car.

Paul Bragg

Almost every human malady is connected, either by highway or byway, with the stomach.

Sir Francis Head

would also be chomping at the bit to let Mr. Whitless and his mechanic know the simple truth of the situation, that his new car needed to be given pure, unadulterated gasoline and oil that was appropriate for its particular needs. (Sound a little like any natural health food enthusiasts you might know?)

Hopefully, by now you are beginning to see the parallels between this parable and what is currently going on with regard to our bodies. We have, in this country and increasingly in many other developed countries, come to a place of denial about the role food plays in our health and what the real needs of our bodies are. Glitzy advertising from food manufacturer's and fast-food chains, as well as our acclimated taste buds, have taken control when it comes to what we eat, overruling common sense itself. Never underestimate the power of what you eat and the effect it has on your body. There is a reason the natural foods industry is one of the fastest growing industries in the world today — eating healthy food works. If Mr. Whitless started giving his car the proper fuel, don't you think it would start running better and have less parts breaking down?

An accompanying belief has to do with how we perceive current standards of health in America. Because for many decades our country enjoyed a high standard of health relative to the rest of the world, many people believe that we still do. As a result, many people have adopted a cavalier attitude when it comes to taking adequate care of themselves, especially with regard to what they eat. The truth is that the United States ranks low when it comes to health standards, very low. At the turn of the century America ranked number one in health among the major industrialized nations. In contrast, according to a recent World Health Organization report, today the average ranking of 13 countries are as follows: Japan, Sweden, Canada, France, Australia, Spain, Finland, Netherlands, U.K., Denmark, Belgium, U.S., and Germany. In other words, we come in 12th in a line of 13 industrialized countries when it comes to overall health standards.

This myth of high standards of health goes hand-in-hand with how we, as a society, view modern medicine. Before the advent of modern technology, people were more conscientious about their eating and lifestyle habits. Lacking the reassurance that the latest medical procedure was available to bail them out if

> The great enemy of truth is very often not the lie - deliberate, contrived, and dishonest – but the myth – persistent, persuasive, and unrealistic.
>
> John F. Kennedy

things got bad, they were afraid to get sick and generally speaking, took better care of themselves. There is a laissez-faire attitude toward taking care of oneself that has developed over the last few decades that is due in part to the belief that if you get sick, modern medicine will take care of you.

This belief has been fostered by massive ad campaigns by the pharmaceutical and over-the-counter drug companies, to the degree that people immediately think of, or suggest to one another, a popular brand of drug to take at the mere mention of a symptom. We have literally come to translate a headache, stomachache, pain or any other *dis*-ease in the body as a need for aspirin, antacids, ibuprofen, or some other drug, rather than as a need to make better food choices, reduce our stress level or something else we could have done to prevent the condition in the first place.

Although the modern medical field deserves to be heralded for its advances and contributions in the treatment of acute trauma, it is not without its problems and limitations. The *Scary Statistics* clearly make a statement about its inability to address chronic, degenerative *dis*-ease. And statistics taken from an article published in the July, 2000 issue of the Journal of the American Medical Association (J.A.M.A.), which are also pretty scary statistics, speak to some of the problems and risks involved when relying on the medical field for health care. This article identifies medical errors as the 3rd leading cause of death in America (heart disease being first and cancer second). It states that over 250,000 Americans die per year as a result of iatrogenic (physician induced) causes. The death toll broken down is as follows:

- *12,000 - die from unnecessary surgeries.*

- *7,000 - die from medication errors in hospitals.*

- *20,000 - die from other errors in hospitals.*

- *80,000 - die from infections they get in the hospital.*

- *106,000 - die from adverse effects of medications.*

This only accounts for those incidents that were reported, and says nothing about the numbers of people who suffer from disabilities and various other complications resulting from

> In spite of all the bravura and ballyhoo about our "great medical progress," when, in the enlightened future, the true medical history will be written, the twentieth century will be known as the dark ages of the healing art.
>
> Paavo Airola,
> How to Get Well

medical mishaps. For those who throw caution to the wind when it comes to the notion of prevention, believing that as Americans we enjoy a high standard of health, and that if you do get sick, modern medicine is going to take care of you, this data is as an eye-opener. This issue of medical misdeeds has claimed much media attention recently and is a reminder to all of us that ultimately health care is self-care.

I do not want in any way to discount or diminish the many amazing technological feats the medical community is now able to perform. What is available to us in the arena of acute trauma care is nothing short of miraculous. When it comes to degenerative *disease*, however, although modern medicine can be very effective in addressing acute situations related to chronic conditions, in the long run it falls short, and has been unable to successfully turn things around in this arena. Realistically though, how can doctors be expected to do what only people can do for themselves, such as eating right, exercising, and managing stress? There is no surgery, drug or procedure that can do what is your responsibility to do. The same is true of natural therapies, such as acupuncture, herbs, and other supplements. We will explore the topic of self-care further, but first, let's look to history and continue to explore how these and other modern belief systems arose.

> If mankind profits from its mistakes, we have a glorious future ahead of us!
>
> Unknown

fast food for a fast nation

The industrial age drove massive numbers of people to urban areas and marked the beginning of a whole new chapter in food production and distribution. This burgeoning urbanized environment required that enormous amounts of food be brought in from the outlying hinterlands. Over the years, the ever-increasing demand for cheap, abundant food led to the development of what we know today as the food manufacturing industry and high-tech agribusiness. But the demand for cheap abundant food wasn't enough for the post-industrialized era. It demanded that food be made available *fast* and *tasty* as well; thus, the birth of the fast-food industry in the 1960's. Fueled by the entry of women into the workforce in record numbers, fast food is now one of the largest segments of the overall food industry. The resultant combination of agribusiness, processed food manufacturing and the fast-food industry has completely

adulterated food

Although many additives are used in very small amounts, it has been estimated that the average American consumes about five pounds of food additives per year. If you include sugar - the food industry's most used additive - the number jumps to 135 pounds a year.

Prescription for Nutritional Healing

70% of all antibiotic drugs in the U.S. are being fed to farm animals as growth promoters or production aids, reducing the effectiveness of these drugs in humans and increasing the spread of resistant bacteria. This practice is now starting to be banned in Europe.

Union of Concerned Scientists

No milk available on the market today, in any part of the United States, is free of pesticide residues.

U.S. Congressional Hearing

reformulated and adulterated what the majority of post-industrialized populations have come to know as food.

The high-tech agricultural business dramatically added a whole new dimension to the meats, fish and fresh produce we ate in the past with the introduction of pesticides, herbicides, ripening and coloring agents, growth-hormones, antibiotics, genetically modified organisms (GMOs), and the like. Add to all this, the extensive processing and additives (i.e. preservatives, refined sugars, artificial sweeteners, colorings, flavorings, anti-caking agents, flavor enhancers, etc.) the food manufacturers and fast-food industry then throw into the mix, and you've got something the likes of which no humans have ever consumed before. A hundred years ago, the overwhelming majority of what makes up the *Standard American Diet* today literally did not exist. Most of the food being consumed today has been so drastically altered that it can no longer be considered *real* food, but has been effectively rendered pseudofood or fake-food items.

Because these fake-food items have been made widely available and popularized over the last few decades, it has become normal for people to eat them regularly and consider them acceptable food. For many, it is the only thing they eat. While it may have become *normal* to eat pseudofood rather than real food, it is certainly not *natural* or healthy to consume these products, as evidenced by the far-reaching deleterious health consequences their introduction has had. Rampant consumption of high-fat-sugar-sodium content foods and chemical-laden pseudofoods on a massive scale has led to tremendous numbers of people being sick, fat and tired on a regular basis, and the proliferation of chronic disease to epidemic proportions, which is subsequently considered *normal* these days as well.

If you think back to the analogy of Mr. Whitless and his car, you can see that a very similar scenario has unfolded. Nearly everyone is eating bad food that is not appropriate fuel for their bodies; nearly everyone is subsequently having different body parts breaking down; nearly everyone is ignoring, denying, diminishing or oblivious to the effects this pseudofood is having on their human vehicles, and nearly everyone has come to think of this is as normal.

Although there are multiple factors at play, massive advertising that includes less than scrupulous marketing tactics has played the most significant role in formulating and perpetuating this charade.

mass marketing & the media

In 1962 Rachel Carson author of *Silent Spring*, a ground breaking book that first awakened the public to environmental issues wrought by industrialization, wrote that the rise of toxic pesticide usage pointed to "an era dominated by industry, in which the right to make money, at whatever cost to others, is seldom challenged." This statement may certainly be said of the rise of the food industry as well.

The food industry has been phenomenally successful in making poor quality, overly processed, chemical-laden fake food into highly profitable fodder for the masses in this country and increasingly in every corner of the world. Such a feat has only been possible due to the development of mass communication, most notably the integration of commercial television into every home in America, which has taken advertising and marketing to an unprecedented level. The impact television and the media have had on shaping our cultural environment over the last few decades is undeniable, and is especially pronounced when it comes to the food we eat.

As the food industry emerged as one of the most profitable businesses, individual corporations learned to cover all bases when it came to initiating, maintaining and expanding their place in the market. In an attempt to achieve widespread name brand recognition, the food industry spends more on advertising via television and radio commercials, print ads, billboards, etc., than any other industry, with the drug companies running a close second. Coca-Cola and McDonald's are among the top ten big spenders when it comes to advertising and are also, not surprisingly, the top two brands recognized worldwide. Ronald McDonald is the world's second most recognized character, with Santa Claus being the first. But slick advertising isn't enough in this competitive market; other marketing strategies must be employed as well.

advertising

In 1993 the National Cancer Institute spent $400,000 promoting the 5 servings of fruit and vegetables a day for better health campaign, whereas the Kellogg company spent $34 million promoting its highly processed and sugared Frosted Flakes to the public in 1992.

Nutrition Action Healthletter

"5 A Day" is the federal government's biggest effort to educate the general public about healthy diets. Yet its budget is minimal. McDonald's spends more every 12 hours to promote unhealthful burgers and fries than the National Cancer Institute spends in a year on "5 A Day" to get people to eat more fruits and vegetables. Consider these annual advertising budgets:

- McDonald's – $1 billion
- Coca-Cola – $770 million
- General Mills – $598 mil.
- 5 A Day – $1 million

C.S.P.I.

widespread availability

Widespread availability of their products is another strategy the food industry has employed to capture the attention of the public. Go anywhere in America today and you will encounter an abundance of fast-food havens, convenience stores, chain restaurants, vending machines and the like, all offering the top brands of fake-food items and beverages. This phenomenon has become so pervasive people don't even give it a second thought.

When one group of participants in an *Eating-for-Health* program was asked what they would do if that Burger King on the corner, for example, wasn't available for them to drive through and pick up dinner on the way home, one woman responded, tongue in cheek, "I would drive through the Taco Bell across the street." This quick-witted response gave us all a good laugh and brought home the point that as a culture we are now surrounded by unhealthy food enticements virtually everywhere we go.

This lively group then started reminiscing about their first-ever trip to the first-ever fast-food franchise that opened in their area when they were young, like 90-year-olds reminiscing about how much the world has changed since the good ole days. But these people weren't senior citizens, these were people in their 40's and 50's who have watched the fast-food industry grow exponentially within just the first half of their lifetime.

It was the mid-60's when I made my first-ever trip to the first McDonald's to open in my neighborhood in Wheaton, Illinois, a suburb of Chicago where I lived as a child. It was a big event. We all piled into the family station wagon, took our cardboard trays filled with paper-wrapped cheeseburgers, fries and drinks, and sat outside beneath the golden arches sporting multi-colored flags flapping in the summer breeze to announce the grand opening. After a few bites of those delicious French fries and a few slurps of that sweet, creamy milk shake, I thought I had died and gone to heaven, and those golden arches were the pearly gates themselves.

That first set of golden arches to make my acquaintance that day loomed from the landscape as a lone pioneer of things to come. Today, like most other main thoroughfares in America, these same golden arches are now lost amidst what has become an almost uninterrupted strip of other popular fast-food emporiums,

We first make our habits, then our habits make us.

John Dryden

with their signs bodaciously competing to be seen emblazoned against the horizon.

In addition to the vast number of fast-food restaurants that now dot our landscape from coast-to-coast, convenience stores packed with junk food are now attached to virtually every gas station, and vending machines spilling out even more junk food, are now lurking at the end of every public hallway. While most people can't help but be aware of the strategic placement of junk food-bearing vending machines, what most people are not aware of, is the often manipulative contracts that accompany them.

I was first struck by this phenomenon one evening while preparing to teach an *Eating-for-Health* program at my local YMCA. I was in the staff lounge making photocopies when one of the fitness coordinators came in swinging a large red thermos jug with a push-button spout. She placed it in the sink and began filling it with tap water. It brought to mind another evening when I forgot my water bottle and with no alternative available, was unhappily forced to buy a bottle of water from the vending machine that had a list of funky-sounding chemical additives an inch long. It seemed like a strange oversight on their part not to have water dispensers available at a health and recreation facility, not to mention a cumbersome task for the coordinator who was now struggling to maneuver the large jug in the not-so-large sink. So, I decided to interject an inquiry about the matter into the friendly chatter we had started.

"Why don't you guys just get a bottled water service and put a couple of dispensers in the fitness rooms?" I asked. "Seems like it would be a lot easier and healthier."

"Well, umm," the coordinator began hesitantly, "we have a contract with Coke that prohibits us from having water dispensers. Since the patrons are always complaining, this is my little way of skirting around it."

I was speechless.

This is a perfect example of the universal availability and easy accessibility that has become an insidiously effective method of inducing mass consumption of poor quality pseudofoods, especially in the frequently deliberate absence of healthier choices. These coercive efforts have quickly made reaching for the unhealthy products abundantly churned out by the food industry a socially conditioned response.

fast food

On any given day, one out of four Americans opts for a quick and cheap meal at a fast-food restaurant, without giving either its speed or its thriftiness a second thought. Fast food is so ubiquitous that it now seems as American, and harmless, as apple pie. But the industry's drive for consolidation, homogenization, and speed has radically transformed America's diet, landscape, economy, and workforce, often in insidiously destructive ways.

In 1970, Americans spent about $6 billion on fast food, in 2000 they spent $110 billion. Americans spend more on fast food than on movies, books, magazines, newspapers, videos, and recorded music – combined.

The average American spends 90% of their food budget on processed foods of low nutritional value.

Eric Schlosser,
Fast Food Nation

super-sizing, pricing & flavoring

super-sizing

A standard serving of soda in the 1950's was 6.5 ounces. Today the standard is 20 ounces. In the U.S., one study found that participants consistently labeled as "medium" portions that were double or triple the size of recommended portions.

World Watch Inst.

Many food manufacturers have adopted *supersizing* portions as another way of magnetizing customers. Supersized sodas, burgers, cookies, candy bars, etc., that far exceed recommended portion sizes, lure people into believing that they are getting more for their money. Similarly, *superpricing* encourages people to consume larger servings by offering these portion sizes at proportionately cheaper prices. Both supersizing and superpricing result in greater profits for the food manufacturer, often at the expense of the consumer's health.

Faster delivery to meet the needs of our fast-paced society has also evolved as a popular marketing strategy. Fast-food restaurants offer drive-thru services. Highly processed, packaged foods that require little to no preparation fill the majority of space in our grocery stores. Convenience foods boasting that you can "just pop it in the toaster or microwave," or better yet, "just open the package and eat it," are common fair. But while convenience, supersizing, superpricing and slick advertising may initiate the first purchase, taste is what will keep 'em coming back for more. Thus there is the emergence of yet another vast industry within the food industry; the business of flavoring.

super-pricing

At Cineplex Odeon theaters, a 20 oz. small drink costs $2.50, while a 44 oz. large, which is 120% larger, costs only 30% more or $3.25.

Nutrition Action Healthletter

Because highly processed food products made from the cheapest ingredients are also lacking in good taste (no pun intended), the food manufacturers have spent a great deal of time, money and effort to overcome this obstacle. Since 90% of taste is attributable to the sense of smell, the same processes that are used to make well-known brands of perfume are also used to develop enticing artificial flavors that have now become the counterpart of what past generations considered as familiar as grandma's apple pie. Flavor additives usually consist of a long list of chemical compounds that are lumped together under the phrase *artificial* or *natural flavorings*.

super-flavoring

Monosodium glutamate (MSG) is a popular flavor enhancer that causes people to crave more of the food to which it is added. Over 60% of processed foods now contain this neurotoxin, despite the fact it has been proven to cause brain damage and is accordingly not recommended for use in baby foods.

nomsg.com

Adding artificial flavors and flavor enhancers, that are often toxic to processed foods as a means of capturing the public's taste buds has increased dramatically over the last few years and is a significant example of the changing face of our food. Canned soups are a case in point.

When this innovative method of processing and storing food first came out, there were no chemical flavors added. Today, with the exception of brands that outwardly proclaim their *all natural, no chemical additives* status, most major brands of processed canned soup now contain artificial flavors (sometimes under the guise of *natural* flavors mentioned earlier) and flavor enhancers. They also now include a host of other chemical additives (such as preservatives and artificial colorings), the number and amounts of which have increased right along with them. In addition to artificial flavors and chemical flavor enhancers, raising the sugar, salt, oil and poor-quality fat content is another profitable way companies have increasingly used to enhance the flavor factor, and the subsequent *dis*-ease causing factor of their foods as well.

According to the U.S. Department of Agriculture, added sugar in processed pseudofoods has increased by 30% since 1983. Similar numbers apply when it comes to the addition of sodium. As for poor-quality fats and oils, fast-food and chain restaurants are notorious for serving extraordinary amounts of these unhealthy, albeit tasty substances to their often unsuspecting customers. For example, a study by the Center for Science in the Public Interest revealed that a mushroom cheeseburger at TGI Friday's contains approximately 1800 calories and the same amount of fat as five strips of bacon, four chocolate frosted donuts, three slices of pepperoni pizza, two banana splits, and a Big Mac combined.

And as if widespread name brand recognition, and bigger, faster, tastier products weren't enough to maintain an existing product's position or to elbow a new product's way into the American pop food culture, a few other insidious strategies have also been added to the list of the most aggressive marketing schemes over the last couple decades.

> Food companies will make and market any product that sells, regardless of its nutritional value or its effect on health.
>
> In this regard, food companies hardly differ from cigarette companies.
>
> Marion Nestle, Food Politics

more aggressive marketing schemes

Because food preferences, much like personalities, are developed in the formative stages of life, targeting children has become the primary aim of many food manufacturers. Tantalizing commercials and appealing toy prizes catalyze innocent children to torment their parents to purchase processed candy, cereals, and fast-food kid meals. Then, the added fat, sugar, artificial colorings and flavorings make the food look and taste so good, children acquire a liking for them, often to the degree that they actually

target: children

Advertisers dispro-portionately target children in order to establish lifelong habits. In the U.S., the average child watches 10,000 commercials each year, more than any other segment of the population. 90% of these ads are for sugary cereals, candy, soda, or other junk food.

C.S.P.I.

McDonalds operates more playgrounds than any other private entity in the U.S. It is also one of the nation's largest distributors of toys.

Fast Food Nation

In November 1997, the Colorado Springs, Colorado, school district signed a ten-year deal with Coca-Cola for $8 million, and more if it exceeds the "requirement" of selling 70,000 cases of Coke products annually.

Feed Your Kids Bright

One contract prompted a school district to push Coca-Cola consumption in the classrooms when sales fell below contractual obligations.

Hunger, Escaping Excess

start begging for these unhealthy food items and refuse to eat anything else (sound like any child you know?).

The food industry has also invaded our public schools. In an aggressive effort to increase sales, profits and create lifelong customers, fast-food and soft drink companies have contracts, often worth millions of dollars, to provide food service and vending machines, at more than 5,000 U.S. schools to date. As the *Scary Statistics* reveal, acquired tastes and regular consumption of high fat-sugar-sodium, processed and fast-food items are leaving children and adults prone to obesity and *dis*-ease at increasingly younger ages.

In addition to having people enjoy the flavor, getting them biochemically addicted to their food is another sure-fire way for food manufacturers to gain repeat customers. This is one of the latest in a long line of marketing strategies that many food manufacturers have adopted in recent years, designed to hook children as well as adults. Reminiscent of ploys undertaken by the tobacco industry, adding excessive amounts of caffeine, sugar and some neuro-toxic flavor enhancers and artificial sweeteners — all known or suspected biochemically addictive substances — has become all too commonplace for processed and fast foods. Anyone who has tried to wean themselves off popular soda drinks or their favorite food items containing these substances, can attest to the biochemical hold these foods can have on a person.

Another marketing tactic involves food corporations developing sponsorships with leading nonprofit organizations by paying for the use of their logos in advertisements. For example, a popular ice cream sandwich company paid the American Diabetes Association to use its logo in ads for its artificially sweetened line of products to give the impression of endorsement by this health-oriented organization. This was done in spite of the fact that these dessert products contain high levels of total and saturated fats, which is a risky choice for diabetics who are prone to obesity and heart disease. These kinds of sponsorships can be deceptive and serve as justification for people to continue poor eating habits.

Similarly, more and more independent professional organizations, researchers, and consumer groups receive funding from the food industry, something many fail to disclose when they talk to journalists and journalists fail to report to the public.

For example, The American Council on Science and Health, which bills itself as a nonprofit consumer education organization, has been funded, in large part, by PepsiCo, Coca-Cola, Dow, Exxon, and other corporations. Big food companies also fund the objective-sounding International Life Sciences Institute and the International Food Information Council.

To counteract the food industry's hidden influence, The Center for Science in the Public Interest (CSPI), a legitimate public interest organization, has created the Integrity in Science Project, which exposes conflicts of interest and encourages journalists to disclose industry funding of research and organizations. In one example, the CSPI revealed a conflict of interest involving the American Dietetic Association (ADA), which publishes "Nutrition Fact Sheets" that defend fast foods, the fake fat Olestra, and starch-filled baby foods, and a position paper that gave sugar a clean bill of health. The ADA has acknowledged that McDonald's, Procter & Gamble, and Gerber underwrote these Nutrition Fact Sheets, and that one of the co-authors of its paper exonerating sugar was a scientific advisor to the Canadian Sugar Institute.

media manipulation

In an additional effort to capitalize on the trend in the direction of eating healthier that has been struggling to emerge, food manufacturers use media news reports as yet another way to manipulate people into buying their products. This is primarily done through what marketing moguls call the *third person* or *expert opinion* approach.

The well-known written press release that dominated this approach in the past, has now been usurped by its television counterpart. Today, entire news stories are written, filmed and produced by public relations firms and then sent via satellite or the internet to television stations all over the world. These video news releases, or VNRs, are used extensively by the food industry and drug companies to provide a steady stream of stories announcing new medical breakthroughs, and the previously unknown health benefits researchers attribute to whatever product the sponsoring client happens to be offering. By 1991, ten VNR's a day were being produced or about 4,000 per year. Today the number is much greater, although no one has an exact count.

---

added caffeine

In July 1997, on the heels of revelations about how tobacco manufacturers have manipulated the level of nicotine in cigarettes to increase consumption, the Center for Science in the Public Interest (CSPI) filed a petition urging the FDA to force manufacturers to label their products for caffeine content... Joining CSPI ... were 10 health and consumer groups, as well as 34 scientists from Johns Hopkins, Yale, Harvard, Duke, the University of Michigan, the University of California at Berkeley, and other institutions. John Hughes of the department of psychiatry at the University of Vermont organized a coalition of scientists concerned about caffeine, and in a separate action, the American Medical Association has called upon the FDA to require caffeine-content labeling.

Stephen Cherniske
Caffeine Blues

Note: Although the FDA was obliged to act within 6 months, as of 9/01 (4 years after the petition was filed), they were still evaluating the issue.

To see these VNRs in action, all you need to do is flip through the TV channels during the prime time news hour and watch for the same reports to be repeated on different channels. It is important to be aware that these are staged reports with the doctors and experts being *paid* by the sponsor to divulge information in the interest of generating more sales of their products. The food industry's top priority is their bottom line, not your bottom. Similarly, the media frequently chooses to run these VNR's and corporate press releases because it's easy and profitable for them to do so. They like to highlight stories that grab your attention, not necessarily those that make you healthier. More often than not, information in these stories is not verified and the source is not revealed, leading readers and viewers to believe that the information is legitimate news.

Given that the average person receives 90% of his or her information regarding health and nutrition from television viewing, it is easy to see how the *third party, expert opinion* approach especially in the form of VNRs, can be most effective for the advertisers, and at the same time, most deceptive and confusing to the unsuspecting viewer. In fact, this is one of the major hindrances people face today when it comes to knowing what is a healthy food choice and what is not. It seems that as soon as the implications of the latest dietary study starts to sink in, whether legitimate or manipulated, another one comes along to contradict it. Some prime examples include: eggs are bad for you, eggs are good for you; margarine is better than butter, margarine is worse than butter; fiber is good, fiber doesn't matter, etc. After being bombarded with so many contradictory reports regarding what is beneficial for them to eat, a recent survey showed that the more confused people were about dietary recommendations, the more likely they were to eat poor quality foods and fewer fruits and vegetables.

To say that mass marketing and advertising by the food industry, with the assistance of the mass media, have something to do with what we have come to know as the *Standard American Diet* would be an understatement. They are, in fact, the primary cultivators of American popular food culture. Their influence has been so strong that today an estimated 91% of the U.S. population ignores the government's recommendation of eating 5 servings a

...you will find that a surprising number of seemingly scientific assertions – perhaps even many in which you devoutly believe – are complete nonsense.

Robert Youngson
Scientific Blunders

day of fruits and vegetables, opting instead for highly processed, chemical-laden, high-fat-sodium-sugar content pseudofoods.

Every branch of the food industry has burgeoned in the last few decades. The soft drink industry alone has grown nearly ten-fold in just over 50 years. With the exception of the natural foods segment of the food industry, they are all guilty of dishing out questionable fake-food products that are unquestionably the primary cause of the deteriorating health of the public. And with the exception of some segments of society (we self-avowed health food nuts for one), this trend of poor eating and the resultant epidemic of chronic *dis*-ease shows no sign of abating. On the contrary, it's growing and spreading.

the american way — and spreading!

Poor eating has gone from being an occasional occurrence to a socially acceptable trend, to the daily dietary protocol for 91% of the population. Eating crappy food, as one of my clients would say, has become as American as baseball and apple pie.

The food industry has been so successful in executing marketing campaigns geared toward promoting widespread, lifelong consumption of high-fat-sugar-sodium content foods and highly processed foods that most people today are so hooked they don't even know or care that they are eating poor quality *dis*-ease causing pseudofoods. People have become so disconnected from their food source and the processes that govern it that poor nutrition has literally become the American way. Soft drink consumption is just one clear example of how consuming foods and beverages that were initially approached with caution when first introduced to the public (and rightfully so) are now consumed on a daily basis, frequently multiple times a day, by the vast majority.

For decades health officials have warned against the health risks posed by consumption of soft drinks with their high-sugar and caloric content and low-nutritional value. The addition of artificial colors and sweeteners, preservatives and caffeine in recent years has made them even more detrimental to one's health. Soft drinks, also known as liquid candy, have been associated with a host of adverse health conditions, including malnutrition, weight problems, diabetes, calcium deficiency, hyperactivity, and learning difficulties.

manipulation

In Feb. 2000 Dennis Avery was the featured expert for an ABC 20/20 story by John Stossel, which speculated that "buying organic could kill you." Avery is the in-house expert at the Hudson Inst., funded by agrichemical heavyweight corporations such as Monsanto, Dupont and Dow.

Avery alleged that people who ate organic and natural foods were 8x more likely to contract a deadly new strain of E. coli than those who ate foods grown using synthetic pesticides. He claimed this data came from the U.S. Centers for Disease Control, a claim the CDC adamantly denies...

Stossel's piece made no mention of Avery's affiliation with the Hudson Institute or its corporate funding. In addition, Stossel claimed that 20/20's own laboratory tests had found as many pesticide residues on organic produce as on the conventionally grown variety – a claim the network later retracted when its researchers admitted that no such tests had been conducted.

Trust Us,
We're Experts

Despite their status as an unhealthy food, consumption of soft drinks has skyrocketed in the last few years, especially among children and teenagers. The average American child drinks nearly 800 cans of soda every year, which is more than twice as much as 25 years ago. (It's interesting to note that soda consumption and obesity rates for children have both doubled in the last 20 years.) As for teens, they drank almost twice as much milk as soda twenty years ago, while today the opposite is true. They now drink twice as much soda as milk.

Because food industry advertising budgets far exceed the public-service campaigns promoting the consumption of healthful foods and beverages, many young parents today who grew up on soft drinks and pseudofoods themselves, either ignore or are not fully cognizant of the health risks involved with regular consumption of these substances. Once considered an occasional snack or treat, soft drinks and junk food have now become a standard part of daily life, and replacing healthy meals with highly processed pseudofoods has become the social norm.

Just because poor eating has become the social norm in this country doesn't means its effect on our health is any less damaging. This new age of rampant poor quality and processed food item consumption is, thus far, a mere blip on the historical screen of humankind. Nevertheless, thinking back to the *Scary Statistics* listed earlier, during its relatively short duration this culturally ingrained habit of poor eating is having a catastrophic effect on our health as a nation that is rapidly spreading around the world.

The United States has long prided itself on being a champion of impoverished countries and has frequently come to the aid of the malnourished and *dis*-eased. As a result of the flourishing American popular food culture, however, we have now actually *become* a nation of malnourished and *dis*-eased.

The concept of malnutrition encompasses not only those who are *under*weight, *under*fed and *under*nourished, but also includes those who are *over*fed and *over*weight, yet lacking in proper vitamins and nutrients. The latter group is the biggest challenge the United States is facing today, to the degree that the numbers of overfed and malnourished have now reached epidemic proportions in this country. Not only that, but we are spreading this phenomenon throughout the world.

With the help of aggressive advertising by U.S. food corporations, overeating the wrong foods and subsequent malnourishment has become an established problem for other wealthier nations, and is now starting to grow rapidly among the middle class and wealthier segments of poorer nations as well.

In both rich and poor countries malnutrition has become an impediment to development. Hunger and obesity on an individual level, increases the risk for chronic and acute *dis*-ease, reduces physical fitness and shortens lifespan. In addition, whether due to a lack of food or from eating too much of the wrong foods, children deprived of adequate nutrients during the developmental years can suffer from permanently reduced mental capacity. On a national level, poor eating decreases economic production, educational performance and general well-being. It also creates a tremendous burden on health care systems. This problem of malnutrition now results as much from those who overeat as from those who are underfed.

In its annual report, entitled *State of the World 2000*, the World Watch Institute, an independent research organization in Washington, revealed that for the first time in history the number of people who are overfed, overweight and malnourished, now rivals the number who are underfed, underweight and malnourished. According to the World Health Organization (WHO) overeating poor quality food is the fastest growing form of malnourishment in the world today. As one might expect, all the associated chronic degenerative *dis*-eases are also increasing in these countries.

It appears that the poor eating habits and associated chronic degenerative *dis*-eases that have become the American way, are quickly becoming the way of the world. Following the trail of obesity and *dis*-ease left in its wake, I'd like to think that a trend toward *Eating for Health* is right on its heels. This won't happen, however, until the veil is lifted regarding pseudofood and its relationship to *dis*-ease, and people clearly see what is happening. This is a challenging task because it is not a popular viewpoint among the vast majority of people. As has been demonstrated, it challenges their very lifestyle, social conditioning and much of what they have come to believe. In addition, accurate information and education are greatly lacking and often distorted when it comes to eating healthfully, as we have seen.

The body must be nourished, physically, emotionally and spiritually.

We're spiritually starved in America and not underfed but undernourished.

Carol Hornig

The weight loss industry, which has ballooned right along with the food industry, offers inadequate, often skewed approaches to making changes in diet. It singles out affected individuals offering fad diets, diet drugs and herbal supplements that are geared toward losing weight often at the expense of one's overall health. It fails to promote prevention and education about healthy alternatives and how to steer clear of heavily advertised processed food.

As mentioned, healthy eating guidelines and educational programs established by organizations and agencies such as the Centers for Disease Control, have funding that pales in comparison to the enormous advertising dollars of the food manufacturers. Their recommendations don't stand much of a chance when in the public schools, for example, children are taught healthy eating guidelines in the classroom, but then poor quality processed food items in the cafeteria and vending machines are what is primarily, and sometimes exclusively, made available to them.

In addition, much like drug addicts, alcoholics, or chronic smokers, over the last few decades people have developed taste buds, biochemistries and lifestyles that are so acclimated to eating poorly they adamantly cling to this familiar, albeit detrimental, behavior. As a culture we are unquestionably addicted to bad food.

Similar to how we felt as third party observers to Mr. Whitless and his car troubles, quite often well-meaning and informed people who see clearly what is going on in this country are anxious to bring it to the attention of those who are either ignorant or in denial. They are frequently met with ridicule, opposition and sometimes even hostility, much like the little boy who announced that the emperor wasn't wearing any clothes. Whereas it was once the socially accepted norm to eat healthy and take care of oneself, now people who do so are few and far between.

On the other end of the spectrum, many well-informed health conscious people like to blame and criticize the food companies for the food-related problems that plague our society today. In all fairness, they were just responding to the demands of the time. People's top priorities in our fast-paced society created the demand for bigger, faster, tastier food. That's the

As Big Medicine took over the responsibility for health, the voices that spoke of obvious connections between lifestyle and *dis*-ease were drowned out by the thundering stampede to junk food and irresponsible lifestyle.

Jon Matsen
Eating Alive

reason this industry has been able to thrive. Americans placed the order and the food industry and fast-food restaurants delivered it.

The proliferation and spread of poor quality food and the accompanying problems associated with it, are not inevitable. If there weren't a demand for processed and fast food, there wouldn't be a market for it either. Like any industry, it is consumer driven. As the public's priorities shift and the demand for healthier food increases, the food industry and fast-food restaurants will shift in response.

As a society we can no longer afford to blame others or keep our heads in the sand regarding the current epidemic of malnutrition due to over consumption of poor quality fake foods, and the concomitant epidemic of chronic degenerative *dis*-ease. As a part of our growth as a society we have gotten off track and now it is time to reset the course. Riddled with *dis*-ease and obesity, a growing segment of the society is now realizing that something is indeed wrong with the eating habits that have become the American way and they are rethinking their priorities.

More and more savvy consumers are starting to cast their vote in the direction of health being a top priority when it comes to what they eat. I'd like to think this is a new trend that is emerging; a trend that puts the health and welfare of individuals, their loved ones and the generations to come as the top priority. In order to bring such a trend to fruition, comprehensive education aimed at unraveling the myths and confusion that have evolved in this arena is key.

I'd like to think that if you are reading this book you have a desire to be a part of this trend, for that's how trends begin, one person at a time. Which brings us back to the original question…

> When a small but significant number of individuals move into new levels of awareness and significantly change their behavior, that change is felt in the entire mass consciousness.
>
> Shakti Gawain

why me, why now?

It is clear that chronic *dis*-ease is rampant in this country and that poor nutrition has played *the* major role in creating this debacle. We as a society have stuck our finger in the proverbial light socket when it comes to what we eat. It would be wise to acknowledge this, pull our finger out of the socket, and start repairing the damage. Poor eating habits are not exclusive to sloppy, weak-willed individuals as once thought, but are, in fact, a cultural epidemic that must be understood in order to be uprooted.

If you grew up in mainstream America, unless you've been living in a remote log cabin somewhere, you have no doubt been greatly influenced by the popular food culture that surrounds you, frequently without even knowing it. If you currently have atrocious eating habits as a result, don't beat yourself up about it. It doesn't matter where you are or where you have been. What matters is which direction you are going. It is never too late to be what you might have been, or do what you might have done.

From this chapter you have gained an understanding of where we are today as a society and the history that has brought us here, which puts you a leap ahead of the crowd already. Awareness truly is key. This alarming look at the bigger picture, however, may be a relief on the one hand, but a bit ominous and overwhelming on the other. Which leads to another factor to consider when pondering this question of *Why Me, Why Now?*, one that goes beyond you as an individual.

People are often more inspired to take action when there is a cause greater than themselves involved. That is certainly the case here. If we don't take action now, collectively and as individuals, the deterioration of the quality of our food will continue to affect not only us, but also our children and subsequent generations. It's literally about shaping the future on a global scale.

Think globally, act locally is a motto that fits well here. As an individual you cast your vote with your actions, by being an example, and by where you spend your dollars. We must counter advertising and marketing strategies with education, and support one another in family, community and school settings to return to a healthy, nourishing diet and have it become the norm once again.

If after all you've just read you are still not inspired or are hesitating to eat for health, that is certainly your choice as well. However, I would like to make one final plea and encourage you to go deep within and consider what that says about your relationship with yourself. People go searching the whole world over for their life partner, when all the while they are walking around every day with what is first and foremost their all-time life partner, their body. Why would you choose to abuse the one and only partner guaranteed to be with you for your entire life's

Man is
the sole and
absolute master
of his own
fate forever.

What he has
sown in the
times of his
ignorance, he
must inevitably
reap; when
he attains
enlightenment,
it is for him
to sow what
he chooses
and reap
accordingly.

Geraldine Coster

journey? Your body is the vehicle that carries you through life, without it you wouldn't be here.

For many years I was a pseudo- and junk-food-oholic, smoker, and binge drinker, whose idea of exercise was walking a block to the convenience store on the corner to pick up a six-pack, a liter of Pepsi, a jumbo bag of Doritos, and a pack of cigarettes. There are few people out there who could rival the unhealthy habits of my past. I used to brag that I could *eat anything*, that nothing bothered *me*. This immature bravado of invincibility and careless ways led me to a place where I literally couldn't *eat anything*, as you'll recall from *The Beginning*. I learned the hard way the unpleasant consequences of this behavior, as the health problems I divulged earlier turned out to be the mere tip of the iceberg of what was to become chronic, possibly life-threatening *dis*-ease.

There are many excuses people use to justify making poor lifestyle and food choices on a regular basis. Believe me, I have heard and used every excuse there is, and I can tell you from personal experience that eating poorly will lead to much more pain than any of the supposed consequences of the excuses you can drum up.

Having made significant and lasting changes in diet and lifestyle over the years, I have much to offer in the way of strategies, practical tools, and information that can help you override any excuses or stumbling blocks and make your journey easier. *Strategize!* and *Make It So!* are two upcoming sections devoted entirely to providing you with the psychological tools and practical know-how you need to succeed. Think of the process of making changes in the way you eat as an adventure, rather than a difficult chore. And remember that it is a process, not an overnight event.

If loss of health is the greatest deprivation, then *Eating for Health* is the greatest gift you can give to yourself, as it will maintain and restore your health. Don't deprive yourself of this gift. You are worth it. You deserve it. Don't let the voices of the world drown out your own inner voice when it comes to making decisions about what you eat. Let your inner voice ring out and guard your precious health.

You can now start thinking for yourself and make your own choices when it comes to the food you eat, choices that arise

> How would your life be different if you learned how to love and respect your body as though it were your own precious creation, as valuable as a beloved friend or child?
>
> How would you treat yourself differently?
>
> Dr. Christiane Northrup

from the whole of you, not just your culturally trained taste buds; choices that arise from an informed and conscious frame of mind, rather than tantalizing commercials, manipulative marketing ploys, or social pressures; and most importantly, food choices that value your personal health and well-being.

In final answer to the question *Why Me, Why Now?*, it is clear that there is a human *need* for you to eat for health, a need that is evident now more than ever.

So, take a deep breath and give yourself a big gold star for having reviewed some unpleasant, albeit vital information. Then continue on and begin to fulfill this human need by learning the five simple guidelines for *Eating for Health*. Guidelines that are guaranteed to help you feel better, have more energy, lose weight (or dispel gas, as the case may be!) and create a brighter future for not only yourself, but for the world at large.

Be the
change
you want to
see in the
world.

Mhatma Ghandi

the guidelines

Five Eating-for-Health Guidelines Everyone Can Agree On

Whenever I first start working with a client or teaching a program, everyone immediately wants to know what is the basic philosophy of what I call *Eating for Health*. They want to know if I am a vegetarian, and what I think about that; what I think about daily calorie and nutrient intake requirements; what I think about different popular diets such as the blood-type diet, low-carb, low-fat or high protein diets. So, I am guessing that you want to know the same. Of course, this is what the whole book is about and I will go into greater detail later. But just to briefly address the questions many people may be curious about up front, I will tell you this:

No, I am not currently a vegetarian. I was for about ten years and started eating animal protein again in the mid-90's. On average, I currently eat about 1-3 servings a week. I will express my views on the topic of vegetarianism in the description of the fourth guideline. In the meantime, for those of you who are vegetarians, although there is carnivorous information and recipes contained in this book, there is also information that you will find helpful and I personally wish someone had told me when I was a vegetarian. It would have made my experience much different. As

The best effect of any book is that it excites the reader to self-activity.

Thomas Carlyle

you will see, the principles set forth here apply to everyone, even those who follow a vegetarian diet.

As for calorie and nutrient intake requirements, I honestly don't pay much attention to them. I've seen people put a highly processed, chemical-filled food next to a whole, natural food and compare the nutrient and calorie make-up between the two. It's an irrelevant comparison. Besides, if you ask ten different people, they will each have a different answer depending on their training and particular school of thought on the topic. People will argue about these numbers and none of them really knows *the* answer anyway. It gets very confusing and ends up clouding the real issue at hand. So why bother yourself with such information? (Remember what Clive said in the *Introduction*?) By the end of this book, you will have a strong base understanding of what is appropriate for you to eat, without having to remember a bunch of numbers and calculations. The upcoming *Eating-for-Health Guidelines* and *The Basics* are applicable to everyone and will cover all your basic nutritional needs. If, after learning and applying these universal recommendations you want to further dissect your food into calories and nutrient counts, go for it! But don't lose sight of a deteriorating forest, as many people do, because you're micro-focusing on the minute details of the trees.

With regard to the many popular diets out there, I believe they all contribute something to the overall understanding of nutrition. Some you might readily recognize as undesirable, while others offer some valuable pieces of the puzzle that can be very beneficial. In addition to the popular diet programs and books, there are also many other books with the similar intention of this one, providing more general, time-tested information on whole, natural foods. Each has something to offer through its own variations, thereby contributing to your overall understanding, experiences and body awareness. Different books resonate with different people at different times. There is a whole list of books that I have found to contain valuable pieces of the nutrition puzzle in the *Resources* section, for those who want to do further study.

On that same note, although I think it is wise to consult with and learn from external authorities and experts on nutrition, it is important to remember that an expert is merely someone who knows a lot about something. That something is usually one piece or a few pieces of the overall puzzle, rather than the whole puzzle.

When it comes to what you eat, the ultimate authority is the wisdom of the ages coupled with the wisdom of *your* body.

K.H.

Nature is very complex and no one could know all of the pieces of the puzzle, their individual nuances, and how they interact with one another. This is especially true when it comes to the human body and nutrition. As evidenced by the vast discrepancies between theories, and all the disagreement and controversy, the field of nutrition is clearly an exploration rather than an exact science. Certainly there are things to be learned from scientists and experts in the field, but in the long run you must consult the ultimate authority. When it comes to what you eat, the ultimate authority is the wisdom of the ages coupled with the wisdom of *your* body. That is the underlying philosophy of *Eating for Health*.

The wisdom of the ages has been to look to Mother Nature for nourishment. Considering there are over 6 billion people occupying the planet, our ancestors must have been doing something right. Some may argue that technology must be taken into account, that our ancestors *had* to rely on Mother Nature for their sustenance, because they had no other choice; but now things have changed and we have other choices. The problem is, the human body didn't change. When it comes to what kind of food is appropriate, the human body has remained basically the same. Regardless of technological advances in food manufacturing, the human body was never designed to eat processed, chemical-laden fake foods. It was designed to eat the pure food that Mother Nature provides. That's not to say that some day the human body may not have evolved to accommodate overly processed, chemical-laden foods high in sugar, fat, and salt without negative consequences. However, this clearly has not happened yet.

While the wisdom of the ages gives us a general layout for what is nourishing, the wisdom of our bodies gives us messages as to the specifics. Our bodies speak to us constantly, expressing their particular needs at any given time. Intuition is the body's subtle voice, while its loudest gestures come in the form of symptoms and *dis*-eases. This communication is crucial in guiding us to eating what truly serves us. It is important to learn to recognize what is appropriate for your body at this particular time in your life, and to know that its dietary needs will vary to some degree throughout your life. The *Eating-for-Health Guidelines* apply for the duration of your lifetime as they are based on universal

Believe only your own experience.

There is no fact like a fact learned from your own life.

Aristotle

principles that have built-in flexibility for individualization within them.

flip the switch

Contrary to what many researchers would have us believe, in order to eat healthfully we don't have to know all the scientific complexities of the body, nutrition and how everything works. Although sometimes helpful, knowing how many calories in this, or nutrients in that just isn't necessary. More often than not it creates confusion for the average person and as indicated earlier, becomes counterproductive. Humankind has sustained itself quite well for centuries without knowing any of this. (Actually, our ancestors did better than us in this regard, when you consider the epidemic proportions of chronic *dis*-ease caused by the poor eating habits of today.)

It's not possible at this stage of our evolution and scientific knowledge to accurately assess every nuance of human nutritive requirements. To date, we have only scratched the surface when it comes to understanding the vitamins and nutrients required for human function, let alone the intricate interplay between them all and in relationship to each biochemical unique individual. There are countless nutrients that work together in a magically complex process, a process about which we know so little. But Mother Nature knows. She is complex so we don't have to be. We just eat what she provides. It's all been figured out for us. Follow the guidelines, which are a return to a natural way of eating that has stood the test of time, and let your body be your guide.

You don't have to know how to electrically wire the house in order to turn on the lights. You just have to know where the switch is, how to operate it and then switch it on. *Eating for Health* is much the same. You just need to know what a wise food choice is, how to prepare it, and then eat it. It's really very simple.

easy as A, B, C

The business of *Eating for Health* may at first appear complex because much of the information will be new to you. For reassurance, remember when you were first learning the 26 letters of the alphabet, with their different sounds, long vowels, short vowels, consonants, etc. That all seemed complex and a little

> It will be decades before we have identified all of the complex compounds in food and even longer before we truly understand how they interact with one another and what they do in our bodies.
>
> Dr. Walter Willett
> Harvard School of Nutrition

overwhelming in the beginning as well. Rest assured that with a little time and active usage, just like the alphabet is for you now, the language and practice of *Eating for Health* will become as easy as A, B, C. Remember too, that you didn't learn the alphabet and how to read overnight. You learned the basics first, then how to build on the basics, and you did so over a period of time. You may have gotten exasperated at times, but you never gave up because you wanted to learn to read; a valuable skill that has served you for a lifetime.

It is wise to approach the process of *Eating for Health* the same way. You will get discouraged at times, but don't give up, because like reading, *Eating for Health* is a valuable skill that will serve you for a lifetime. The upcoming chapters offer specific tools and techniques that will help you make and integrate changes step-by-step, while the guidelines provide the underlying foundation needed to implement them.

The *Eating-for-Health Guidelines* are designed to inform, guide, and alleviate nutritional confusion. They act as steering mechanisms for making food choices that are nourishing and supportive to *your* body at this time in your life. Rather than rigid rules to be followed, they help guide you in the direction that you want to go, providing enough flexibility so that you remain the captain of your ship. The simple guiding statements are easy to remember and apply, while the descriptions provide a comprehensive understanding of their meaning and what they represent. In brief, the five easy guidelines for *Eating for Health* are:

eating-for-health guidelines:

1 ~ if it's not food, don't eat it!
...and if you do, wait a long time before you do it again so your body can recover.

2 ~ eliminate or relegate stimulants to rare occasions
...the more distant and rare the better.

3 ~ eat an abundance of whole, fresh, natural foods
...and little to no processed foods.

It is best to follow the ideas of someone who has a balanced health program, a balanced food program, proven over years of actual use by thousands of people.

We should not follow confusion, but wisdom in this matter.

Dr. Bernard Jensen

4 ~ account for food allergies & sensitivities
...when making wise food choices.

5 ~ account for ailments
...when making wise food choices.

"Eat plenty of fruits and vegetables" is timeless advice that science is only now catching up to.

It is a simple, easy-to-remember, and tasty morsel of excellent dietary advice that ranks high on the list of smart and healthy nutritional habits.

Dr. Walter Willett
Eat, Drink & Be
Healthy

As you read through the following detailed descriptions you will discover that these guidelines interweave, intertwine, overlap and acquiesce, while still providing a structure, much like nature itself. Although the *Eating-for-Health Guidelines* are simple unto themselves, a true understanding of them addresses many issues and serves many purposes. They will help make it easier for you to decide what to eat, as well as what *not* to eat. They will bring clarity by providing user-friendly meaning to words and phrases such as processed foods, whole, fresh, natural foods, etc., which for many have become confusing buzzwords.

When making food choices you can use each of the guidelines as a cue for asking yourself: Is this item a *real* food or is it a pseudofood or stimulant? Is this food *whole, fresh* and *natural* or is it processed? Does this food agree with my system or is it something to which I have a sensitivity or allergy? Does this food support, or work against any health conditions or ailments I am currently experiencing? How to answer these questions will be made clearer as you read through the descriptions.

In addition, the guidelines provide a more in-depth understanding of food and it's relationship to your health, state of mind and life in general. Armed with this greater understanding, you will be less likely to make sweeping generalizations about food that can adversely affect your ability to make wise choices. For example, it is very popular in our culture for people to refer to this or that food as being either healthy or unhealthy, good or bad without regard to whether or not this is actually true for *them*. This is a limited perspective and often proves counterproductive rather than helpful. Similarly, using phrases such as "everything in moderation" or a "balanced" diet is also very popular and equally as counterproductive. Without quantifying these terms, they are open to wide interpretation, hence rendered meaningless. They are also frequently used, often unconsciously, to justify and continue poor eating habits.

After becoming familiar with the *Eating-for-Health Guidelines*, you will feel more confident, clear and empowered, as opposed to confused when making food choices, thereby increasing the possibility of making wise and appropriate food choices regularly.

slowly I turned, step-by-step...

To genuinely integrate the guidelines and make *Eating for Health* a lifelong habit, it is wise in the beginning to focus on one guideline at a time until you feel you understand the guideline, and you are implementing it on a regular basis. That doesn't mean that you ignore the others, as they are all interconnected, but that you prioritize and give most of your attention to the one that will best serve you at this time. For those of you already well versed in the guidelines, use them to further refine your already established habits and take yourself to the next level. *Eating for Health* is a lifelong process and we can all continually raise the bar in this arena. You may also find that you are reminded of something that you already knew, but may have forgotten, and seeing it again is just what you needed to get you back on track. As you read through the guideline descriptions you will get a sense for which of them would be most beneficial for you to focus on initially.

> The secret of getting started is breaking your complex overwhelming tasks into small manageable tasks, and then starting on the first one.
>
> Mark Twain

Once again let me remind you that for many the *Eating-for-Health Guideline* descriptions may seem like a lot of information. This is necessary to give you a thorough understanding of the overall picture, as well as to accommodate many different levels of knowledge and understanding. You may also feel a little overwhelmed at the prospect of making the kinds of changes that they suggest. Don't worry. Remember that subsequent chapters will reinforce your understanding and assist you in adopting healthier eating habits step-by-step. Eventually you will no longer feel as though you are overlooking Niagara Falls, but instead you are navigating with map in tow and the path ahead is getting clearer and easier with each step.

eating-for-health guideline #1

_____

if it's not food, don't eat it!
> *...and if you do, wait a long time before you do it again so your body can recover.*

This is a life changing guideline. At least it has been for me and the many other people who have adopted it as a regular part of their lifestyle. In addition to quelling a plethora of lesser symptoms, I also have clients and students who have followed this first guideline religiously, and subsequently have not had a seizure, asthma attack, or migraine headache since. This guideline makes a crucially important distinction which most health advocates either neglect to mention or fail to adequately emphasize, thus leading to a lack of adequate understanding on the part of the average consumer. In addition, it is a guideline that is relatively easy to implement once you get it and get into the habit of doing it.

I discovered the wisdom and impact of this first guideline through a first-hand experience that was to become one of the most significant milestones in my quest for healing. It occurred well into the third year of actively making healthy changes in my diet and lifestyle. I had quit smoking. I had quit eating sugar. I had quit drinking coffee, soda, and alcohol. I was practicing yoga and meditating daily. Given that I was doing all the right things, or so I thought at the time, I subsequently found it frustrating and baffling as to why I was still sick and tired all the time. I had recurrent headaches that were excruciating, depression, brain fog, irritability, mood swings, and frequently had *extreme* fatigue after eating lunch and dinner — so extreme, I often literally could not stay awake.

It was after one of these unavoidable after-lunch-napping episodes that one of the primary causes of my woes was revealed. A co-worker was sent to look for me because I was noticeably late coming back from my allotted hour long lunch period. She found me in the break room out cold. I was quite embarrassed when she woke me up out of what felt like a drunken stupor. Fortunately, she was a compassionate woman who had been on a natural healing path of her own for several years and had much knowledge and wisdom to share. When she asked if I was all right, I willingly expressed my puzzling plight, but doubted she would have any helpful answers, as no healthcare professional had been able to help. I told her how it had become literally impossible for me to keep my eyes open after I ate lunch and dinner, and how I would have splitting headaches on a daily basis, which was making it difficult for me to function. She listened attentively, then smiled and picked up the bottle of popular brand salad dressing sitting alongside my empty lunch containers.

"What do you expect?" she quipped looking at the ingredients label. "This dressing is loaded with MSG, chemical preservatives, and a bunch of other toxic garbage. That'll not only give you headaches and put you to sleep, honey. After awhile it'll kill ya!"

"MS…what?," was my response. I was essentially clueless. She went on to explain that MSG (monosodium glutamate) is an artificial flavor enhancer that acts as a neurotoxin and is notorious for causing a host of symptoms and sometimes very severe reactions in addition to contributing to the development of chronic conditions. She further explained that in general, chemical additives can accumulate in your system as they exceed your body's ability to process them, causing a person to react to things they had been able to neutralize in the past; and that a host of chronic *dis*-eases such as cancer can be related to their long-term consumption as well.

Although I had heard some of what she was telling me before, that was the first day I fully understood the powerful impact that chemical food additives can have on a person. Since then, I have learned how to avoid MSG and other chemical additives as much as possible. As a result, I have not had a migraine headache or any of the other severe symptoms associated with what many refer to as *MSG syndrome,* except on rare occasions when I have inadvertently ingested this toxic substance at a restaurant or social gathering. Because I am now able to recognize my symptoms as being caused by the ingestion of MSG, I am able to take appropriate and effective action in remedying the acute reaction.

Learning this significant piece to the puzzling *dis*-ease I had been experiencing was one of the first times I distinctly

barrage of chemicals

Since the 1950's over 3500 man-made chemicals have found their way into manu-factured food. Nowadays in the U.S. alone we consume every year a staggering one million tons of food chemicals In addition, 50,000 chemicals are released into the environment by industry and 2.6 billion pounds of pesticides and herbicides are sprayed onto food and pastures.

Patrick Holford, Optimum Nutrition Bible

remember thinking, *why hadn't anyone told me?* And my second thought was that there shouldn't have been a need for anyone to tell me, because *dis*-ease causing substances shouldn't be in my food in the first place!

As a result of this experience, I had a profound insight. I realized that instead of something being really wrong with me, which is what I had been led to believe, there was something really wrong with the food I was eating. Millions of people have had very similar experiences, discovering that one or more chemical food additives is the culprit in an acute or chronic condition they have been grappling with, sometimes for years, and once they removed the offending substances from their diet, their symptoms and *dis*-eases went away. I shudder to think of the many others who are needlessly suffering from the same, yet unaware of the cause of their distress. This has become a very prevalent phenomenon, but because of its historically recent inception and the current cultural food climate discussed in the previous chapter, it is consequently one that many have yet to realize or understand.

it's not food

The obvious first step in understanding this first all-important guideline would be to define what is food and what is not. For the purpose of *Eating for Health*, food is defined as anything Mother Nature created that is *nourishing* and supportive to the human body. Anything that is *not* created by Mother Nature and is *not* nourishing and supportive to the human body is *not* food. This would include, but not be limited to, any of the following:

- *Any synthetic or chemical food additives such as preservatives, artificial sweeteners, artificial flavorings, artificial colorings, anti-caking and thickening agents, flavor enhancers, or any other chemical added to food for whatever purpose.*

- *Any synthetic or chemical substance that has found its way into food by vicarious means, such as growth hormones and antibiotics fed to livestock, pesticides sprayed on produce, and tap water that contains toxic chemicals such as chlorine, lead, arsenic, etc.*

- *Any substance that may have once been considered food,*
  but which has subsequently been processed to the degree
  that the chemical makeup is so greatly altered that it can no
  longer be considered a real food according to any reasonable
  standards (white refined sugar or flour, high fructose corn
  syrup, highly refined oils, etc.).

In addition to these three categories, I would like to offer some further clarifications. The reformulated end product of any processed food that contains any of the above substances would no longer be considered a real food either. It would be considered what I refer to as a pseudofood, fake food, or food item. Likewise, any food that has been derived from natural sources, but has been processed to the degree that it is no longer natural or nourishing to the body, would also be considered a pseudofood.

For example, the phrase "natural flavoring" is a catch-all phrase for what is frequently a lengthy list of chemicals, which can include MSG. In order to be labeled a *natural flavoring*, the ingredients must be *derived* from natural sources, but that doesn't mean they are natural anymore. In fact, once processed, they often have the exact same chemical make up as artificial flavorings once put on the market. (Remember that many dangerous street drugs were once derived from natural sources as well.) If people actually saw this list of ominous chemicals that go into *natural flavors* they would probably think twice before ingesting them.

Another question that may be raised here is whether or not genetically engineered foods (also referred to as genetically modified organisms or GMO's) would be defined as food. In my opinion, based on the preliminary findings that are emerging, I do not personally consider them to be real food or a wise choice for consumption. There are a variety of problems surfacing regarding these substances; the inability to contain them and allergic reactions being just two of them. Mother Nature rules when it comes to the food we eat. As history has demonstrated we are not capable of foreseeing all the possible future ramifications associated with such colossal endeavors. We will talk more about this topic later and, as with diet and nutrition in general, I invite you to do further research on this topic for yourself.

As you can see, and will find with most of the other *Eating-for-Health* guideline descriptions, things are not always cut and

Unhappily we must remind ourselves that scientists today, and always, accomplish little without a sponsor.

Official scientific facts are expensive to come by.

William Dufty

You are what you eat. And you are also what you don't eat.

Conventional Wisdom

dry. There are often areas that overlap and intertwine, as mentioned before. I have established the guidelines in the particular fashion in which they are presented, so as to provide a framework within which to make it easy to work. For example, stimulants, which are discussed in the second guideline, are considered by many not to be foods as well. However, I have chosen to include a separate guideline on stimulants in an effort to further dissect the information. This makes it easier for people to absorb and be able to make identifications and distinctions for themselves; and also offers an opportunity to provide additional understanding as to how they operate in the body.

why this guideline

As for why I formulated this first guideline and have singled out the above-mentioned substances, it's simple. In addition to my own tangle with at least one of these menacing substances, in general, there is no mystery or controversy about the fact that chemical-laden processed foods, pesticides, synthetic growth hormones and antibiotics that show up in our foods are chemicals, not food. Not only are these substances not nourishing or supportive to the human body, they are actually harmful to us and our environment in a variety of ways known and not yet known. This is one point that all reasonable health advocates seem to agree upon. Aside from their contribution to mass production and higher profits, even the food industry has great difficulty defending their usage.

Regardless of whether or not they cause an immediate reaction, *all* chemicals when taken into the body from our food, water, air and even over-the-counter and pharmaceutical drugs, act as *anti*-nutrients. They are defined as such, because they rob our bodies of essential nutrients in several ways. Anti-nutrients can block nutrients from being absorbed, cause nutrients to be excreted, and burden the body by expending nutrients in an effort to process and detoxify them. Furthermore, they displace the nutrients that a person would otherwise derive from quality, nutrient-rich foods.

As for the safety of individual chemicals that, in addition to being anti-nutrients, are also known or suspected to be carcinogens or neurotoxins, such as MSG, aspartame, nitrates, nitrites, etc., all of which have been in the spotlight in recent years

How much more health effective and cost-effective it would be if more emphasis were placed on prevention – on keeping harmful materials out of the air, water, and soil – and out of our people.

Douglas Costle
Administrator, EPA

— why take the chance? Let food companies, health advocates, doctors and scientists quibble about who fed what to which rat for how long. If you are not eating it, you don't have to worry about it. Much better to be in the position of not having eaten it, than to be one of the sorry lot who regrets having done so when the conclusive study is released, whether from researchers or the public laboratory, confirming that one specific substance or combination of these substances causes cancer, strokes, heart disease, Alzheimer's, Parkinson's, etc. *If it's not food don't eat it* and you don't have to try to keep track of all the latest findings, which depending on their origin, are often questionable anyway.

When in doubt, do without is an appropriate adage to apply here. There is no reason to put these substances in your body, especially when there are bountiful whole, fresh, natural foods available that you can be confident are not going to harm your body and will, in fact, nourish and strengthen it. In addition, there are now an increasing number of processed foods available that do not contain these toxic anti-nutrients.

A few would still contest this wisdom by saying that chemical additives contained in foods are in such small amounts as to be rendered harmless, and that if they weren't safe, they wouldn't be on the market. It is not my intention here to offer specific evidence in defense of the commonly held notion that the above-mentioned substances are toxic and detrimental to our health. It would take another whole volume to do so. However, for the sake of greater understanding on everyone's part, it would be beneficial to briefly explore these contentions in general. For anyone who is interested in specifics, I encourage you to do your own research by reading publications and reports that are widely available from both camps. Having done so, based on my own findings while delving into these issues, chances are you will come out more doubtful and suspicious, as opposed to confident about the safety of what is being added to our foods.

on safety patrol

The business of mass food production and all that it entails is a multi-faceted and complicated topic, a discussion of which cannot be adequately covered in this book. However, touching on a few issues can help you to feel somewhat better informed and, therefore, able to make better food choices.

The ways in which food industry practices distort what Americans are told about nutrition – and compromise food choices – raise serious issues that are worth consideration by anyone concerned about nutrition and health.

Marion Nestle
Food Politics

To start, it is important to understand that when something has been approved by the U.S. Food and Drug Administration (FDA), it means that the FDA is allowing it to be put on the market in this country. *Not* that the FDA has done its own independent research and testing to establish or confirm a food or drug's eminent safety, as many believe. The burden of proof regarding the safety of chemicals used as food additives is left to the manufacturer. Common sense would tell us that relying on someone to provide objective information when they have a lot of money riding on the outcome wouldn't be the smartest thing to do. Unfortunately, because the FDA currently has neither the staff nor the budget to do the required testing itself, we all must rely on the information provided by the manufacturer. Consequently, when a company touts that a particular chemical additive has been approved by the FDA, this doesn't hold a lot of weight with those who are well informed, and still does not take away from the fact that it is an anti-nutrient.

We have already seen how the food industry provides the media with manipulated research for dissemination to the public. Can it really be trusted to provide the FDA with credible studies on chemical food additives when it has a vested interest in having them proven safe?

Similarly, it is wise to be aware that when it comes to suspicious substances that make their way into the marketplace, the food industry performs public relations antics similar to those used in its marketing and advertising campaigns. In response to anecdotal evidence that surfaces for example, many companies defend questionable additives contained in their pseudofood products by stating that "there is no *evidence* that it causes _____" (fill in the blank with cancer, Alzheimer's, multiple sclerosis, etc.); because something has not been conclusively proven guilty in a clinical study that has never been done, it is automatically innocent. That defies logic, but unfortunately because of its deceptive wording most people believe it.

Furthermore, the FDA with its limited resources fully recognizes that it is incapable of regulating the thousands of food and drug manufacturers and the millions of products they produce today. As for the substances that have been given the FDA's seal of approval, can we really trust this approval status? Distant and very recent history would tell us we cannot. One doesn't have to look too far for examples of consumer ingested products that have been approved by the FDA, only later to be taken off the market due to complications, including many deaths. In the last 2 years alone the FDA has pulled more than 7 drugs from the market because of their deadly side effects that have left thousands of others with adverse health conditions and disabilities. So, if you think that something is safe just because it has been approved by the FDA, think again.

After doing a little digging into the arena of research and studies, you will find that there appear to be many questions that do not have solid answers when it comes to the safety of the chemical anti-nutrients mentioned above, which are now rampant in our food and environment. Clinical studies have so many variables to consider and may be manipulated in so many ways, it is prudent to follow the money to see who initiated the study in the first place and to be confident about the validity of the testing before adopting the resultant information as something you want to believe or act on.

There are an escalating number of harmful chemicals involved in modern food production, including over 3500 chemical food additives, and tens of thousands of pesticides, hormones and antibiotics. We can't rely on science to account for all the variables involved with these chemicals when it comes to human consumption. It literally isn't possible to adequately test all of these chemicals, in combination with a host of others, fed to humans every day, usually multiple times a day, over a number of years, which is what is happening with the average American today. As mentioned, the validity of the tests and studies that have been done are often inadequate or suspect. For example, many tests done on chemical food additives are decades old. Most studies are performed on specific substances in isolation of the numerous other chemicals with which they are usually combined, and the relevancy of many studies is often questionable as well. In addition, there are many studies that have been done *proving* the harmful effects of a substance, which have subsequently been ignored.

One of the clearest examples of the above involves the previously mentioned flavor enhancer, MSG. Continuous consumer complaints led the MSG industry to conduct numerous studies that were later revealed to have included intentionally

Although testing of the effects of food additives on the liver, brain, kidneys, blood-forming organs, and excretory and reproductive systems is required under the Color Additive Amendment of 1960, it is impossible to test every additive, every pesticide, every herbicide, or every other chemical in the environment.

It is even more impossible to test the combined effects of these chemicals.

Carol Simontacchi
The Crazy Makers

faulty testing

In one case, where the researcher used soup in the (MSG) study, the researchers obtained the soup from Ajinomoto in Japan (the world's largest producer of MSG)... In these controlled studies, some subjects always react to MSG, but large numbers of subjects also react to a placebo. These studies conclude that since the subjects react to both MSG and placebos, it "proves" that it is not the MSG that people are reacting to...For years, I could not figure out why large numbers of subjects in MSG industry-sponsored studies were reacting to placebos which, by definition, should be made up of inert, non-reactive material. Finally, in 1993, we found the answer. The placebos contained aspartame!... Aspartame is far from inert and non-reactive...Indeed, MSG-sensitive people suffer similar adverse reactions from aspartame, providing that they ingest amounts that exceed their tolerance levels, and vice versa.

Jack L. Samuels
Truth In Labeling

irrelevant testing criterion geared toward throwing the results in favor of MSG usage (see side bar). In other credible studies done on small animals, MSG has been proven to cause brain damage in the young due to their undeveloped protective blood brain barrier. As a result, considerable pressure was put on the food industry to remove MSG from baby food. However, no official action has been taken by the FDA to outlaw MSG in baby food. In fact, there are junior food products and baby formulas on the market that contain MSG. Ironically, many of the formulas for allergic infants contain larger amounts than the regular formulas. In addition, there are many infants and toddlers who eat table food that contains MSG.

Other studies have revealed that MSG causes obesity (it is actually used to fatten laboratory animals without increasing their food intake) and when fed to pregnant rats or mice, the offspring suffer from learning disabilities. In general, neuroscientists agree that MSG is a neurotoxin, killing brain neurons by exciting them to death. The leading reaction to MSG is migraine headaches, a fact well recognized by headache clinics throughout the country. Many other symptoms, including depression, irritability, fatigue, mood swings and reproductive dysfunction have also been reported. According to the *Consumer's Dictionary of Food Additives*, in 1980, over 20 years ago, MSG was added to the FDA's list of additives needing further study due to the uncertainties that exist. Despite this fact, the use of MSG has not abated. Quite shockingly, it has actually escalated in this same time period and is currently estimated to be contained in over 60% of processed food products on the market today. Given that 90% of the food people eat is chemically processed, that would put regular consumption of MSG at a very high range. Aspartame is another common neurotoxin with equally detrimental side effects.

FDA approval and the subjective research and studies orchestrated on behalf of food manufacturers are clearly not something you can rely on. However, if you look at anecdotal evidence and the public sector, which has essentially become a laboratory of sorts, the study that has been taking place over the last few decades in the public laboratory clearly indicates that eating fake foods is detrimental to people's health. Unfortunately, the most obvious display of the effects these toxins and pseudofoods are having, is on the most vulnerable segment of the American population, our children.

Today's school-aged children are the first generation to eat these substances in the amounts and frequency with which they do for the first time in history. In only two decades, in addition to obesity rates having doubled, when you look at the skyrocketing numbers of learning disabilities, ADD, ADHD, autism, depression, suicide and psychosis among our children, it becomes apparent that something is wrong. These are complex issues that, no doubt, have multiple factors coming into play, toxic chemicals in the environment being another primary culprit. However, the fact that chemical anti-nutrients and pseudofoods in combination with a lack of proper nutrients is compromising our children's development and having a catastrophic effect on their general health and well-being, is indisputable.

Although a growing number already exist, we don't have to wait for objective, conclusive clinical studies to confirm what we already know in our hearts and minds to be true. It is wiser to err on the side of caution given the burgeoning physical and mental health problems among both children and adults in this country by sticking with natural foods that have stood the test of time and which we *know* do not cause harm. Reflecting back to our earlier analogy involving Mr. Whitless and the inappropriate fuel he puts in his car, by doing so one effectively goes from being a Whit*less*, to being a Whit*more*.

While there is a possibility that modern technology will advance and that humans may evolve as a species to accommodate chemical-laden pseudofoods with little to no nutritional value, from the way things look today, we're not there yet and we may never be. In the meantime, the best defense for ourselves and our families against these substances, and the best offense in terms of influencing food manufacturers to mend their ways, is to regularly implement this number one guideline: *if it's not food, don't eat it!*

Since processed, packaged, highly refined foods containing chemical non-foods account for most of what people are eating today, "What are we supposed to eat?" is a common response to this guideline. In short, the answer is: an abundance of whole, fresh, natural foods, fish, meat and dairy products that *do not* contain synthetic growth hormones or antibiotics whenever

Understand that when the word *processed* is used, it refers to procedures that ultimately undermine your health.

It is a term that you can easily and accurately interchange with the word *destroyed*.

Processing is the practice of taking a perfectly good food, one that contains the nutrients necessary to prolong life, and stripping it of everything and anything of value and then offering it up for sale.

In other words, processing is making something to put into the human stomach that no longer resembles what nature produced and intended for consumption.

Harvey & Marilyn Diamond, Fit for Life II

possible, as well as processed foods that *do not* contain chemical additives.

make the transition

Unfortunately, avoiding anti-nutrient pseudofoods essentially means staying away from all highly refined, processed and packaged foods containing chemical additives, including fast foods and much of the food served at chain restaurants. Fortunately, this is becoming increasingly easier to do because of the growing popularity of the health food, or natural foods, industry. Once considered a hippie fad consisting of small store fronts with dusty shelves full of foods that resembled and tasted like cardboard, the health food industry has emerged as big business and is now one of the fastest growing industries in the world. Even a few mammoth food corporations have jumped on this bandwagon by creating health food divisions within their companies. This is not surprising, given the public's growing awareness and concern with what they consume.

A dish can
only be
as good as
its worst
ingredient.

Dr. Andrew Weil

Anyone can easily make the transition from eating large amounts of anti-nutrient foods by merely switching the brands of foods they regularly eat to natural food brands. This is the very least that anyone can do for themselves in terms of *Eating for Health* and is a cinch to do once you have become familiar with what to buy. The health food industry now provides a growing supply of organic produce that is grown without toxic pesticides and herbicides; free-range and organic meat, fish, poultry and dairy products without synthetic growth hormones and antibiotics; and processed foods that do not contain chemical preservatives, additives, or hydrogenated oils. They can be found at recognized natural foods stores, and at an increasing number of regular chain grocery stores usually placed in sections designated as "natural" foods.

Or, if you like, you can carry around the definitive guide to food additives when shopping for foods, along with a magnifying glass so you can check the ingredients labels. However, in the interests of your time, stress level and sanity, make life easier by buying natural food brands that do not contain chemical food additives. In addition, every time you purchase a brand that does not contain harmful chemicals you strike back at the profit-minded food manufacturers who do use them, and at the same time reward those that do not.

The number of health food companies and brands that are now available have become too numerous to list (see side bar for partial list of natural food brands). The best thing to do is to visit your local natural foods store or health food section of your regular grocery store, and familiarize yourself with the brands that are available. You can make this transition a fun adventure by exploring new brands and discovering which ones you like.

Keep in mind that taste is acquired and if you've been eating brands that contain chemical additives, especially artificial flavorings and high amounts of sodium, sugar, etc., your taste buds have acclimated accordingly and may be burned out to some degree. Whereas some of you may not be excited about the taste of a natural food brand counterpart when you first try it, over time you will acclimate to them and start enjoying them more and more. Eventually you will find the former foods offensive. This can take some time. Learning the new brands and making a transition to having them become a regular part of your diet is an adjustment and takes time as well. It may be a little challenging at first for some, but give this process the attention it deserves and you will be rewarded. Many of you will like the taste of the natural food brands right from the start, sometimes even better than the fake-food brands you had been eating! Either way, countless people who have made this one simple change in their diet have come back to me later and testified that they have more energy, mental clarity, balanced moods, have lost weight, are in less pain, are sleeping better, stopped having headaches, and more.

Nevertheless, I realize the thought of making this transition may still be a little uncomfortable for some people. Many have confided to me that they have never been in a health food store or are not familiar with natural food brands and, consequently, find the whole business a little intimidating. If you are among those who feel this way, get creative and courageous. Enroll a friend, child or family member to embark on this adventure with you (preferably a willing one). Many natural foods stores arrange store tours. Call your local store for details. You can also ask a friend or family member who is a self-avowed health food nut (I'm sure you know at least one) to accompany

natural food brands

Some popular natural food brands include, but are not limited to:

Alta Dena

Amy's

Annie's Naturals

Arrowhead Mills

Barbara's Bakery

Bearito's

Breadshop

Cascadian Farms

Eden Foods

Fantastic Foods

Garden of Eatin'

Hain

Health Valley

Horizons

Imagine Foods

Kettle Chips

Knudsen's

Lundberg Farms

Newman's Own

Pamela's

Seeds of Change

Shari's Organic

Shelton's

Spectrum Naturals

Westbrae

you on your first trip to the health food store. Most would be thrilled to help you.

If you do not have health food brands available in your town or the selection is limited, there are a variety of options for you to explore. Once again, get creative. First, look to the surrounding areas and consider driving a little distance. Plan ahead and stock up on non-perishable items. You can then supplement with fresh produce and meats from your local grocery store. If your local grocery store doesn't carry any of the additive-free brands mentioned, request that they do. Given enough requests, they are bound to start carrying at least some of them. Some food can be purchased online such as bulk grains and organic produce. Wild Oats and Whole Foods Markets, two of the largest natural foods store chains, used to have shopping online, but they have both discontinued this service due to lack of adequate response. Once again, if enough people started requesting this service they might be persuaded to reinstate it.

If you don't have a health food store in your area, chances are you live in rural America. If that is the case, start asking around for farms in your area that have antibiotic and hormone-free fresh meats, poultry, eggs and dairy products that they make available direct to consumers. Remember *Eating for Health* is an adventure. You will be meeting new people, going new places and otherwise creating a whole new life for yourself in unsuspecting ways. It really can be fun and you never know to what other opportunities this adventure may lead.

food for thought

Because what you eat is equally as important as what you don't eat, an approach to making a transition away from anti-nutrients and pseudofoods is two-fold. You'll want to consider foods that are best avoided as well as the desirable foods you'll want to replace them with. The upcoming chapter *Suggested Foods* is an easy reference that is very helpful when it comes to specifics and works in combination with the general guidelines given here. Of equal importance is the psychological mindset with which you approach making changes in your diet and lifestyle. After reading the *Eating-for-Health Guidelines* for the first time, some people may react by thinking, "Gosh, I can't eat anything!" Watch yourself on this one, it is simply not true. We have grown accustomed to

Many of us think of people who lobby for pure water and pure food as food faddists or health nuts.

We call a section in our local supermarket the "Health Food Section."

What is the rest of the store called, the "Death and Disease Section"?

Carol Simontacchi
The Crazy Makers

eating a very small percentage of the foods available to us. Once again, turn to the *Suggested Foods* chapter and see all the things Mother Nature has provided for your sustenance and enjoyment. The list of foods to avoid is quite small in comparison.

Reflecting upon the essence of the first guideline, *if it's not food, don't eat it*, conjures up thoughts of basic human survival skills. We can all hear the voices of well-meaning adults the world over, grimacing as they tell a small child to take something out of its mouth because it isn't food. This first simple guideline embraces this same notion, addressing what has become a culturally acceptable propensity to eat substances that have been passed off as food, but in fact are not. I believe that following this first guideline to *Eating for Health* is the very least that we can do for ourselves and our families; for to do otherwise, is surely the equivalent of eating for *dis*-ease.

When you look at the ingredients of a packaged product labeled "All Natural" and see several words with more syllables than you can count on both hands, it's not *natural*!

Harvey & Marilyn Diamond
Fit for Life II

implementing guideline #1

_____

if it's not food, don't eat it!
...and if you do, wait a long time before you do it again so your body can recover.

- Avoid all packaged and processed foods containing chemical food additives.

- Avoid all highly refined pseudofoods (i.e., white refined sugar or flour, high fructose corn syrup, refined oils, etc.)

- Eat mostly whole, fresh, natural foods.

- When you do eat processed foods, eat only additive-free natural brands, and check the ingredients list.

- Buy organic produce whenever possible. Wash fruits and vegetables with produce wash to reduce pesticide intake.

- Buy organic, free-range or otherwise antibiotic and hormone-free meats, fish, and dairy products.

- Eat in restaurants that serve natural foods.

- Drink purified, filtered water only.

eating-for-health guideline #2

eliminate or relegate stimulants to rare occasions
…the more distant and rare the better.

"How can you be so wide awake?" Karen asked at the start of another lengthy day. "You always have so much energy and never seem to get tired, while I just can't wake up in the morning and can hardly keep my eyes open by the middle of the afternoon. What's up with that?"

Karen and I had become instant, inseparable friends after being paired together as roommates for an intensive 7-day seminar. We had eaten every meal together for the previous few days, so I knew exactly what she had been eating.

"Well, only because you asked, I have noticed that like most Americans today, you eat sugar every day, all day," I responded. "That's undoubtedly the cause of your lack of energy and probably other problems as well."

"What? I hardly eat any sugar," Karen protested. "I've only had two cookies and one Danish all week. What are you talking about?"

Like many people, Karen only associated sugar with the likes of sweet treats such as candy, cookies, cakes, and ice cream, until I explained further.

"Yes, but there is a lot of refined sugar contained in many of the foods you have been eating and you also eat a lot of refined carbohydrates in the form of white refined flour, which is basically sugar as well," I explained. "For example, for breakfast you usually have a bagel or croissant, which are refined carbohydrates, with Smucker's jam and Dannon yogurt, both of which are loaded with sugar. Then for lunch and dinner you have a plate of pasta made from white refined flour, or basically, more sugar. And the iced tea or fruit drink you've been drinking is loaded with high fructose corn syrup — or more sugar, once again. The cookie or Danish you have is just icing on the cake."

The look of confusion on Karen's face began to fade, so I continued. "If you cut back or completely cut out all the refined carbohydrates in your diet, replace them with whole grains, a bit

…coffee, tea, chocolate, white sugar, alcohol, artificial sweeteners and preservatives and salt and tobacco.

It takes little awareness to realize that the effect of most of these is as stimulants, not nutrients.

They are used to whip an overloaded liver and/or stressed adrenals into one more round of struggle.

Unfortunately, their end result is to cause further weakness of these organs as well as thoroughly irritating the stomach.

Jon Matsen, N.D.
Eating Alive

of fruit, lots of veggies, and a little protein, you'll not only have more energy, your whole life will change," I assured her.

Karen was open to the possibility that what I was saying was true, but was still skeptical. Over the next few months she drilled me with questions via long distance phone calls and told me of different things she had read on nutrition in general, and refined carbohydrates in particular. I finally advised her to forget about intellectualizing the issue to find the answer. Instead I challenged her to go off refined carbohydrates for 30 days and see for herself what would happen. That was the end of that particular conversation for a while, until a few months later when she called unexpectedly. Karen told me that she had finally taken me up on the challenge to stop eating refined carbohydrates. It had now been a little over a month and she was nothing short of amazed at what had transpired.

"I can't believe how much energy I have. I hardly ever get cranky or tired, my concentration and focus have improved incredibly, and I didn't even know my period was coming this month. Usually I get really bad PMS with severe headaches, bloating, and extreme irritability, but this month it just all of sudden came and I had no symptoms whatsoever!"

"But what's amazing is that I didn't have any menstrual cramps." Her voice began to choke up as she continued, "Since I was young, pretty much my whole life, I have had excruciating pain and discomfort for a few days every month, taken a bunch of drugs that didn't help, and missed so many days of school and work. I've always felt like a helpless victim to this monthly suffering. I thought it was normal and something I had to live with for the rest of my life. I can't believe that all I did was quit eating sugar and refined carbohydrates and it completely went away. But what I really can't believe is that no one told me this before. There are so many women out there suffering needlessly. Why aren't we told that it's our diet that is causing all these problems?"

Karen's story is just one among many. She was lucky that sugar and other refined carbohydrates were her only nemesis as far as stimulant foods are concerned. Many people, in addition to sugars and refined carbohydrates, are also under the spell of caffeine, chocolate, salt, alcohol, or all of the above, compounding the burden on their body-mind system even more. Each stimulant

Once you decide to kick the sugar habit, you'll notice that your taste buds will start picking up flavors and sensations you may have never experienced before.

Everything you eat will start to taste better and more alive in its flavor.

Marilu Henner

can bring about different physiological reactions that can alter the body-mind system in a variety of ways, but there is one thing they all have in common…

phhheeeeeeooooow – boom!

All stimulants or extreme foods send your body's chemistry soaring out of balance, then crashing in the opposite direction in an effort to restore balance. *Phhheeeeeeooooow — boom!* really is the best sound effect to describe what takes place in the body when stimulants are consumed, and a good thing to keep in mind when making the decision whether or not to indulge in them. In terms of foods and beverages, stimulants include, but are not limited to:

- *Sugars – including refined carbohydrates (high fructose corn syrup, white refined flour, etc.) and all concentrated sweeteners*

- *Refined Salt*

- *Caffeine & chocolate*

- *Alcohol*

These extreme foods are anti-nutrients that act more like drugs than food in the body and as such, could also easily be included in the first *Eating-for-Health Guideline*. Like drugs, they are notorious for being addictive in nature and the dramatic biochemical upheaval they induce can cause acute and chronic reactions ranging from mild to severe. In general, stimulants are the biggest robbers of energy, mental clarity, and your taste buds. You won't believe how much better food will taste once you have been off them for awhile. They also alter your natural instincts, causing unnatural cravings. For example, no one would even think about sitting down and eating a whole bag of apples or slamming six glasses of water, but how many of you have ever eaten a whole box of cookies, or drank a six-pack of beer in one sitting?

In addition, all stimulants have a dehydrating effect on the bile, blood, and digestive juices, which can interfere with all bodily functions. But most importantly, regular consumption of stimulants over time weakens and degenerates the body, the manifestation of which can develop into a variety of chronic symptoms and *dis*-eases. Depending on the stimulant(s) of choice,

stimulated nation

About 80% of American adults drink 3-4 cups of coffee each day.

Stephen Cherniske
Caffeine Blues

Americans consume 10 times the sodium of our ancestral diet.

Patrick Quillin
Beating Cancer with Nutrition

The average American eats 39 teaspoons of refined sugar a day.

Gary Null
PBS Anti-Aging Program

this includes but is not limited to the following: lowered immune function, adrenal exhaustion, fatigue, anxiety, depression, mood swings, PMS and menopausal symptoms, cancer, heart disease, high cholesterol, sinusitis, allergies, edema, inflammation, arthritis, tooth decay, kidney and liver problems, hypoglycemia, digestive disturbance, candida (yeast over growth), headaches, high blood pressure, and on and on. If that's not reason enough to eliminate stimulants altogether or only have them on rare occasions, I don't know what is!

Although the concept of eliminating stimulants from your diet might be pretty straightforward, the actual process of eliminating them may not be as easy. In fact, out of all the guidelines this may be the most difficult to implement for the majority of people for three main reasons.

Everything
in excess
is opposed
by Nature.

Hippocrates

First these extreme foods are often the focal point of social functions, such as cake and ice cream at birthday parties, cocktails and salty snacks before a holiday dinner, doughnuts and coffee during a business meeting, etc. Second, most people are addicted to one or more of them, which makes going off of them a process they don't understand or never get around to. And finally, people frequently underestimate the toll stimulants are taking on their health and energy, and, consequently, have no desire or motivation to eliminate them from their diets. I guarantee, however, that if you do eliminate extreme foods or have them only rarely, like Karen, your life will change in ways you never thought possible.

go for the ferris wheel

Imagine for a moment that you were forced to ride the high speed, thrills-'n-spills roller coaster over and over again every day a few times a day. You could get confused, exhausted, irritable, or sick to your stomach just thinking about it, and those are only the immediate effects. Yet that's exactly what people do when they regularly consume stimulants, as we have discussed.

Now imagine if instead, you rode on an even paced, old-fashioned Ferris wheel each day. You rode around only once in a 24-hour period, and the easy ebb and flow of the ride coincided with your natural sleep/wake cycle, feeling tired when it was time to go to bed, sleeping soundly through the night, awakening refreshed and feeling energized throughout your day, until the evening when your energy naturally began to taper off. This is the kind of ride you can expect when you either eliminate stimulants altogether, or when you keep the stimulants in your diet under control instead of letting them control you.

People frequently dismiss the notion of cutting out the extreme foods in their diet because they mistakenly believe these stimulating substances are giving them energy. In fact, they are what is depleting many people's energy in the first place. Carole is one such example. When she first came to an *Eating-for-Health* program, Carole announced that she wanted to increase her energy and lose at least 5-10 pounds. She had revealed earlier that she drank a cup of coffee every morning "to get her going" and drank 1-2 caffeinated sodas to "get her through the day." When I suggested that letting go of these beverages would restore her energy and also help her to lose the weight she had desperately been trying to lose, she vehemently opposed the idea.

"Are you crazy?" she blurted out. "There is no way I am giving up my coffee or soda. They are my only source of energy. If I don't have them every day I can barely function I'm so tired. And since when does cutting out coffee or soda help with losing weight? I never heard that before."

I explained to Carole that she was riding the double-whammy roller coaster of sugar and caffeine, and that the longer she continued on this ride, the worse she would feel over time. Once again I encouraged her to forget about intellectualizing the matter and put it to the test instead. I challenged her to go off the coffee and soda for one week, starting on a Friday so she would have the whole weekend to lay on the couch as she would undoubtedly need to do, while her body withdrew from these drug-like beverages. I promised her that if she pushed through this initial withdrawal period that by Monday or Tuesday she would be feeling better than she had felt in years.

Not totally convinced, she said she'd think about it.

When Carole walked into the room for class the following week I could tell by the look on her face that she had done more than think about it. She kept smiling at me and could barely contain herself when it was her turn to give her report for the week.

"Well," she began, "I took the challenge and quit drinking coffee and the colas. By Friday night I thought I was going to die.

Just 2 cans of soda can suppress the immune system by 92% for up to 5 hours.

Dr. Kenneth Bock

The only thing that kept me from having a soda to get some relief was that I kept remembering you saying that I might feel this way, and to just drink a lot of water, rest as much as possible, and go through it to get to the other side. By Sunday I started feeling better and then, oh my gosh! Ever then I have had so much energy I'm driving my whole family crazy cleaning and doing things! You were right, I feel better than I have in years. But what's even more surprising is that I lost five pounds! I have been doing everything under the sun to lose five pounds for the past four years and nothing has worked. I just can't believe it!"

Inspired by the results of quitting caffeine, the following week Carole decided to quit eating refined carbohydrates. She did this by simply switching from the *white stuff* (i.e., white sugar, bread, and pasta) to the *brown stuff* (i.e., whole grain bread, pasta, and natural sweeteners). After just one week she felt even better and lost the other five pounds she had been trying to lose. Like Carole, most people are excited to discover that they can regain their health and energy, and lose weight without having to resort to restrictive fad diets they could never maintain, and often compromise their health in the long run.

In addition to lack of energy and excess weight, the other common consequence of extreme food consumption that people are often not aware is lowered immune function. Many have taken me up on the challenge to significantly reduce or cut stimulants out of their diet completely and haven't had a cold, flu, hay fever, sinus infection or other immune-related condition since. One such person was a woman who came to me because she was having recurrent bouts of bronchitis and wanted to boost her immune system. She had a relatively healthy diet compared to most, eating a wide variety of whole grains, vegetables, and organic animal proteins. Her one downfall, which is common, was sweets. Although she made most of them at home with whole grains and natural sweeteners, it was the fact that she was consuming them daily that concerned me. It's important to understand that even natural sweeteners can be detrimental to the body. As per my recommendation, she went off the sweets and, not surprisingly, got rid of the bronchitis. She also gained two unexpected bonuses: the hay fever she'd had since she was a child never showed up that Spring and she lost ten pounds.

Refined sugar, coffee, tobacco, tea, chocolate, alcohol, drugs, and emotional excitement can raise the blood sugar levels and help us to feel good.

The problem is that the pancreas and liver will immediately try to decrease the sugar to a lower level.

The resultant drop in blood sugar results in a craving for more sweets, coffee, alcohol, cigarette, drugs or emotional tirades.

Jon Matsen, N.D.
Eating Alive

Another woman who took this challenge was a Harvard Medical School professor who once attended a *Food Fitness by Phone* program I offered. She was astonished at her firsthand experience of this phenomenon. Although her medical training had, of course, mentioned that refined carbohydrates suppressed immune function, she had never given it much thought. After all, refined carbohydrates are as commonly accepted as paper napkins in America today. Not even doctors have been able to escape from this pervasive aspect of our popular food culture. After a class in which I talked about the immuno-suppressive nature of refined carbohydrates and encouraged the program participants to put my assertions to the test, she decided to try it for herself.

"I didn't have any refined carbohydrates for a whole week," the professor reported to the class. "Then on Friday, I decided to have my usual bagel before my morning run. It was amazing. I could actually feel my immune system weakening as I ate it! I ate it anyway, but it changed my perception of refined carbohydrates forever." Her highly prized Harvard education rightfully provided her with this same information, but it was her own body's experience that spoke to her the loudest, as is usually the case.

Although we have talked a lot about the effects of sugar in this section, it is important to remember that *all* stimulants create a severe imbalance in the body and deplete the body of vital nutrients; and are subsequently capable of causing the same, or similar symptoms and *dis*-eases in the body. That's why it is crucial, whether you want to reverse an undesirable condition in your body or head one off at the pass, that you implement this all-important guideline to *Eating for Health*.

switching gears

Because of their stimulating nature and powerful ability to dramatically alter one's blood chemistry, as mentioned, stimulants can be highly addictive due to the body's need to continually bring balance to the severe imbalance they create. For this reason, whether it's sugar or other refined carbohydrates, coffee, chocolate, alcohol, refined salt, or any combination of the lot, going cold turkey in a calculated manner is usually the best way to break such addictions. *Chapter 9 ~ Clear the Way* outlines detailed recommendations to help you through the process.

---

america's sweet tooth

Americans consume 53 teaspoons of caloric sweeteners per day, the equivalent of a 5-pound bag of sugar every week and half – 75% more than in 1909. In Europe and North America, fat and sugar count for more than half of all caloric intake.

World Watch Institute

The average American consumes 53 gallons of soda pop per year. Americans drink more soda than any other beverage, including water. Regular and diet cola are what Americans choose 69% of the time.

CBS News

In a nutshell, you will want to give yourself at least a couple of at-home days to rest, alert all household members, throw out any temptations (people who are serious about breaking their addictions do not leave a stash in their cupboard!), drink lots of water, and sweat it out. For some, the withdrawal process will be uneventful. For others, it may be rough for anywhere from two days up to a week or two depending on the severity of the hold these addictive substances have on you. You may feel extremely tired, nervous, irritable, and have stomach or headaches during the withdrawal phase. However, I guarantee that you will be so glad that you went through it, because increased energy, mental clarity, a heightened sense of taste and loss of many symptoms (including weight loss) await you on the other side. Isn't experiencing a few days of withdrawal symptoms better than an ongoing life of miserable symptoms and no energy?

Once you have restored balance to your body, you may be able to consume stimulants on rare occasions. I use the word *may*, because many people may not be able to for quite some time, if ever, as it will send them spiraling back into their imbalanced addictive state. Notice also that I did not use the popular, yet meaningless term, "in moderation" here. I used the word *rare*, which has a different meaning altogether and is important to clearly define.

According to my dictionary, "rare" is defined as: *1. infrequently occurring, uncommon, unusual. 2. highly valued due to uncommonness, special.* When it comes to translating the word *rare* on a personal level with regard to the consumption of stimulants, use this definition to guide you while simultaneously taking into account your own personal tolerance level to each individual stimulant. Everyone's tolerance level will be different depending on their weight, overall constitution, level of activity, and current state of health. If symptoms start to return, you have exceeded your tolerance level. In which case, going back off the stimulants before they take over your energy and your life is the best plan.

48 hours

Unfortunately, many people believe that they are not being affected by the stimulants they consume regularly. They believe that stimulants either don't pose a threat in general, or that they personally are somehow immune to the ravages of these health-

Studies show conclusively that caffeine contributes to anxiety, irritability, panic attacks, depression, and anger.

With high levels of caffeine in your blood, even the small annoyances of life can gain tragic proportions.

...what you get from caffeine is really not energy; it's metabolic and neurological stress.

Caffeine is, after all, a psychoactive drug, (which) is poisonous.

Caffeine is considered harmless simply because it is so widely used.

Stephen Cherniske
Caffeine Blues

robbing substances. If you are one of these people, forget about all the studies you may have read in favor of their consumption, or even anything I have said here, and let your body speak to you. It is there that you will uncover the most powerful evidence one way or the other. In order to do this, take the 48-hour test. For 48 hours eliminate all stimulants in your diet: caffeinated foods and beverages, sugar (including natural and artificial sweeteners), chocolate, salt and alcohol, and any foods that contain them. Remember that sugars and caffeine have been increasingly added to foods, so check labels carefully. Or better yet, eat only whole, fresh, natural foods that don't sport man-made labels. If after 48 hours of being stimulant-free you feel worse rather than better, one or more of these buggers is undoubtedly running you.

If, on the other hand, you do not experience any noticeable difference in how you feel, keep in mind that whether or not you are currently exhibiting any effects, stimulants are not good for any*body*. They undermine health over the long haul and it's probably just a matter of time before regular or excessive consumption of one or more of these decadent delights catches up with you. Remember that food is something that is *nourishing* to the body. Stimulants are not foods, they do not nourish the body. They are, in fact, damaging and depleting to the body-mind system. As the body weakens and the adrenal glands become exhausted from imbibing in these extreme substances, it takes more and more sugar, cups of coffee, shots of alcohol, and bars of chocolate to get the same high you used to get with just a little; until eventually you won't get a high at all, but will instead be in a constant state of down and out.

For more information on individual stimulants, including healthier alternatives, see *Chapter 8 ~ Suggested Foods: Getting to Know Natural Foods to Enjoy & Things to Avoid*. Once again, at first these healthier alternatives may not have the same pizzazz as the real stuff, but give them a chance. Your taste buds will soon adjust to the natural flavor of foods, and the old junkie foods you used to hanker for will lose their appeal. The health, energy, and sense of well being that you will experience once you are stimulant-free will be well worth any adjustments you may initially have to undergo.

Any food that makes you feel good is bad for you.

Foods don't make you feel good – drugs do.

Heroine and cocaine will make you feel good too.

Gary Null

implementing guideline #2

_____

eliminate or relegate stimulants to rare occasions
...the more distant and rare the better.

- Free yourself from dependency on any of the stimulants by eliminating them completely until balance is restored.

- From then on, relegate extreme stimulant foods to rare occasions in accordance with your personal tolerance.

- If symptoms return, eliminate completely once again to restore equilibrium. To expedite the process, drink plenty of water and do a cleanse for a day or two (see *Chapter 9*)

- Switch from the health-robbing "white stuff" (refined carbohydrates) to the nutrient-rich "brown stuff" (complex carbohydrates).

- To satisfy a sweet tooth, substitute fruits and natural sweeteners for refined sugars and artificial sweeteners.

- Substitute herbal teas or roasted grain beverages for coffee or caffeinated tea (see *Beverages*).

eating-for-health guideline #3

_____

eat an abundance of whole, fresh, natural foods
...and little to no processed foods.

At first glance this guideline seems easy enough. However, as mentioned earlier, in our contemporary urbanized culture most people have become disconnected from the source of their food, which has resulted in a great lack of knowledge about what they're ingesting. At first it may seem ridiculously simplistic to go through and define terms such as whole, fresh, natural, and processed. My experience in working and talking with people, however, is that the overwhelming majority are confused when it comes to these terms with regard to food. The business of clarifying these terms is imperative when you consider the truth in the saying, "if you don't know any better, you can't do any better."

> The whole is more than the sum of its parts.
>
> Goethe

By reading through these definitions you will soon learn to easily identify and distinguish between foods that are whole, fresh, and natural compared to those that are processed. In a nutshell, the easiest way to know if a food is whole, fresh or natural is to ask yourself if you could find it out in nature. If you took a walk in the jungle or on a farm would you see it? Have you ever heard of a Tator-Tot tree or a bagel bush? If the answer is no, then it's a processed food. Basically any food item that is not whole, fresh or natural is a processed food.

whole

It is interesting to note that the words *wholeness* and *health* have the same meaning and same root in the English language. Identifying a whole food is easy. Just think of any food that is completely intact just as Mother Nature made it. Any produce, such as apples, broccoli or potatoes, whole grains such as brown rice, millet, or quinoa, vegetable proteins such as beans and legumes, animal proteins such as eggs, a piece of fish or meat. That's pretty much it, any food that is in its whole form containing all of its parts and nutrients. Any food that has been ground, separated, processed, refined, and stripped of its parts and many, or all, of its valuable nutrients, would not be considered a whole food.

I frequently hear people say that they eat whole grains regularly because they buy whole wheat or whole grain bread. Certainly whole grain bread is a better choice and may be closer to whole than white bread, but don't be fooled into thinking you're eating whole grains. Bread is not a whole grain. It is bread. And bread is a processed food no matter how you slice it. It may be processed without chemical additives (check the label to be sure!), but it is processed nevertheless — ground, baked, mixed with other ingredients, etc. Also, notice that I said it "*may* be closer to whole than white bread." A peek at the ingredients label of many breads claiming a whole grain status list white refined flour as the first ingredient. Many have added sugar as well. Mother Nature doesn't put labels on her foods. If a whole food happens to be packaged for convenience, the ingredients label will simply say "brown rice" for example (which *is* a whole grain, by the way); rather than a long list of words both mysterious and unpronounceable.

fresh

The concept of fresh comes in a close second to the principle of whole, when it comes to simplicity. If food has been cooked, processed or preserved in any way, it is not fresh. Of course there are degrees of freshness to consider as well. For example, produce trucked in from the farm to your local store is going to be less fresh than produce picked from your garden (which is as fresh as you can get!), but still much fresher than frozen, canned, or dried produce. The same may be said of meats, poultry and dairy products.

Mother Nature has been very helpful to us by installing in her food products an automatic expiration date system. It's called rotting! Something that doesn't ever rot or takes a very long time to rot (excepting properly stored grains or legumes which have a naturally long shelf life) would obviously not be considered fresh and should be given at least a second thought before eating, and preferably not considered at all.

The fresher food is, the more alive it is, which means the more enzymes and life-force energy it contains. Most Americans have a deficiency of vitamins, minerals, and enzymes because

---

Generally speaking, time is an opponent of flavor and nutrition.

The closer you get to a tree-ripened fruit, the more satisfying it will be.

Shoppers Guide to Natural Foods

they do not eat a large enough variety and quantity of fresh, raw fruits and vegetables. Enzymes are not only contained in fresh, living (raw) foods, but also produced in the body. The combination of the two sources of enzymes work together for proper digestion, assimilation, and elimination of the foods you eat. Unfortunately, most Americans eat very little fresh, living food. Consequently, their body's digestive and metabolic enzyme stores are exhausted from consuming an excessive amount of cooked or processed (dead) food, which require double or more enzyme activity to make up for those provided for by fresh, enzyme-rich foods.

natural

The principle of natural is a little trickier and the topic of some debate, at least among the FDA and food manufacturers who have to adhere to agreed upon usage of the word natural when it comes to labeling. Getting into that topic could be another whole volume. So to make it easy, for our purposes here, we will define natural foods as those that Mother Nature has provided us (as opposed to a manufacturer), are not refined or processed or minimally so, and do not contain any artificial or chemical additives, such as colorings, preservatives, flavor enhancers, etc.

Once again with each of the preceding definitions, it becomes clear that there are degrees to which a food may be considered natural. For example, a store bought can of tomato sauce that *does not* contain any preservatives or chemical additives would be more natural than another brand that *does* contain preservatives and additives. While a fresh batch of tomatoes from the garden or produce section cooked down to tomato sauce would be more natural and fresher than either of the canned products.

Two other important considerations on the topic of natural have to do with *how* we eat our food. First, many people who advocate an all raw, or a predominately raw foods diet believe that cooking food is not natural. On the other hand, fire is a natural element as well, and has been used to cook foods since humans resided in caves. As a result, I tend to agree with the more moderate position of including a combination of both raw and cooked foods in the diet. Most Americans could, however, benefit from eating more raw foods. The problem is, because

Living under conditions of modern life, it is important to bear in mind that the preparation and refinement of food products either entirely eliminates or in part destroys the vital elements in the original material.

U.S. D.A.

most have been raised on overly processed, refined and primarily cooked foods and little to no raw foods, their weakened systems are often not accustomed to digesting and eliminating raw foods. This is evidenced by the abdominal discomfort, gas, bloating, and disturbed bowel function that those who fit this profile sometimes experience upon introducing raw foods into their diet. If this is the case for you, starting with steamed vegetables and gradually integrating more raw foods into the diet over time is the wisest thing to do.

In addition, eating big plates of many digestively incompatible foods at one sitting is considered by many to be unnatural and can be very disruptive to the digestive system. So as not to confuse our simple definition of natural, we will leave that particular topic for a later discussion on food combining in the upcoming chapter, *The Basics*. Another matter that we will discuss here has to do with something else that is often considered natural for humans to consume. It has to do with a specific food, loathed by some and gorged by others, and begs the question...

to eat or not to eat — meat?

Probably the most hotly contested debate regarding the human diet is that of the meat-eaters versus the vegetarians. In one corner are those who believe that eating meat is as natural as humans being a member of the animal kingdom. In the other corner are those who believe that eating meat is an aberration, that humans were never meant to be carnivores, and doing so goes against our natural biological make-up.

As with any issue that seems to be extremely polarized, myself, along with many others, tend to believe that the truth lies somewhere in the middle. If we look to the wisdom of the ages for guidance and imagine how early humans lived off the land before the domestication of animals, it is very probable that there would be times when animal protein was scarce and people would not eat it for days at a time. On the other hand, there would most certainly be times when schools of fresh tasty fish swam in the nearby stream, and edible animals, large and small, roamed the prairie and populated the forests. It is very unlikely that a hungry human would pass by this abundant source of food. In fact, his or her very survival probably depended on it. Based on this observation, common sense tells me that it is natural and

It is the unnaturalness that deceives the tongue and appetite, leading to over consumption.

Today, we're so sophisticated, and our food is so corrupt, that our sophisticators have us believing doubletalk.

Does our food need to be "fortified" or "enriched"?

Why refine flour and then enrich it?

The refinement process strips many vital elements from the grain.

William Dufty
Sugar Blues

healthy for humans to eat animal protein on some days and to abstain from eating it on others, thereby simulating the natural order.

This conclusive observation has clearly not resulted from the latest high-tech clinical or anthropological study. However, given that there exist such studies that *have* produced evidence that supports *both* a vegetarian diet and a non-vegetarian diet, it is my opinion that the common sense observation that it is natural to do both, is of equal validity. Whether you agree with this or not is your choice. Recommendations put forth in this book allow for both a vegetarian and a non-vegetarian diet.

Furthermore, I believe that it is wise for people who have been observing one extreme or the other for a long period of time with regard to the eating or not eating of animal protein, to adopt the opposite extreme for a period of time in order to restore balance to an ailing system. In other words, a vegetarian who has not been eating any animal protein for a lengthy period of time and who is feeling very depleted and out of balance (especially those who have very weakened immune systems and are hypoglycemic) may benefit greatly from consuming a bit of animal protein until their system is stronger. While a voracious carnivore who has been eating animal protein without reprieve for a number of years would benefit greatly by abstaining from it for a period of time.

The most important thing is that you discover what is right for your body at this time in your life and be honest with yourself about whether or not something is working for you. Letting go of a long held belief or position that is not working for you may be the best thing you could ever do for yourself.

How do you know whether or not it's working for you? An objective assessment of your energy level and how you look and feel is the best place to start. Also take into consideration that Americans in general eat *way* too much animal protein. Most Americans are eating animal protein 2-3 times a day, which is excessive. Cutting animal protein consumption down to 3-5 times a week (including dairy products) is a much healthier range for both humans and their environment.

over eating processed foods

Highly processed food is, of course, usually soft and requires very little chewing. One is thus led to enjoy the initial taste of the food (which is enhanced by artificial flavoring) to swallow the bite, quickly by-passing the off-flavors, and to rapidly get another mouthful of food. In this manner a large number of calories are eaten in a short period of time, but one experiences little of the satisfaction that should come from normal chewing and tasting. Not feeling satisfied, he is tempted to continue eating far beyond his needs or capacity. People are sometimes heard to say, as they push away a box of processed tidbits which they have just half-emptied, "These things are habit forming!"

Dr. Randolph Ballentine, *Diet & Nutrition*

little to no processed foods

We have already covered a great deal on processed foods, so we won't spend much time here except to stress a couple of important points.

Whole, fresh, natural foods are completely intact, and contain all of their original enzymes, life-force energy, and nutrients, thus supporting, strengthening, and nourishing the body. Processed foods have lost many, and sometimes all of these vital elements. Consequently, not only do they not provide complete nourishment, they rob the body of nutrients through the effort of processing them. As discussed, this renders them *anti-nutrients*, which deplete and degenerate the body. Don't be misled by processed foods with labels touting that they have been 'enriched' or 'fortified.' The synthetic chemicals added to masquerade as vitamins and minerals are anything but natural, and do nothing for the devitalized food products to which they are added, as they are still devoid of most enzymes and fiber. In addition, most big brand processed foods on the market today contain toxic chemical additives that further contribute to numerous symptoms and *dis*-eases in the body as we have also discussed.

Processed foods, like stimulants (which are often one in the same) also alter the body's natural instincts, causing unnatural cravings. This is especially important for those who struggle with their weight and fall prey to emotional eating. Often what is referred to as emotional eating is not that at all, but rather an addiction, if you will, to a processed or extreme food that has gotten a strangle hold on your whole body-mind chemistry. Such addictions also greatly influence your moods and emotions, which can lead to *real* emotional eating. It's a vicious cycle, which we will talk more about later. There's nothing like a stimulant food or toxic neurotransmitter, such as MSG or artificial sweeteners (aspartame in particular) to upset your emotional balance and cause mental fogginess and confusion (to name just a few of the side effects). Understanding this can prove to be invaluable in making changes in this area. As with stimulants, when you wean yourself off these substances, you will restore your energy, gain mental clarity, lose excess weight, and relieve or eliminate symptoms.

The bottom line is that we don't need new gimmicks or fake foods in order to have healthy diets.

Dr. Walter Willett
Eat, Drink & Be Healthy

There is a vast difference between foods that have been processed with chemical additives and those that have not. Naturally processed foods can be a great transition or occasional item, but they are still processed foods and wisely kept to a minimum as well. If it comes in a box or a wrapper, it's not whole, fresh, or natural, even if you bought it at the health food store. It may be *more* whole, fresh*er*, and *more* natural than other choices, but it is still not your best choice. For most people cutting processed foods out completely would be a major feat in our fast-paced world. Instead, focus on cutting out the chemical-laden pseudofoods, then gradually reduce the percentage of time you eat natural brand processed foods, and all the while increase the percentage of whole, fresh, natural foods in your diet. This is a sure recipe for better health as a couple that came to an *Eating-for-Health* program demonstrated.

On the first night of the program as we went around the room and introduced ourselves, the husband shared, "For the past year my wife and I haven't eaten anything that comes in a box, can, or package. As a result, I have lost 40 pounds and my wife has lost 35. Both of us feel better, have more energy, sleep better and all of my wife's previous digestive problems have disappeared."

He went on to tell us that they came to the program because they wanted to learn more and gain continued inspiration for what they had begun, and make it an enduring lifestyle. The endeavor this valiant couple undertook was impressive even to me. You don't have to go to this extreme of *never* eating *any* processed foods as they did, however. (Although I highly recommend it, especially if you want to make big changes in your body quickly as we will discuss in the next chapter.) You can still get many of these same benefits just by *reducing* processed foods and *increasing* real foods in your diet. And contrary to popular belief, eating an abundance of whole, fresh, natural foods has gotten even easier these days. Bagged carrots and salad greens, rice cookers, vacuum sealers, food processors and other kitchen gadgets can all help cut down on time spent in the kitchen.

Wholesome food is one of the causes of the growth of living beings and unwholesome food is one of the causes for the growth of diseases.

Charaka

implementing guideline #3

———————

eat an abundance of whole, fresh, natural foods
...and little to no processed foods.

- For a treasure trove of ideas on how to include more whole, fresh, natural foods in your diet please see *Chapter 10 ~ Be Prepared: Quick, Easy Tips for Healthy Food Preparation & Meal Planning.*

eating-for-health guideline #4

account for food allergies & sensitivities
...when making wise food choices.

"One man's food is another man's poison" best describes the topic of food allergies. The problem of food allergies and sensitivities is quickly gaining in recognition and understanding as it has become widespread, and is associated with a multitude of symptoms and adverse health conditions.

In *Food Allergies Made Simple* the authors site an article linking food intolerances to 60% of human illness. Other experts estimate that one out of three people suffer from one or more food allergies, the majority of which go undiagnosed. I believe that these are very conservative estimates, as they primarily take into account full-blown food allergies. Many people are eating foods, especially wheat, dairy, soy and sugar, that are causing them digestive problems, constipation, inflammation, congestion and sinus problems, depression, and otherwise upsetting the body-mind system as a result. Although these people may not show an allergy to these foods, they are nonetheless sensitive or intolerant to them on other levels.

My personal struggles with food intolerances pale in comparison to the story of Mike, a lifelong friend of my former husband. I first met him while visiting my husband's hometown. At the time, this once healthy young man shared with us that he was experiencing a variety of physical and emotional difficulties. He was severely depressed, his hair was falling out in clumps, he had lost a considerable amount of weight, and he was having severe headaches and digestive disturbances, just to name a few. Although he had followed the recommendations of a couple different medical doctors, who prescribed one drug after another and advised him to seek psychological counseling, he just kept getting worse.

At that time I was not yet a nutrition and health coach (it's stories like these that inspired me to become one!), but I knew a great deal about natural healthcare, so I gingerly suggested to Mike that he might try consulting with a holistic nutritional consultant or natural healthcare practitioner and have them check

food allergy symptoms

Common symptoms associated with food allergies and sensitivities include, but are not limited to:

acne
anxiety
arthritis
asthma
attention deficit
autism
bedwetting
bronchitis
candida (yeast)
chronic fatigue
Chron's disease
celiac disease
colitis & diarrhea
depression
dermatitis
diabetes
ear infections
gallbladder problems
hay fever
headaches/migraines
hormonal imbalance
hyperactivity
inflammatory bowel
learning disorders
mental fogginess
mood swings
multiple sclerosis
PMS
schizophrenia
sinusitis
skin disorders
sleep disorders
tonsillitis

most common food allergens

The most common food allergens include, but are not limited to:

alcohol

artificial additives

artificial sweeteners

chocolate & cola

citrus *(esp. oranges)*

coffee & caffeine

corn & its derivatives

dairy products

eggs

nightshades *(eggplant, potatoes tomatoes, etc.)*

peanuts

preservatives

colorings

sugars *(esp. refined)*

shellfish

soy

strawberries

wheat & refined flour

yeast

Note: *Allergies to beef and dairy products sometimes result from the antibiotics and hormones fed to the cows. After switching to organic products some people's sensitivities subside.*

him for food allergies. Unfortunately, my suggestions were initially dismissed. Mike couldn't fathom, at first, how the problems he was having could be related to something as simple as a food allergy. After all, he had been seeing top-notch medical doctors in New York city and none of them had suggested this as a possibility. Instead he decided to consult with yet another medical specialist shortly after we left.

A few weeks after returning home from our visit, we received an emergency phone call informing us that this dear friend was in the hospital in critical condition. He had suffered a *grande mal* seizure brought on by a strong anti-depressant drug prescribed by his new doctor. Fortunately he pulled through, and as a result of this brush with death, a short time later Mike finally decided to follow my promptings and explore the natural route. He consulted a natural foods nutritional consultant and discovered that he was allergic to wheat and other gluten grains. After just a few days of eliminating foods containing wheat and gluten he started feeling better than he had in years. Within a few weeks his hair had grown back and all the other symptoms had disappeared as well. He literally had a new lease on life.

Knowing this story and those of numerous other people, myself included, I can't help but wonder how many other people suffer needlessly on a daily basis or have had similar crisis situations that could have been avoided by a simple change in diet. By checking out food allergies and sensitivities as a possibility, you have nothing to lose and you may have *literally* everything to gain. It is definitely worth exploring. Be aware, however, that identifying and eliminating food sensitivities can be tricky business, and a medical doctor is usually not the place to go for help.

tricky business

When most people think of allergies, they think of breaking out in hives, a rash or having some other immediate or dramatic reaction. That is sometimes the case with food allergies, but more often it is not. The nuances of food allergies are not completely understood, but we do know that there are essentially two different kinds of reactions. One is said to be a classic allergic response in which the body exhibits an immediate antibody reaction. The other is often referred to as a food sensitivity, in which the immune system is also triggered but in a slower, less dramatic way. As mentioned earlier, it can also happen that a person does not have an immune response to a food at all, but that particular food is nevertheless wreaking havoc on their body.

Scientific distinctions aside, to make things easy to remember for our purposes, as has become common practice, the terms food allergy, sensitivity, intolerance or reaction will be used interchangeably and will refer to any one of these three scenarios. Once again, let the doctors and scientists quibble about these distinctions. The bottom line for our discussion here is that no matter what you choose to call it, we are talking about foods that don't work for your body.

People's responses and the time it takes to respond to food allergies can vary widely. Some people will develop sinus problems in reaction to an offending food, while someone else will experience a headache or stiff joints in response to the same food. Similarly, a reaction to a food may not show up in the body until a couple of days after consuming the offending food. This can throw a person off track; not ever thinking that the symptoms they are experiencing could be related to something they ate a couple of days before. This is especially true of some foods or additives such as my old friend, monosodium glutamate (MSG). MSG is known to cause severe symptoms, including migraine headaches, fatigue, and irritability often not until one to two days after consumption.

Another problem is that quite often people eat the foods they are sensitive to on a daily basis and their symptoms become chronic. This is one reason people develop sensitivities to certain foods in the first place: they are *over* eaten in our culture and people develop intolerances to them as a result. Run down the list of common food allergens on the preceding page and you have a pretty good profile of the typical American diet. Most Americans eat an abundance of difficult to digest, non-organic dairy products and the same refined, overly processed foods (pasta, breads, cereals, pastries, baked goods, etc.) with very little nutritional value, every day, frequently three or more times a day. Their digestive and immune systems degenerate as a result and sensitivities to these and other foods develop. It's the body's way of trying to tell you "I am *sick* of this food" — literally!

The fact that we tire of eating the same food meal after meal and day after day is a part of body wisdom, and guides us in the direction of diversity.

Roger J. Williams
Nutrition Against Disease

Unlike food allergies – which involve the immune system – food intolerances affect up to 45% of people and are caused by the body's inability to properly digest certain foods. The most popular is lactose intolerance, but any food can be the culprit.

York Nutritional Laboratories

Blanket statements such as "whole wheat is good for you," "milk is good for you" or "soy is good for you" are commonly parroted and accepted statements. Unfortunately, these statements don't take into account the fact that these are some of the most common food allergens, causing problems among increasing numbers of people today. These foods are certainly *not* good for those who are allergic or sensitive to them. And whether you currently show signs of being sensitive to them or not, it is not wise for anyone to consume these common food allergens daily, as doing so can cause intolerances to develop.

constant craving

The body tends to *crave* foods to which it is sensitive. This occurs because the biochemistry of the body has become dependent on the offending food, much the same way as a smoker craves nicotine when trying to quit. Food cravings can be a form of withdrawal symptom and as such, are great indicators of food sensitivities. What foods do you crave? What foods cause you to become irritable or anxious when you go for any length of time without them? These are foods to which you are probably allergic and addicted.

In addition to becoming aware of the foods you crave and eat most frequently, the most accurate and effective method for identifying food allergies is an elimination diet. In a nutshell, an elimination diet involves eliminating common food allergens from your diet long enough to clear them from your system, then introducing them one at a time, noting any reactions or the return of symptoms (more on this in *Chapter 9 ~ Clear the Way*). Blood tests, scratch tests, and kinesiology, or muscle testing, are other methods available from various healthcare practitioners. These tests can be inaccurate and costly for a variety of reasons. For example, they may not identify foods you have difficulty digesting or those that affect your blood sugar. When done properly, the elimination diet is the best way to go. It doesn't cost you a thing, gives your digestive system a rest, and is usually all you need to get an understanding of what foods are causing you problems. Allowing your body to speak directly to you is most convincing. It also inspires you to avoid the offending foods, as you gain a clear association between your symptoms and the cause.

alternatives to...

dairy products:
goat's milk/cheese
coconut milk
rice, almond, or
oat milk & cheese

wheat:

non-gluten grains
amaranth
millet
quinoa
rice

gluten grains
barley
buckwheat
kamut ®
oats
rye
spelt
triticale

refined sugar:
agave
barley malt syrup
brown rice syrup
fruit sweeteners
honey
maple syrup
molasses
stevia
xylitol

chocolate:
carob

caffeine:
See Beverages *in*
Recipe *section*

When seeking *solutions* to the problem of food intolerances, the *causes* are what provide the most important clues. As mentioned, over consumption of specific foods is one factor that plays into people developing food sensitivities. Other causes include regularly consuming overly processed foods laden with toxic chemical additives; constant exposure to pesticides and other harmful chemicals prevalent in our environment; an overloaded, toxic, and weakened digestive and eliminative system, lowered immune function, and, in women especially, a deficiency in the vital hormone progesterone. It is clear from this interrelated list of causes that food allergies are essentially an indicator of a weakened body that has been thrown out of balance. Once balance is restored, the food sensitivities subside or disappear altogether. So, *once a food allergy, always a food allergy*, is frequently not the case.

The elimination diet is a useful tool not only for identifying food allergies, but for reducing and clearing them as well. In this case, an elimination diet is implemented over a period of time, followed by rotating the offensive foods every four days or so to avoid re-triggering reactions. *Chapter 9* outlines a basic elimination diet that anyone can easily follow and is a great place to start. There are a multitude of books on the topic of food allergies that also include protocols for an elimination diet. One book I find to be helpful is *The False Fat Diet*, by Dr. Elson Haas. This book lays out plans for four different variations on the elimination diet so you can choose the one that best suits you. Although it focuses on the relationship between food allergies and the inability to lose weight, these plans can be used by anyone who wants to clear or identify food sensitivities, whether you want to lose weight or lose symptoms and *dis*-eases, or both. Whatever you decide to do, however, be sure to follow an established elimination diet protocol to the letter, or you run the risk of producing inaccurate or non-existent results.

It is important to note that most people have multiple food allergies, not just one. All too often today, people who discover they are allergic to dairy, for example, substitute soy products instead. Because soy is one of the most notorious food allergens, by doing so a person is substituting one food allergen for another; and consequently, frequently exchanging one set of symptoms for another. Sometimes these symptoms show up immediately and

You can't count on a food's ingredient list to keep you safe. Some allergens are hidden in "natural flavors," and others may end up in foods by mistake. In a new study, a quarter of the food-processing plants checked by government inspectors in the upper Midwest were producing foods that contained allergens not listed on the labels.

Nutrition Action Healthletter

sometimes they don't develop until later. They usually show up one way or the other, however, because people who are prone to food sensitivities have a weakened digestive and immune system and they cannot tolerate such a highly allergenic food. Unfortunately, because many people think they are doing themselves a favor by switching to soy, when new symptoms show up or the old ones cease to subside, they never make the connection. (For more on soy, see *Foods to Limit* in *Chapter 8*.)

I cannot stress enough the importance of discovering whether or not you are suffering from food allergies and sensitivities. After going over the food allergy information segment in an *Eating-for-Health* class, a woman once made the comment that no one in her family had any *known* food allergies. This same woman had earlier listed a whole litany of symptoms that she and her family had collectively — digestive problems, headaches, joint pain, and more. As I told her, if you are about to discount this information, thinking it doesn't apply to you, and yet you are experiencing *any* of the conditions listed associated with food allergies (refer to previous sidebar) or even those that aren't, do yourself a big favor, think again!

If you are having any of these *dis*-eases, your system could greatly benefit from following an elimination diet for a few days anyway. While you're at it, you might as well test for at least the most common allergens if you eat them regularly, especially dairy, wheat, soy, and sugar. As a result, you will most likely be very surprised to discover the effects these foods are having on you. At the same time you'll give your body a little cleanse and rejuvenation, so you win either way.

Similarly, another woman once came to an *Eating-for-Health* class with multiple symptoms, the most prevalent being a persistent cough. For three years she had sought help for this condition from numerous healthcare practitioners who gave her drugs and nutritional supplements. None of these solved the problem and she had grown weary having spent much time and money trying to get relief. When she told me this, the first thing I asked was if she drank orange juice, a notoriously mucous producing food to those with allergies. (Normally I would have first asked if she consumed dairy products, but I wrongly assumed this had already been checked.) She said no, she only

Dr. Lendon Smith, retired pediatrician and author, attributes many behavior disorders to food sensitivities and places dairy products at the top of the list of offenders.

He believes that between 50-70% of the children in America are allergic to milk.

Dr. Smith also found that of the 6,000 hyperactive children he treated, more than 75% got better just by changing their diets...

The Solar Flair

drank milk and water. To which I replied, "There's your problem right there."

Of course, she didn't believe me at first either, thinking certainly the allergist would have come up with something that simple. Finally, I told her I would give her $100 cash if she quit drinking milk and her cough didn't subside. She came back a week later and I could tell just by looking at her that she had quit drinking milk. The bags and dark circles under her eyes, a common indication of food allergies, had diminished. When the time came, she shared with us that she had, in fact, not drank milk that week, that her cough had all but gone away and that she was really pleased that she had finally gotten to the bottom of this longstanding problem. She also expressed anger that she had consulted, at great expense, more than one medical doctor, including a top allergist, and they were unable to uncover the root of this persistent coughing.

"Why didn't anyone tell me?" she lamented. "If only I had known." I reminded her that I had tried to tell her earlier, but she didn't believe me. She responded that she was very grateful for my persistence and that she had finally heeded my recommendations to account for food allergies and sensitivities. (Hint, hint.) When she returned the following week, she reported that she had taken her son off milk, too. As a result, the symptoms he was having in response to this common food allergen, including bed wetting and hyperactivity, had begun to subside.

As this woman's experience with her son demonstrates, accounting for food allergies and sensitivities is especially important for children. So remember to include them as well when implementing this critical guideline. There are so many little ones who spend the first few years of their lives suffering needlessly from a host of symptoms and *dis*-eases, including recurrent ear infections, colds and flu, skin rashes, behavior problems, digestive disturbances, and much more, which could be easily remedied by eliminating offending foods, especially wheat, soy, dairy and sugar. Please educate yourself and get help if you need it. Be sure that you and your family are receiving the most appropriate foods for your precious bodies and avoiding those foods to which you are intolerant. As we will discuss next, proper nutrition is the first line of defense in preventing *dis*-ease, as well as the first line of offense in reversing it.

When you conquer your food reactions, your appearance, your health, and your zest for life will improve immeasurably.

Elson Haas, M.D.
The False Fat Diet

implementing guideline #4

---

account for food allergies & sensitivities
...when making wise food choices.

Be aware of the causes of food allergies, sensitivities, and intolerances:

- Weakened digestive function (diarrhea, constipation, gas, bloating, leaky gut syndrome, etc.)

- Over consumption of the offending foods.

- Overtaxed immune systems due to poor eating habits, lack of exercise, stress, and environmental pollutants.

To relieve and eliminate food allergies, sensitivities, and intolerances:

- Follow a basic elimination diet by eliminating known food allergens from your diet until your system is cleared and strengthened.

- Deep clean your tissues and organs, especially your liver/gallbladder and colon, with an intensive cleansing protocol that's appropriate for you, and do regular maintenance cleansing thereafter.

- Minimize or eliminate toxic chemicals in your environment (i.e., household cleaners, paints, skin care products that contain mineral oil, harmful chemicals, etc.)

- Reduce stress and exercise regularly.

eating-for-health guideline #5

account for ailments
...when making wise food choices.

There isn't any condition in the body that can't be improved by improving your diet. There isn't any condition in the body that can't be improved by improving your diet. No, the cut and paste button on my computer didn't get stuck. This is a line I rattled off during a seminar one day, a line I think is worth repeating.

It is a line worth repeating because the simple truth of it has either been lost, forgotten, or never understood amidst the high-tech, commercially-oriented mumbo jumbo of our world today. As illustrated earlier, the highly processed pseudofoods laid out by giant food corporations have contributed enormously to the abysmal standards of health in this and other countries, which has in turn contributed enormously to the burgeoning pharmaceutical companies and medical industry. Indeed, on closer examination, they would appear to be feeding off of one another. Eat our bad food, get indigestion, go to the doctor, take our over-the-counter or prescription antacid, etc. All the while ignoring the original cause. This turn of events over the past few decades has led to a warped perspective of health and how to restore and maintain it. It is a warped perspective because it is based on misinformation and disillusion with regard to the real causes of *dis*-eased conditions and what to do about them.

One example of this warped perspective has to do with the way in which we have been lulled by the medical industry into believing that we can take this or that drug to eradicate this or that condition. And the natural healthcare industry isn't much better. Many alternative healthcare providers perpetuate the 'taking this for that' mentality by substituting natural supplements for drugs, sending people off with a bag full of them, without ever addressing, or adequately addressing the diet and lifestyle from which the person's problems emanate.

The fact is, with rare exception, *dis*-ease in the body is caused by poor eating and lifestyle habits that then create a compromised, degenerated internal environment. It is by reversing this damage and at the same time, discontinuing the

There is little the doctor can do to overcome what the patient will not.

Dr. Mark Percival

habits that caused it in the first place, that we can bring about true healing. In the case of infants and young children who seemingly have not been around long enough to develop *dis*-ease, their bodies are merely a product and perpetuation of the poor condition of the parents who bred them. In either case, taking drugs or natural supplements without changing the dietary and lifestyle habits that are *causing* the condition is like rearranging the furniture on the Titanic, or putting water in a bucket that has a hole in it.

Certainly there are many natural supplements that can contribute to the restoration of health and wellness, but these remedies are the icing on the cake, not the cake itself. The cake itself is what you are putting into and doing, or not doing with your body and mind on a regular basis. All *truly* holistic healing approaches to health include altering the diet and lifestyle habits that contributed to, or caused the health problems to begin with.

> Drugs may change the blood chemistry, but they can not rebuild or replace tissue. Only foods can do that.
>
> Dr. Bernard Jensen

Food is the most effective, and yet most neglected healing tool. Food recreates your biological condition on a daily basis, either building it up or breaking it down. Many people go doctor and healer hopping, spending oodles of time and money searching everywhere for the magic panacea that will cure what ails them, never realizing that the cure doesn't reside in a bottle or procedure, but rather in their kitchen and unhealthful living habits. If you are in search of assistance in relieving or eliminating symptoms or *dis*-eases, you can save yourself a tremendous amount of time, money, energy and frustration by following this and all the other *Eating-for-Health Guidelines*.

My personal experience is that out of all the drugs, tests, medical procedures, herbs, supplements, healing modalities, etc., to which I was subjected, the single most powerful influence in my recovery from chronic illness was FOOD! As I have continued to eat predominately for health and refine my individual dietary needs, I keep getting stronger, healthier, clearer, and have more and more energy. Scores of other people have had similar experiences.

Doctors, drugs, herbs, vitamins, or other supplements do not heal the body. The body heals itself. The foods you eat either help or hinder this healing process. A longstanding poor diet over a number of years, which has become the norm in our modern Western world, is the root cause of the overwhelming majority of symptoms and *dis*-eases people experience. Therefore, if you are experiencing *any* health conditions or afflictions, no matter what they are, the best thing you can do to help your body heal itself and restore a balanced state of well being is to implement this fifth *Eating-for-Health Guideline*. By doing so you are giving your body every advantage possible in its quest to heal, at least in the nutrition arena. Reducing stress, exercising, making amends with the past, enjoying loving relationships, and having a sense of purpose in life are all, of course, tremendously helpful to the healing process as well. Making improvements in your diet, however, is usually the first step necessary before a person is able to implement these other elements.

For example, it's difficult to exercise when you have no energy, or to enjoy loving relationships when you are sick, tired, and irritable. As you start improving the quality of your diet, you will start feeling better, and other areas of your life will start improving as a result. Health is your natural state of being. If you want to restore it or prevent it from being lost, pay particular attention to this final guideline: *account for ailments when making wise food choices.*

> Medicine is only palliative.
>
> For behind disease lies the cause, and this cause no drug can reach.
>
> Dr. Weir Mitchell

diet & *dis*-ease

There are three primary recommendations to consider when accounting for ailments when making wise food choices. Each plays an important role in the relationship between diet and *dis*-ease. These three primary recommendations are:

1 ~ follow the eating-for-health guidelines

First, you will want to follow the first four guidelines to fully support your body in functioning optimally. Often, this is enough to completely clear a condition. I can't tell you how many clients I have had who eliminated chemically processed pseudofoods from their diets and haven't had symptoms since, including severe conditions such as seizures, migraines, and asthma attacks. Equally as many others have identified and eliminated their food sensitivities or freed themselves from an addictive stimulant, and likewise, have become symptom-free. It may take some time and detective work, but by eliminating these foods, even if they are not directly related to your specific affliction, you are creating an internal healing environment that will give your body a chance to work its magic. When the body is out of balance and *dis*-eased, one food is usually not to blame, but the array of foods that make up a poor eating lifestyle. As you improve your diet, you will experience a concurrent improvement in your overall health.

2 ~ eliminate and include specific foods to address particular conditions

In addition to adopting the other guidelines, you will also want to hone in on specific foods that may be exacerbating your condition, as well as those that can aid in the healing process. For example, if you have kidney or gallstones, you may want to stay away from spinach, which is high in oxalic acid and can contribute to these problems. At the same time you could incorporate a lot of apples and pears and their juices in your diet as they are known to help dissolve the stones.

In the natural healthcare realm, arthritis is known as the "junk food" disease. Consequently, people who suffer from arthritis would do well to improve the overall quality of their diets in general. In specific, they could also benefit from avoiding vegetables in the nightshade family, including tomatoes, eggplant, potatoes, and chili peppers, which are known to exacerbate arthritic conditions. In many cases children with ADD, ADHD, or autism have cleared these conditions completely just by going off pseudofoods and the common food allergens, and supplementing their diets with cod liver oil or flax oil. Similarly, people who have chronic sinus or bronchial congestion have cut out wheat and dairy products, the two most notorious mucous-producing foods, and are now able to breathe freely. Sugar, soy, and oranges are also known to produce mucous and should therefore be avoided by people who are congested as well.

This is just a sampling of the many specific considerations to be taken into account. It is not the focus of this book to offer specific recommendations for individual maladies, as that would encompass another whole volume. For more information, you may want to consult a whole foods nutritional consultant who is familiar with your particular malady, or do some research on your own. There are also some great books that list multiple conditions and nutritional recommendations, such as:

Of all the knowledge, that most worth having is the knowledge about health!

The first requisite of a good life is to be a healthy person.

Herbert Spencer

- *How to Get Well*, by Paavo Airola
- *Foods for Health & Healing*, by Yogi Bhajan
- *Healing with Whole Foods*, by Paul Pitchford
- *Healthy Healing*, by Linda Page
- *Prescription for Nutritional Healing*, by James & Phyllis Balch

And other books entirely devoted to specific ailments or systems, such as:

- *Digestive Wellness*, by Elizabeth Lipski
- *How to Eat Away Arthritis*, by Lauri Aesoph
- *Preventing & Reversing Arthritis Naturally*, by Raquel Martin
- *The Yeast Connection*, by Dr. William Crook
- *Sinus Survival*, by Robert S. Ivker & Todd H. Nelson

Let thy food be thy medicine.

Hippocrates

There are many other books available on the market today. Peruse the book store to find what will help you.

3 ~ cleanse, clear, & rejuvenate your system

Finally, you will want to take into consideration that symptoms are often the mere tip of the iceberg to an underlying body-mind system that is weakened, congested, and out of balance. This *dis-eased* internal environment frequently requires more than a change in your daily diet to bring it back to a state of health and well-being. Cleansing, clearing, and rejuvenating the organs and systems of the body are usually necessary to restore balance, strength, and optimal function. The road to good health is paved with good intestines — and liver, and kidneys, and spleen, and all other internal organs. There are a variety of ways to do this, from mono-diets to juice fasting, to herbal teas and remedies. Once again, volumes have been written on the topic of cleansing. The elimination diet and other information in *Chapter 9 ~ Clear the Way*, is a great place to start.

Although it is not the focus of this book to offer specific recommendations for individual maladies, there is one health condition that is of growing concern to millions of people that I would like to briefly touch on, the problem of excess body weight.

finding your natural weight

Maria was 280 pounds when she began a *Basic Food Fitness by Phone* program, which focuses on the preceding five *Eating-for-Health Guidelines*. When I spoke with her five months later, she had lost 50 pounds at an average rate of ten pounds per month, by implementing what she had learned in the program. But what was most heartwarming to hear was what she told the group during the final class of the program.

"I have done a zillion different diets throughout my life, and obviously gained it all back every time," Maria shared. "But for the first time in my life I feel like what I have learned in this program is something I can actually do for the rest of my life. For the first time I feel really hopeful about the prospects of being able to keep the weight off that I have lost, because I'm not on a diet. Instead I am developing an eating lifestyle that I can live with for the long haul."

Maria had *Strategized* a personalized program, which you will learn how to do shortly. For her program she primarily focused on implementing the first two *Eating-for-Health Guidelines*. More specifically, all she did was switch from pseudofood brands to natural food brands, and started eating nothing sweeter than fruit, except on special occasions that she planned in advance, such as her birthday and Easter. She was enjoying the new foods she was discovering and no longer craved the sweets. In fact, when her birthday came around, she was pleasantly surprised to find that she didn't really want the cake and ice cream she had planned to indulge in.

Don't underestimate the power of any one of these *Eating-for-Health Guidelines*. People get obsessed with their weight and go in search of special weight loss diets and products to no avail. Instead, get obsessed with your health and creating an *Eating-for-Health lifestyle* that you can live with, and your weight will take care of itself, as Maria's story illustrates. There are, however, a few specific tidbits regarding weight loss worth mentioning here.

things to consider in finding your natural weight

1 ~ Strategies focused on losing weight immediately conjure up the idea of eating less, hunger and deprivation, sometimes at the expense of overall good health and well-being. Although very

I think we place too much emphasis upon the weight loss issue and too little emphasis upon health and wellness for the mind, the body and the spirit.

Dr. Pamela Peeke

common, this is not the wisest approach and is often fleeting and unsuccessful in the long haul. It's wiser to focus on finding your natural weight by restoring health and balance to your body, rather than losing weight. Many people believe that in order to lose weight they will have to deprive themselves of foods they love. This fear of loss alone can prevent them from achieving their goal. Start adding natural, healthy foods into your diet and put your focus on *gaining* these new additions into your life rather than *losing* something.

2 ~ There are some things that are important to lose, however, like foods that contain MSG and aspartame. As previously mentioned, in addition to the other problems associated with MSG, it can also contribute to weight gain by causing those who eat it to crave foods. That's one of the reasons manufacturers put it in their products. It keeps you coming back for more! MSG is a neurotransmitter that affects the hunger and weight control centers of the brain. It is actually fed to laboratory animals to fatten them up for research. These animals become obese without increasing their food intake. Review the list of names under which MSG may be disguised in the *Things to Avoid* segment coming up, and otherwise avoid this neuro-toxic substance by following the first *Eating-for-Health Guideline*.

3 ~ Aspartame, the chemical component of artificial sweeteners such as Nutra-Sweet, should also be avoided if you are trying to lose weight. Contrary to popular belief, there is nothing diet about these toxic sweeteners. Aspartame is addictive and causes people who consume it to crave junk foods, snack foods and more artificially sweetened foods and beverages. There are many other adverse symptoms and conditions associated with aspartame as well, much like MSG. Once again, educate yourself about this substance. It is not a food, it is a chemical and it is wise to completely avoid it. For more information on both artificial sweeteners and MSG, there is a fabulous book I highly recommend you read: *Excitotoxins: The Taste that Kills*, by Russell Blaylock.

4 ~ Another often little known factor that can interfere with the ability to lose weight has to do with food intolerances. For this reason it is vitally important to identify and clear food allergies

After having been consulted by thousands of overweight people suffering with problems concerning the liver and/or metabolism I can assure you that aspartame will not help you in any way, indeed it will help you to gain unwanted weight.

Sandra Cabot, M.D.
The Liver Cleansing Diet

and sensitivities as recommended in the fourth guideline. Many people have lost significant amounts of weight just by eliminating wheat or dairy from their diet, for example. *The False Fat Diet*, by Dr. Elson Haas cited earlier is a good resource for more specifics on this particular topic. Remember that you must also follow the other *Eating-for-Health Guidelines* at the same time to ensure success.

5 ~ There is a lot of hoopla about eating a low-fat or no-fat diet these days which is, frankly, just silly. Our bodies need fat to function. The 'good' fats that is. The real problem is that people are eating mostly 'bad' fats and not getting any 'good' fats. Not getting the essential fats your body needs compromises every function in the body, including digestion and elimination, hormonal balance and production, brain function, the immune system, even metabolism. Switch to a 'no-*bad*-fat' and 'adequate-good-fat' diet and your health will increase while your weight decreases. More on good fats and oils coming up. High-protein diets are equally as silly. Sure you can lose weight, but often only temporarily, and also at the risk of your overall health. Balance, combined with persistence, and patience are always the key to establishing and maintaining your natural weight.

6 ~ Stevia is a natural sweetener that actually helps you lose weight by reducing cravings for sweet and fatty foods. It also increases digestion, which is important in finding your natural weight as well as your overall health. As a bonus, it regulates blood sugar and is recommended for diabetics. Some people find certain brands of Stevia unpleasant tasting. Don't let this discourage you. Try different brands until you find one you like.

7 ~ Using *natural progesterone* (not *progestin*, the harmful synthetic drug) is known to help women lose weight by bringing the hormones into balance. I know of women who have lost weight by going on natural progesterone without even changing their diet. It also has proven to be effective in preventing and reversing osteoporosis and many other women's maladies as well. This is an important topic for all women to educate themselves about, whether you are overweight or not. Read any one of Dr. John Lee's books devoted to this topic for more information. There are many other health conditions that can contribute to the inability to

> Also, keep in mind that no evidence exists to suggest that using artificial sweeteners helps anyone lose weight. So why use them – especially if safety concerns exist?
>
> Dr. Andrew Weil

lose weight that need to be addressed as well. In his book, *The Mind-Body Makeover,* Michael Gerrish refers to these conditions as "UFO's." He offers questionnaires for identifying what your UFO's may be, and helpful tips for overcoming them.

8 ~ Cleansing and clearing your internal environment is an important part of any healthcare regime, and that includes restoring and maintaining normal weight. Detoxifying the organs and systems of the body will help improve digestion and elimination, reduce food cravings, and increase metabolism, all of which add up to a trimmer, healthier, more energetic body. See *Chapter 9 ~ Clear the Way* for more on cleansing.

eat well, be well

Whether you are currently overweight or experiencing any ailments or not, you will want to pay attention to the tenants of this last *Eating-for-Health Guideline*. If you don't make your body a priority, your body will do it for you. So start now and lessen the chances of developing health problems later. And if you ever do find yourself in a state of symptomatic *dis*-ease, remember: *there isn't any condition in the body that can't be improved by improving your diet* :-)

> If you strive for thin, you'll never win.
>
> Strive for health and thin will follow.
>
> Elson Haas, M.D.
> The False Fat Diet

---

implementing guideline #5
account for ailments
…when making wise food choices.

- Follow all five *Eating-for-Health Guidelines* to allow your body every opportunity to restore and maintain health.

- Research recommendations for including foods in your diet that can help heal specific conditions, as well as identifying those that may be causing problems.

- Cleanse, clear and rejuvenate your system to restore health and energy. See *Chapter 9 ~ Clear the Way* for help.

no arguments here

After reading this section, I'm sure you would agree that the *Eating-for-Health Guidelines* are basically common sense with which few could argue. No health advocate would argue with the wisdom of reserving stimulants for rare occasions or eliminating them from the diet altogether. None would argue that it is wise to eat whole, fresh, natural foods and little to no processed foods. None would argue that it is wise to know what, if any, food allergies or sensitivities you may have and to avoid those foods accordingly. None would argue that it is wise to know what, if any, foods may be aggravating or contributing to any current ailments you may be experiencing and to avoid those foods as well. And finally none would argue, unless they had an ulterior motive such as sales of their products, with the number one guideline: *if it's not food, don't eat it.*

Some might dispute certain specific details outlined in these basic guidelines, but don't get caught up in that. The guidelines themselves are universal. Educate yourself and experiment to find the specific details that work for *your* body at this time in your life. In most cases, you are the only one who is going to be able to do that anyway. A great place to start is by assessing where you are currently in terms of your eating habits, and then devising a next step for where you want to go, which we will do next.

For some, the information contained in this chapter is more than they wanted to know, while for others familiar with the information, it may not be enough. As previously mentioned, there are volumes written on each of the topics the *Eating-for-Health Guidelines* address. For those of you who would like to learn more, consult the resource list at the end of this book.

Adopting the guidelines as a regular part of making food choices will initially cause you to at least *think* about *Eating for Health,* rather then letting your ingrained habits, taste buds, or social pressure dictate your actions. Coupled with the suggestions in the following chapters, you will more than likely start to increasingly and consistently make food choices that are healthier for you and begin to experience the fruits of your actions as a result.

The food processing industry created the modern Western diet.

As this devitalized diet was adopted, the incidence of heart disease, colon and breast cancer, diabetes, osteoporosis, and arthritis all increased right in step.

Just because everyone else goes on eating this harmful Western diet, you don't have to.

Lauri Aesoph, N.D.
How to Eat Away Arthritis

eating-for-health guidelines ~ quick reference

1 ~ if it's not food, don't eat it!
...and if you do, wait a long time before you do it again so your body can recover.

2 ~ eliminate or relegate stimulants to rare occasions
...the more distant and rare the better.

3 ~ eat an abundance of whole, fresh, natural foods
...and little to no processed foods.

4 ~ account for food allergies & sensitivities
...when making wise food choices.

5 ~ account for ailments
...when making wise food choices.

Chapter Three

level with yourself

Taking Inventory & Determining Your Next Step

We have been deluged with an onslaught of often conflicting nutritional information in the last few decades. As a result, many people have very different ideas about what's healthy and what's not when talking about food, while many others remain completely confused. That's one of the reasons diet plans are so popular; they lay out very clearly what to do and what not to do. The problem is, diet plans don't work over the long haul. General phrases, such as "eat a balanced diet" or "everything in moderation" are not very helpful either. What do they mean? Ask ten different people and you will get twenty different answers.

This chapter offers a solution to this problem by delineating *Four Levels of Eating for Health* to get everyone on the same page. It then introduces a simple method for quantitatively assessing your current level of eating, which serves two main purposes. First, it gets you to take what is usually an eye-opening look at what you're actually eating, which helps to increase your conscious awareness, and acts as a springboard for making changes in gradual increments. Second, it creates a baseline level from which you can measure your progress.

What you learn in this chapter can then be combined with what you have already learned and what you will learn in upcoming chapters, in order to devise an individualized plan of action; a plan of action that is appropriate for *you* at this juncture, and can be modified in accordance with the changing needs of your body-mind system throughout your life. It is an important first step in creating lasting dietary changes. Before we get to this more detailed process, however, there is another quick, easy and very effective process I would like to share with you first.

the food continuum

Whenever I give a lecture or seminar on healthy eating, I set up a large food display on a banquet table at the front of the room. This display is divided into three distinct categories. To the far left is a collection of some of the most popular brands of pseudofoods that everyone recognizes. In the middle, is a collection of natural food brands, which are gaining in popularity. And to the far right is a display of whole, fresh, natural foods, including produce, whole grains, nuts & seeds, and a rubber chicken representing free-range, organic meat and poultry. (Actually he's a multi-talented rubber duck, that also doubles as a pseudofood chicken raised in deplorable conditions and pumped full of growth hormones and antibiotics.)

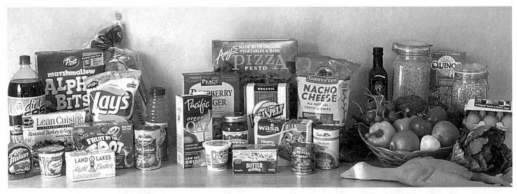

Health-robbing pseudofoods, natural food brands, and whole, fresh, natural foods.

One of the first things I ask the audience is what they notice about the display. Without fail, scanning from left to right they tell me that the far left (pseudofoods) is the worst, the middle is better (natural food brands), and the far right (whole, fresh, natural foods) is the healthiest. Also without fail, many people chuckle as they divulge that they eat the pseudofoods to the far left almost exclusively. This comes as no surprise because, as we have learned, this is where 90% of food budget dollars are being spent.

This commentary leads into a reminder of the fact that since the dawn of humankind, the opposite has been true. People have eaten foods exclusively from the far right category, the whole, fresh, natural foods — *real* foods — for thousands of years. It is only in recent decades that we have made the transition away from these natural foods to the increasingly devitalized fake-food category. An explanation, complete with *Scary Statistics*, of the devastation this transition is causing, follows. I then ask people to consider for a moment what the health standards would be like in America today if instead of pseudofoods, people ate whole, fresh, natural foods 90% of the time. And how would their lives personally be changed if they themselves were eating real foods 80-90% of the time. People are then asked to estimate what percentage of the time they eat in each of the three food categories displayed. I invite you to do this now as well. It is a quick, easy way to generally assess where your eating habits are, relative to what is natural for you to be eating.

Most people admit they are eating the highest percentage of time in the category that has been identified as the worst, the pseudofood category. While they can clearly imagine the health benefits of turning the tables and eating whole, fresh, natural foods 80-90% of the time, for most, this would entail a sizeable learning curve and major lifestyle adjustment; a lifestyle adjustment of such magnitude that it would be a step too big for most to take. Taking smaller steps to reach the length of this bigger step over time, however, is a wiser and more realistic proposition.

For this reason people are then asked to consider what small steps they could take in the direction of eating whole, fresh, natural foods the highest percentage of time, and to once again express this in terms of a percentage. You can do this now, too. For example, think about increasing the amount of real foods you eat by 10-20%. Eating an apple or handful of trail mix as a snack, or having a fresh salad or bowl of steamed vegetables at lunch or dinner. Doing any of these would easily add up to a 10-20% increase in the amount of whole foods in your daily diet, without having any major impact on your lifestyle. Thinking in terms of making changes at 10-20% intervals over the course of a few weeks or months is absolutely doable and highly recommended.

It is wise to adopt any new changes in life in stages in order to truly integrate them into your life, become really comfortable with them, and transform them into lifetime habits, as opposed to overwhelming yourself and having those changes become a short fling that you soon discard out of frustration and longing for your old comfortable ways. This food continuum is a great place to start in assessing where your eating habits are, and determining simple measures to move them in the direction you want to go.

To review, simply estimate the amount of time you eat in each of the categories described, then commit to increasing the percentage of time you eat in either the middle (natural brands) or far right (whole, fresh, natural foods) categories. Consider going a step further by clearly outlining the exact measures you will take to accomplish this (i.e., will have 1-2 pieces of fresh fruit a day, will have whole grain, sprouted bread instead of white bread, will have oatmeal for breakfast instead of sugar-laden bits in a box, etc.) The clearer you are, the more likely you will follow through with your commitment.

While this quick exercise will get you started, the three-step process that follows will help you dig even deeper, in order to successfully devise an individualized plan of action for adopting and maintaining an *Eating-for-Health* lifestyle that will serve you for a lifetime.

daily food diary

The first step is to take a detailed inventory of your diet by keeping a *Daily Food Diary*. Knowing where you are is a logical place to start for determining where you want to go. I highly recommend that you do this exercise. It takes very little time and it is enormously valuable.

For many of you, keeping a food diary may be a scary proposition. You may want to stop right here, or think that you don't need to do it because you already know what it will look like. Listen to all the creative excuses you come up with and then do it anyway! It really is the first step in making lasting changes. You will be surprised. No one else needs to see it. You can write in a notebook, jot in your day planner, or record on your PalmPilot. But whatever you do, just do it! Be sure to keep a copy so that you can repeat this exercise in a few weeks, then months, to see how far you've come.

Financial experts insist that people do a financial inventory as a first step in taking control of their money. There is something about putting it down on paper that makes it real for people. They say that people are always amazed to discover how many little expenses they have (such as coffee money, video rentals, bank fees, etc.) and even more shocked at how much it all adds up to over the course of a month or a year. It's the same with food.

Tracking what you consume by keeping a food diary helps you see things from a broader perspective. It becomes easier for you to pinpoint problem foods and habits, and also to see how an accumulation of little indulgences can have big consequences over the long run. With money, it's financial consequences; with poor quality food, it's health consequences. Once you are aware of what you are truly eating on a regular basis, it becomes much easier for you to make small changes that can lead to huge results. In this regard, the money you spend and the food you eat are much the same.

To get the most out of your food diary, keep track of everything you ingest for at least three days, five days is even better. List all food, drink, and even prescription or over-the-counter drugs and supplements (i.e., herbs, vitamins, etc.). Include all snacks and condiments (i.e., mayonnaise, ketchup, salad dressing, etc.) indicating the brand names when applicable to make it easy to determine if they are pseudofoods or not. Include at least one weekend day if you eat differently on the weekend. Eat what you normally eat. Be honest and objective, with an emphasis on *objective*. Don't beat yourself up about where you are. Where you are headed is what's important.

You may also want to indicate any symptoms you experience at the bottom of the food diary page for each day. Write the time that you first became aware of the symptom. If you noticed a very direct correlation to a food you just ate, make note of that as well. For example, heart started racing, got a headache, fatigued, etc. Keep in mind that sometimes reactions to foods do not show up immediately, but can occur up to 48 hours after consumption.

The food you eat has a powerful impact on you as a whole. View the food diary as an opportunity to be an objective observer and increase awareness of your body, mind and spirit. In addition to physical symptoms, pay attention to all aspects of your life, including sleeping patterns, moods, interactions and relationships with others, self-talk, outlook on life, and reactions to situations. Tremendous insight can be gained by doing so, especially when you start to make changes in your diet. You can then get a clearer idea of what foods are nourishing and supportive to your body and mind, and which foods are not.

the four levels of eating for health

Next, you will want to familiarize yourself with the *Four Levels of Eating for Health* that follow. Then, using your food diary and what you know about your eating habits in general, estimate the percentage of time that you eat in each of the first three levels according to the descriptions given. It is helpful to think in terms of percentages, as this quantifies what you are eating and makes it easier to make changes in a quantifiable way. It also gives you a baseline from which to measure your progress.

As you begin to increase the percentage of time that you consume foods from the higher levels, so too will you experience an increase in your energy, emotional balance, reduction of physical ailments and symptoms, and in your overall health and well-being. If you think back to Betty at the beginning of the book, she was eating at *Level I* zero percent of the time when she first consulted with me. Just by beginning to eat at *Level I* 50-60% of the time she was able to achieve dramatic results in just a short period of time.

Take a moment now to review the *Four Levels of Eating for Health*. If you have already completed your 3-5 day food diary, continue by going through and estimating the amount of time you are eating at each of the levels. Most people will be eating below *Level I* the highest percentage of the time at this stage of the game. Remember that you are taking an *objective* inventory. Balance any negative emotions that may come up regarding your dietary inventory with the positive anticipation of things to come.

level I:

- Follow guideline #1: *if it's not food, don't eat it*. (i.e., foods that do not contain any additives, preservatives, artificial colorings or flavorings, flavor enhancers, artificial sweeteners, etc.) 90-100% of the time.
- Limit stimulants or extreme foods such as sugar and other refined carbohydrates, coffee, salt, chocolate and alcohol to 1-3 servings a week.

level II:

- Follow guideline #1: *if it's not food, don't eat it.*
- Follow guideline #2 : *eliminate or relegate stimulants or extreme foods to rare occasions* (caffeine, alcohol, chocolate, sugar, etc.) Having these substances in the range of 0-4 times a month.
- Rotate food allergens (i.e., foods you have identified or suspect to be problematic for you) having them only once every 4-5 days.
- Limit natural concentrated sweeteners (i.e., honey, maple syrup, fruit juice concentrate, etc.) to 1-3 times a week.
- Limit sodium intake.

level III:

- Follow all five *Eating-for-Health Guidelines* regularly.
- Consume whole, fresh, natural foods 90-100% of the time.
- Eat natural brand processed foods and baked goods 0-10% of the time.
- No concentrated sweeteners.
- No common food allergens (or at least those to which you are sensitive).
- Follow the food-combining principle of separating proteins and carbohydrates (see *The Basics).*

level IV: Cleanse & clear –

Level IV involves adopting a regiment specifically designed for cleansing the body for a short period of time. This includes anything from an elimination or mono-diet to full out fasting. This important topic will be covered in *Chapter 9 ~ Clear the Way.*

begin where you are

Now that you have leveled with yourself and have a clear picture of your current alimentary practices, you will want to use this information as a springboard for determining the next *best* step for you to take. For example, jumping from below *Level I* to *Level III* would not be the wisest move. Taking a dramatic step such as this is not advisable because it increases the possibility of creating the yo-yo syndrome, going from one extreme to the other. The exception to this would be if someone were very ill. In this case, it may not only be wise, but may be critical for someone with a life- or limb-threatening condition to go straight to *Level III* or *IV*; cleansing the body in order to stop the degenerative process and jumpstart the body's healing mechanisms. Much as it would be wise for someone just diagnosed with lung cancer to promptly quit smoking and take measures to start healing their lungs.

For most people, however, it is better to integrate changes in diet and lifestyle gradually, over a period of time. Approaching the matter as the process that it is, rather than an event. This decreases the likelihood of falling back into old patterns and increases your chances for long-range success. This is easily done by upgrading the quality of your daily nutritional intake in small increments of 10-30% every few weeks or so. Don't overwhelm yourself, and be sure that you have integrated an upgrade and it has become routine before taking the next step.

To review the 3-step process outlined in this chapter, take an objective assessment of your current eating habits by keeping a food diary. Go through your completed food diary and estimate what percentage of the time you are eating at each of the *Levels of Eating for Health*. Based on the information you gather, determine your next best step. For example, increase the percentage of time that you eat at *Level I*. In a few weeks, review your original food diary to see how you've progressed. Give yourself a big pat on the back for even the smallest changes in the right direction. And keep moving forward.

It is important to understand that the idea is not to eat at a particular level 100% of the time for the rest of your life. The idea here is to become familiar with the *Levels of Eating for Health* and what is appropriate for you to be doing at any given time. For example, let's say that normally you eat at *Level I* and *II* most of the time, but over the holiday season you ate a lot of poor quality party food below *Level I* for a couple of weeks. For the following week or two it would be beneficial for you to eat at *Level II* or *III* to compensate, and restore balance to your system. You may also consider doing a short cleanse, *Level IV*, for a day or two.

Similarly, whenever you are not feeling well it is wise to increase the percentage of time you eat at *Level II* or *III*, and also consider doing a cleanse to give your body every advantage in dealing with whatever is going on. In the case of chronic *dis*-ease, it is always wise to go to *Level IV* and do a series of cleansing programs over a few months in order to reverse whatever conditions are present, as mentioned. Going to *Level IV* for a few days, cleansing and clearing the body, should ideally be a regular, usually seasonal, part of ongoing self-care as well.

Eating in the range of *Levels I-III* is what is most appropriate for a regular routine, raising and lowering the bar within that range as you see fit. If achieving and maintaining a balanced state of well-being is your goal, eating below *Level I* is never advisable. If you are going to eat below *Level I* anyway, be sure to keep it down to 0-10% of the time. You can get away with throwing in a couple of wet logs on occasion, quickly recover from the assault, and return to the healthful state you have acquired. But any more than this and you run the risk of putting out your internal fire and returning to a state of *dis*-ease. You will have to decide for yourself what to strive for as a general practice, but a good range would be something along the lines of eating whole, fresh, natural foods 70-80% of the time, natural brand processed foods 20-30% of the time, and pseudofoods 0-10% of the time.

This chapter is the first of four, designed to help you take what you are learning and apply it toward making desired, lasting changes. The other practical applications chapters, include, *Chapter 6 ~ Strategize*, *Chapter 9 ~ Clear the Way*, and *Chapter 10 ~ Be Prepared*. These chapters, one in each section, build on and interface with one another to help you move forward comfortably and successfully. But before we get to the next of these all-important chapters, let's first explore and erode the psychological and social roadblocks that can often get in the way.

Section Two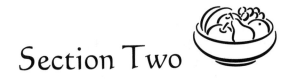

what's the strategy?

Overcoming Obstacles & Designing a Plan that Works for You

An old friend of mine had an arsenal of quick-witted remarks. One of my favorites was the one he used when he observed someone doing, or talking about doing something that was clearly not in their best interest. While most other people would pretend they didn't notice, or hem and haw around the issue so as not to bruise the person's ego, Gene would cut right to the chase. He'd flip his palms up, cock his head slightly, and say with a smirk, "What's the strategy?"

I got hit with this line more than once. It never failed to make me laugh and at the same time realize the foolishness of what I was doing. Perhaps for many of you, if Gene had been looking over your shoulder observing what you had been eating over the past few years, you might have gotten hit with this clever quip as well. As discussed in *Chapter 1*, as a culture we certainly would have. When it comes to what we eat, on a societal scale there clearly is no strategy. Things have run amuck and this has filtered down to us as individuals.

Frequently people are fully aware that the way they are currently eating is not the wisest approach and that they are lacking a strategy in the nutrition department, but at the same time they feel powerless to do anything about it. Over and over, people tell me how confused they are about what they should be eating, that they don't know where to start when it comes to making changes. They also feel there are so many obstacles stacked against them, that they often don't even try.

Whereas a substantial part of this book will give you a good idea of *what* to eat and the associated logistics, this section is solely devoted to helping you with that formidable pile of social and psychological obstacles that may be standing in your way. Having taken a look at our popular food culture on a grand scale, we will now take a look at how this cultural phenomenon is affecting you closer to home. Starting with the way you think.

You've got to dig deep to uncover why you eat the way you do, and unravel the thought processes that have been ingrained in you over the course of your lifetime. These ingrained thought processes and beliefs are at the root of the choices you make. The next chapter, *As You Thinketh*, will help you examine your current thoughts and beliefs around food. This examination will serve as a powerful ally that can help you make conscious, informed choices, choices that reflect what you truly want for yourself rather than falling victim to old, primarily unconscious inner programming and strong outside influences.

Then *Chapter 5 ~ Children & Others*, will help you with those outside influences that can have the strongest hold on you, namely your significant other, your children, and close family and friends. It will address two of the questions I am most frequently asked:

1. *How do I get my family members and others to support my efforts to eat better?*

2. *How can I get my children, spouse or other loved ones to eat healthier, too?*

These are two important issues that often surface when making the transition to a healthier way of eating. Not having the support of those around you, or even worse, having them working against you, can make success challenging or virtually impossible. In addition, once aware of the devastation that our *Standard American Diet* is causing, it is natural to have the desire to help others become more aware and eat well too, especially those who have children. People often feel disheartened and at a loss as to how to deal with these two issues. *Chapter 5* provides insights and communication recommendations that can help.

Another major reason people are unsuccessful when it comes to improving their diets is that they don't make any concrete plans or commitments as to how they're going to do it. Their good intentions are thwarted without a plan of action to carry them through. People will make nebulous statements such as, "I'm going to start eating better," and that's as far as they get. If you really want to succeed, you've got to *plan your work and work your plan*, as the old saying goes, and be as specific as possible about what you're going to do.

Strategizing the process will significantly increase your chances for victory in this arena. And that's exactly what the final chapter of this section will help you do — *Strategize!* The fun and effective techniques this chapter supplies will pull together all that you've learned thus far, and guide you further in designing a personalized plan of action that will work best for you. So if my old friend, Gene, happened to be looking over your shoulder, he'd give you a big thumbs up and say, "Now *that's* a strategy!"

Chapter Four

as you thinketh...

Hurdling Mental Obstacles to Eating for Health

I once heard a woman recount an intimate story about a very difficult period in her life. Her despair was so great she decided to seek professional help. For almost the entire duration of her first therapy session, the woman rattled off a detailed litany of the problematic situations in her life that were causing this despair — from her emotionally abusive relationship, to dire financial straits, to dissatisfaction with her job, to recent weight gain and health conditions. At the end of her saga she sighed deeply and said, "I just don't understand how I got to this place in my life."

The therapist, who had remained silent up until then, replied, "You chose."

This response marked a pivotal moment in this woman's life, she told us. It was the moment in which she first realized the responsibility she'd had in creating the unpleasant situations she found herself in. This realization brought with it a host of mixed feelings. We have all experienced the sting this woman must have felt at that moment, being hit for the first time with the awareness of the role she played in shaping the course of her life. For many of us, it is like the day we found out there was no Santa Claus. We felt disappointed and deceived, and at the same time comfortably relieved because our suspicions were confirmed and so many things began to make sense. It's like a childhood rite of passage of sorts, a crossing over into the adult world.

> Choice,
> not chance,
> determines
> one's
> destiny.
>
> Unknown

Discovering and taking responsibility for your choices in any area of your life is much the same. It is a milestone in the maturation process that brings you a step closer to individual sovereignty and exercising your personal power. For when you come to the realization that you have played a major part in creating unwanted situations, logic would have you simultaneously realize that you can create situations you *do* want as well.

We are all the sum total of our choices. Whether it be how we choose to spend our money, to how we choose to spend our time and with whom, to what foods we choose to put in our mouths, it all adds up to the creation of our environment both internal and external, which ultimately determines the overall quality of our lives. When it comes to diet and lifestyle choices, you either create a balanced state of health and well-being, or an imbalanced state of uncomfortable symptoms and *dis*-eases in the body and mind. In each moment with each choice that you make, whether consciously or unconsciously, you are also choosing the consequences that come along with those choices. You are literally choosing your fate.

Our thoughts are the precursor to any and all of the things we choose for ourselves. First come the thoughts around whatever is being presented, then come the choices and actions we take in reference to those thoughts. Over time those choices determine the course of our lives. Thus, the old saying "as you thinketh, so too shall you become" really is true. This same truth then applies to the food choices you make. Whatever your thoughts and beliefs are about food will determine the food choices you make. In this case the saying then becomes "as you thinketh, so too shall you eat!"

If you want to change the way you eat, you must first change the way you think. And that's what this chapter is all about, exploring your current thoughts and beliefs about food and what you eat, so that you can begin to make informed, conscious choices that are in alignment with your values, rather than being a victim of subconscious beliefs you may not have even been aware existed.

Whatever you have right now in your life is the result of what you thought, felt and did up until this time.

If you want things to be different, to be better, you will have to change what you think, feel and do.

John-Roger &
Peter McWilliams

the biggest obstacles

Over the last few years I have informally surveyed hundreds of people. Consistently they identify the following challenges as being the biggest obstacles when it comes to eating healthier:

1 - it takes too much time
...to plan ahead and prepare healthy foods.

2 - it's too expensive
...I can't afford to buy healthier foods.

3 - it's no fun
...to eat healthy and be deprived of my favorite foods.

4 - it's too hard
...to eat healthy foods when surrounded by a family, friends and a society that doesn't.

Actually, the first obstacle people usually express goes something like, "It's all so confusing, with all the conflicting information out there I don't know what to eat." But because this topic is addressed in-depth in previous and upcoming chapters — and is really the whole reason I wrote this book! — it will not be specifically dealt with here. The others we will explore in detail one-by-one. Doing so will help you begin to unravel your current thoughts and beliefs about food. Many people after reflecting on what follows discover that what they had been picturing in their minds as big, bad insurmountable obstacles were nothing more than thoughts and beliefs that they had held, often unconsciously, for many years; unconscious thoughts that dictated their actions impulsively without regard to their true values. Once they started re-evaluating and changing these thoughts and beliefs, these mental obstacles began to dissolve, and changes in the way they actually ate, naturally and more easily began to follow as a result.

> We can no more afford to spend major time on minor things, then we can to spend minor time on major things!
>
> Jim Rohn

1 - it takes too much time
...to plan ahead and prepare healthy foods.

This is sometimes a very real obstacle and the reason that a whole chapter of this book is devoted to addressing it. (See *Chapter 10 ~ Be Prepared: Quick, Easy Tips for Healthy Food Preparation & Meal*

Planning.) But it is just as often not the case. In fact, making healthier choices can sometimes take even less time than some other less healthy choices. Having a piece of fruit or baby carrots or ready-to-eat salad for a snack, rather than toasting a bagel with cream cheese would be a good example. In this particular example, it is more about acquired tastes and acculturation than time. The same is often true when it comes to preparing meals. For example, it takes the same amount of time to steam some fresh vegetables as it does to pop a frozen entrée in the microwave and wait for it to cook. They both take an average of between 5-10 minutes.

Similarly, the challenge is often not about having the actual *time* involved that is the issue, but rather having the *energy* needed to prepare healthier foods. People, women with families especially, are frequently exhausted by the end of the day and just don't have the mental or physical energy to prepare meals from scratch. This becomes a Catch-22 situation, however, as the quick and convenient fake foods people resort to instead are so devitalized and of low nutritional value that they *cause* a lack of energy and productivity. This can become a vicious cycle that can be challenging to break. However, with a little know-how it can be done more easily than you might think and the rewards you'll reap are well worth it.

In a nutshell, the way to do it is to push through that initial transition period and expend the time and energy necessary to get yourself consistently eating energy boosting, health-promoting foods. If you can eat in accordance with the guidelines set forth in this book, even if you have to drag your behind into the kitchen to do it, you will eventually regain your energy. The length of time it takes will depend on the individual and also to what degree you are actually *Eating for Health*. But if you do it, you can't help but begin to have more energy because you will be adequately nourishing and fueling your body and mind. Having more energy on a consistent basis translates into having more time, because you will be more productive, need less sleep, take fewer naps, and generally feel better. So, when you think about it, eating poorly and the fatigue that inevitably goes along with it is what's really sucking up your time and energy!

To help with logistics, think about ways you can multi-task by combining food preparation and cooking with other activities.

How different our lives are when we really know what is deeply important to us, and keeping that picture in mind, we manage ourselves each day to be and to do what really matters most.

Stephen Covey

One client of mine listens to inspirational and educational tapes while she chops vegetables for the week. Another savors it as a kind of Zen-like meditation time, quieting her mind and reflecting on the events of the day. I like to plug in my headset to my cordless telephone and catch up with long distance friends and family members, or watch Oprah and the evening news programs. Enlisting the help of others can be another way of multi-tasking, especially with children.

People are frequently saying they'd like to spend more quality time with their children. Preparing food together can be just the opportunity. It's only been in recent decades in our modern Western society that we have adopted this idea that children's time should be spent playing or doing their homework rather than doing such things as helping in the kitchen. First of all, given the right attitude and approach, being involved in the preparation of food can be a source of great fun and fulfillment, play time if you will.

In addition, teaching children how to develop cooking and food preparation skills that will serve them for a lifetime is a worthy endeavor that in my opinion is equal to, and sometimes even more important than a lot of the homework they are required to do. One of the primary reasons many people, especially young adults, aren't eating as well as they could be today is because they never learned how to prepare and cook fresh foods. These are essential life skills for proper self care and the care of offspring. Enrolling children and other household members to assist with food preparation and cooking is not only a great way to connect and spend quality time together, but will also cut down on the time you personally have to spend in the kitchen. Yes, it will require some initial time and patience for training, but the rewards are well worth the investment.

Another thing to consider when thinking about the time element involved with the preparation of healthy foods is how you spend your time in general. How you spend your time is a reflection of your values. Take a moment to think about where you might be wasting time that could be freed up in order to take better care of your nutritional needs — chit-chatting, watching T.V., cleaning the spaces between the shower tiles with a Q-Tip?

Next think about prioritizing your time and making nourishing your body a top priority. I once worked with a woman

> The best results are achieved by using the right amount of effort in the right place at the right time.
>
> And this right amount is usually less than we think we need.
>
> Michael Gelb

who initially complained she had no time to cook for herself and her family because of her numerous outside obligations. She was on the board of two community organizations and belonged to at least another three. With all the meetings, fundraisers, and phone calls involved with these organizations, in addition to a successful full time career, she had no time to take care of herself or her family. Or more accurately, she had plenty of time, but she chose to spend it in other ways.

As this woman's health started to deteriorate, she began to value taking care of herself more. Gradually she started to let go of her outside commitments, which certainly would not have been considered a waste of time by any means as they were all worthy causes. However, her ability to fulfill these obligations and maintain a balanced personal life as well was impossible. It soon became clear to her that she was placing a higher value on others than she was on herself, and that she needed to make her own and her family's basic needs a top priority. With more time available, it then became a matter of retraining herself to create and integrate a routine of preparing and eating nutritious foods. Establishing routines is key.

The more you start taking the time to eat healthier foods regularly, the less time consuming and easier it becomes. Think of those things that we are obligated to do as part of being in a human body that just become routine. Most people wouldn't think of going off to work without taking a shower, brushing their teeth, dressing, shaving, putting on makeup, etc. However, many of these same people complain that they don't have time to eat breakfast or pack a wholesome lunch.

Can you imagine walking into work naked and stubbly, with bad breath and body odor on a regular basis claiming you don't have time to get ready? It would never happen. Sure there are days when you leave the stubble, lose the eyeliner, and throw on a baseball cap because you *really* didn't have the time or are taking a day off from the routine. But for the most part, you make the time to take care of these necessities for your benefit and the benefit of others. These hygeinic rituals have become ingrained routines that you automatically schedule in without giving them a second thought. It's just what you do. The same kind of automatic routines for healthy eating can be established as well.

> The single most powerful investment we can ever make in life is investment in ourselves, in the only instrument we have with which to deal with life and to contribute.
>
> Unknown

Initially you will have to go through a short transition period. However, once you have trained yourself to make the time and create routines around regularly eating healthier, you will find that eventually it will become as routine as taking a shower and brushing your teeth every morning. Eventually you won't give it a second thought. It will just be what you do. And in fact, much like the days when you miss your morning shower, start feeling a little grungy and can't wait to take one, as you start to experience the many benefits of healthier eating — looking better, feeling better, having more energy, etc. — you will find that you miss your healthier eating routines when you aren't able to follow them and can't wait to get back to them.

All in all, any time devoted to the preparation, cooking and enjoying of whole, fresh, natural foods is time well spent that serves you in all areas of your life. The same may be said of money spent on nutritious foods, which we will explore next.

2 - it's too expensive
...I can't afford to buy healthier foods.

Values were meant to be costly.

If it doesn't cost much, we probably wouldn't appreciate the value.

Jim Rohn

"Do you know what we call *Whole Foods Market* around our house?" a participant asked coyly when we got to the topic of food costs in an *Eating-for-Health* program, "We call it *Whole Paycheck*!" Everyone laughed and nodded in agreement with this play on the name of the multi-chain natural foods store, including me. I knew exactly what she was driving at. I have felt the bite of exorbitant grocery bills myself. However, over the years that I have been an avid consumer of health food, I have had many thoughts and insights about this common complaint and have come to the conclusion that all factors considered, it just isn't true.

If you think that you can't afford to eat healthier foods, I am here to tell you that you can't afford *not* to. There's nothing more expensive than poor health. And that is certainly what you will get from continually eating poor quality foods. When you look at the bigger picture and consider the costs of doctor visits, drugs, diagnostic tests, surgeries and procedures, and time off work that can accrue due to poor health caused by a poor diet, you can begin to see how a little self-care via nutritious foods could easily pay off. If you were to compare these costs over time with the costs of healthier foods, you would find that prevention through proper nutrition is always cheaper.

When thinking about food costs, in addition to the costs in terms of dollars, it is also wise to consider the costs in terms of quality of life. If you had extreme fatigue, headaches, sinus or stomach trouble on a regular basis, wouldn't you be willing to pay a few cents or a couple of extra dollars or so per day to get rid of these nagging symptoms? That may be what you are doing already by purchasing over-the-counter or prescription drugs to treat these or similar *dis*-eases. Or some of you may be buying a double mocha latte every morning for the caffeine jolt you hope will get you jumpstarted. The problem is, these approaches merely mask the symptoms and ultimately contribute to the perpetuation of any current ailments, in addition to the possible development of new ones, because they tax the body and often have harmful side effects that go along with them. Symptoms and *dis*-eases of the body and mind prevent you from living your life to the fullest. Not having enough energy or feeling well enough to play with your children, participate in recreational activities, or pursue your passions is a much higher price to pay than the little extra you might spend on better quality health-promoting foods.

Not only does how you spend your time reflect your values, but how you spend your money does as well. Take a moment to reflect on where you currently put your dollars. What do you not give a second thought to spending money on? What do you insist upon spending a little extra on to ensure better quality — clothes, furniture, jewelry, a luxury car? Are these conscious choices that reflect what you currently value in life, or have they developed over time and just become habit? How much are these choices influenced by outside forces — society, family, friends, and colleagues?

In our modern society, although we claim otherwise, the care of our bodies and our health rank low when it comes to how we spend our money. Many people, for example, think nothing of spending exorbitant amounts of money every month on a new car and auto insurance payments, yet refuse to pay a few extra pennies or dollars for higher quality foods. They place a much higher value on their automobile than they do on their human vehicle. Frequently, if you ask these same people what they value more, their health and the health of their children or their car, they

> To know what you prefer instead of humbly saying 'Amen' to what the world tells you you ought to prefer, is to have kept your soul alive.
>
> Robert Louis Stevenson

will most assuredly tell you their health and the health of their children. But that's not what their spending habits say. More often than not, this is because they never really thought about it. It's just what people do these days. It's a consumer-driven cultural phenomenon. Similarly, most people are diligent about maintaining the health of their cars by taking them in for regular tune-ups, oil changes and the like, while completely neglecting their body's nutritional needs. As a society we currently spend more money on and take better care of our cars than our bodies.

Which brings us around to the question of how much does it actually cost to eat healthier foods? The answer in a nutshell is: *not as much as you might think.* Many people have the belief that eating health food costs more without having ever fully investigated the matter. Yes, there is no doubt that most health food brands of processed foods, such as salad dressings, pasta sauces, breads, etc., do cost a little more on average than the chemical-laden pseudofood brands. But this is not what you optimally want to be eating in great quantities anyway. If you are eating whole, fresh, natural foods, such as produce, legumes and whole grains from the bulk bins, you will be spending much less than what you would spend on processed foods of any kind and getting much greater nutritional value for your money. Organic produce used to be significantly more expensive across the board, but today it is often no more than, and occasionally even less than the non-organic produce. Check the prices and see for yourself.

Also consider that if you are truly *Eating for Health* you will not be spending money, or will be spending considerably less money, on expensive junk foods such as soda, alcohol, salty and sugary snack foods, coffee, and the like. You will also, no doubt be eating out less and dropping fewer dollars in vending machines. All of which add up to a smaller overall food bill. I could make a whole meal for two with leftovers on what some people spend every morning on their gourmet coffee and pastry to go.

When you take into account all the health benefits you derive and all the money you save on acute and chronic illness care now and in the future, all things considered *Eating for Health* is the best deal going. Put your money where your mouth is, literally! You'll be glad you did.

> The ability to discipline yourself to delay gratification in the short term in order to enjoy greater rewards in the long term, is the indispensable prerequisite for success.
>
> Brian Tracy

3 - it's no fun
...to eat healthy and be deprived of my favorite foods.

Contrary to what many accustomed to the *Standard American Diet* believe, *Eating for Health* doesn't translate into pining for pizza and Krispy Kremes while you struggle to force down natural foods that taste like cardboard. People who have integrated healthy eating as a lifestyle habit aren't walking around feeling deprived of foods they "can't" have and loathing those they do, at least not those that I know. Nor are they individuals who don't enjoy food or eating, as I have heard some people suggest. People who regularly consume natural foods, health food nuts if you will, enjoy food just as much as the next person. They have just come to enjoy and have fun with different foods. And that is the key.

> For everything you have missed, you have gained something else.
>
> Emerson

The idea that it's no fun to eat healthy and be deprived of my favorite foods is, for the most part, a misconception that with a little understanding becomes much easier to uproot and toss aside so that it no longer stands in your way. Yes, it is true that when endeavoring to eat differently as you first begin to let go of foods that are not serving you, some people will be mourning their losses. And at the same time you will be acquiring tastes for new foods, such as vegetables, whole grains and naturally-sweetened treats. During this transition period, depending on the individual and how you go about the process, you may or *may not* feel acutely deprived of certain foods. The most important thing to be aware of here is that this is a *temporary* situation. It will pass.

Soon you'll be just another one of those health food nuts with un-indoctrinated onlookers grimacing in disbelief that you are actually enjoying whatever it is you're eating that is so foreign to them. Ask any health food aficionado. They'll tell you. They've all been through it. And the other thing they will tell you is that the long-term gains they have experienced were well worth any short-term fleeting challenges they had to go through to get them. Many will even tell you that they never experienced any such feelings of deprivation or loss, that their body actually felt relieved as they embraced healthier foods and the nourishment they provided, leaving them feeling truly satiated, often for the first time in their lives. As for the grimacing onlookers, many will eventually come around to learn from you as they develop an interest and desire to eat healthier as well.

As mentioned earlier, it's imperative to really understand that taste is *acquired* and it can be *un-acquired* as well. I guarantee that given the right amount of time, which will be different for everyone, once you start eating natural foods, your taste buds will acclimate to a new level of food discernment and you won't feel deprived. On the contrary, many of you will reach a place of feeling very grateful and experiencing a much deeper satisfaction, a holistic satisfaction if you will, that will be much more gratifying than the ephemeral satisfaction of your taste buds. You'll discover new culinary pleasures (some in the recipe section of this book!) that you will come to love even more because you'll feel good about eating them on all levels, including your taste buds. Trust me on this one. I've seen it happen numerous times.

People frequently come back to me after going through the *Eating-for-Health* program, and thank me for the information and encouragement to persevere. They go on to tell me that I was right. They *don't* feel deprived or miss those things they used to die for (literally!). In fact, most don't even have a taste for them anymore and many have actually developed a *dis*taste for foods they used to think they couldn't live without. Studies show that on average it takes about 8 weeks to change your palate. But everyone is different, for many it can happen much sooner.

For example, Susan committed to giving up her favorite cookies for a couple of weeks during an *Eating-for-Health* class. She had eaten a whole package of these pseudo-cookies every week for as long as she could remember. When the two weeks had passed she decided that she wasn't ready to give them up. When she anxiously bought a package of these old familiar friends that week she was puzzled because they tasted so different from what she remembered. At first she thought the package must be stale. Then she remembered what I had said in class about tastes changing along with changes in diet and concluded that this must be the case. From there, it was much easier for her to replace them with a healthier alternative as they had lost their charm. She transitioned to a new naturally sweetened, additive-free bag of cookies that quickly became her new favorite treat. By doing so she raised the bar on her cookie consumption, taking it up to *Level I of Eating for Health.* By taking this first step, she greatly increased the odds of eventually taking the next step, minimizing her cookie intake altogether by relegating them to occasional treat status.

> Happiness can be defined, in part at least, as the fruit of the desire and ability to sacrifice what we want now for what we want eventually.
>
> Stephen R. Covey

Speaking of treats, they are definitely one of the things people are afraid they will miss if they start eating better. First of all, this is not what *Eating for Health* advocates doing. Instead, see what you can do about progressively upgrading the quality of your treats as Susan did, and also intentionally scheduling them in and having them once in a while, a planned indulgence, if you will. (More about planned indulgences later.)

Secondly, think for a moment of the most scrumptious, no holds barred treat you can think of. How often do you have it? How often do you treat yourself to this treat? Let's just say it's a double hot-fudge sundae with a boatload of delectable toppings. Now, think about having this sugary, crunchy, syrupy delight every day, three times a day. Does it still seem like a treat? Would you even want to do this? When you think of having it this often it starts to lose its appeal, doesn't it?

When you allow yourself to have something every day or on a very regular basis, you are effectively diminishing its special treat status. A real treat is something that is not only a special delight, as my dictionary says, but there is also a frequency of indulgence factor involved here as well. If, for example, you have ice cream and cookies before you go to bed every night, going out for ice cream and cookies is no longer a special treat to look forward to, because you do it every night. You are in essence depriving yourself of treats. Another example of how you may be depriving yourself by *not* eating healthy consistently has to do with your health.

It would be really wise to ponder this whole issue of perceived deprivation that you might encounter on the road to a better way of eating. Really get clear about what exactly you think you are going to be deprived of. People are often attached to certain foods claiming they enjoy them immensely. They will indulge in these terrific tasting foods and feel magnificent for the few minutes it takes to chew and swallow them, then spend an entire day or night with unpleasant symptoms as a result – gas, bloating, stomach upset, sluggishness, headaches, etc. Doesn't sound very enjoyable to me.

And that's only their acute symptoms. They are frequently suffering from an array of chronic degenerative conditions as well, including excess weight, sinus problems and allergies, arthritis, diabetes, depression, heart disease, cancer and more. One of the

Hell begins on the day when God grants us a clear vision of all that we might have achieved, of all the gifts which we might have wasted, of all that we might have done which we did not do.

Gian-Carlo Menotti

greatest human tragedies is when people continually indulge in shortsighted fleeting pleasures for fear of being deprived in the moment, only to find in the long run they have subjected themselves to the ultimate deprivation, the loss of their health. Eating poorly on a regular basis, as we learned in *Chapter 1*, will surely rob you of your health. If you think *Eating for Health* isn't going to be any fun, ask yourself if being unhealthy is any fun? I can tell you from firsthand experience, it is not. If you are not *Eating for Health* you may already be sick or fat or tired or all of the above, and if you're not, that is most assuredly the direction in which you are headed. When you violate the Laws of Nature, you will be humbled not as a punishment, but as a consequence of your actions. It's a simple matter of cause and effect.

I want to clarify here that I do not advocate total abstinence from favorite treats, no matter how decadent they may be. In fact, I think it's not only fun, but also healthy to indulge in what might otherwise be considered unhealthy foods just for the sheer pleasure of doing so. This, however, should be done only once in a while; "once in a while" translating to once a week, once a month or once every quarter depending on the degree of decadence and your tolerance level. The rest of the time it is essential to maintain a certain level of quality and balance to your diet on a regular basis, in accordance with the *Eating-for-Health Guidelines* and *Dietary Basics* outlined in *Chapters 2* and *7*, respectively. Doing otherwise creates an imbalanced state in the body, which is asking for trouble.

There are many people who express the sentiments coined by the old saying, "Eat, drink and be merry, for tomorrow we die." Yes, of course we're all going to die sometime, but let's be optimistic and assume that you are going to live for at least a few more days, or even a few more months or years. Wouldn't you like to be *really* enjoying each of the days before that time and spend them doing the things you love to do? Often the people I hear express this sentiment, that they're "going to eat whatever they want and enjoy themselves while they're alive," are older people that aren't really enjoying themselves at all. They're sick and fat and tired and complaining about all their aches and pains and doctor bills and not having the energy to do anything.

When people are on their deathbeds they most frequently express regret for the things they never did in life. I believe many

It takes a touch of genius — and a lot of courage to move in the opposite direction.

Albert Einstein

people, at least in our modern world, never do many of the things they'd love to do in life because they are too sick, fat, tired or depressed to get out there and do them. Do you seriously think you are going to be lying on your deathbed regretting that you didn't eat more pizza or ice cream or chocolate cake? If you're lying there dying of cancer or heart disease you're probably regretting just the opposite, especially if your age is well below the average lifespan.

The ultimate measure of a man is not where he stands in moments of comfort and convenience, but where he stands at times of challenge and controversy.

M.L. King Jr.

I'll never forget my mother saying to me going into her third week of what turned out to be a six-week unexpected stay in the hospital, "I wish I had taken better care of myself. I probably wouldn't be in here right now." She then vowed that given a second chance she would change her ways and start eating better once she was discharged and would be looking to me for help. It was one of those moments that fanned the flames of my desire to complete this book. Unfortunately, she never got that second chance. What she didn't know then was that initial hospital stay was the first in a succession of lengthy hospital stays she would have to endure until she died almost a year later. In the end, she felt that her neglectful habits had deprived her of precious months, possibly years of her life. This was not fun for her. She was only 63. She had a new grandbaby, a wealth of friends and family that loved her, and an award-winning career as an artist. She wasn't ready to go. She knew she could have eaten better and exercised, and she regretted not having done so when she'd had the opportunity.

If you are reading this book, you still have the opportunity. Seize this opportunity, do it for yourself and your loved ones. *Eating for Health* is much more fun than depriving yourself of the quality and possibly the quantity of life to which you are entitled.

4 - it's too hard

...to eat healthy foods when surrounded by a family, friends and a society that doesn't.

This fourth obstacle people regularly voice is admittedly the most legitimate and challenging. Yes, it can be very hard to adopt and maintain a healthier eating lifestyle when surrounded by family members and coworkers who don't, not to mention having to resist the vending machine down the hall at work, the banquet table covered with unhealthy food at every social gathering, and the drive-thru window of fast-food emporiums that beckon to you from every main street corner. It can be tremendously challenging. There's no doubt about it. That's why I wrote this book, to make it easier. Use what you are learning here and persevere. It will get easier and easier, I promise. Three of the most important elements for easing this burden are gaining support from others, strategizing this lifelong process, and being prepared by making healthy food choices readily available. These elements are so important that an entire upcoming chapter is devoted to each of them. In addition, following are a few other suggestions that can be tremendously helpful.

The first has to do with bringing the subtle, yet immensely operative workings of the food that you eat to the forefront of your mind. If you step out in front of an oncoming train going 100 miles an hour, the consequences you face are clear and immediate. When it comes to the food you eat, however, the consequences of your choices are often neither clear nor immediate. As a result, you often don't make the association between the two. This can be an insidious force working against you when it comes to making changes in your diet. Since the long-term consequences of eating a particular food are not readily visible, going for the immediate gratification of your taste buds is frequently the choice that wins out.

One of the most effective internal tactics I know of to deploy whenever you find yourself entertaining the thought that healthy eating is too hard in order to justify an unhealthy indulgence, is to STOP! and ask yourself, is it any easier to have a headache, stomach ache, arthritis, heart attack, sinus problems or any other symptoms or *dis*-eases you are currently experiencing, or could potentially experience as a result of eating this food? The more that you can train yourself to make a direct correlation between symptoms or *dis*-eases and the foods you're eating, the easier it becomes to make better food choices.

Continuously making poor food choices over the course of many years can result in *dis*-eases that are capable of having an impact on a person's life similar to that of stepping in front of an oncoming train. Remember that people don't just suddenly have a heart attack or get diabetes or cancer. These are chronic

The only difference between winners and losers, is that losers try and fail... try and fail... try and fail... and give up.

Winners try and fail... try and fail... over and over again until they succeed.

Don't give up!

Unknown

degenerative diseases that develop in the body over time due to poor diet and lifestyle habits. The same is true of non-life threatening, albeit equally annoying, conditions such as arthritis, sinus problems, depression and the like. The more that you can keep this in mind and remember it when faced with having to choose between a healthy and not-so-healthy food choice, the easier it will become to make the choice that is best for you.

Take a moment now to close your eyes and think of a food choice that you know you are having too much of and is causing you problems. Now think of the symptoms or *dis*-eases that it is causing in your body. Feel those conditions in your body, pain, bloating, headache, high blood pressure, post-nasal drip or whatever it is. Really feel how these things feel in your body and how much you dislike having them, while continuing to visualize that food choice that is causing or contributing to them. Make that association. Next time you are faced with this food choice and start thinking it is so hard to resist, once again, STOP! Remember how it makes you feel and ask yourself, is it any easier to have _____ , fill in the blank with the symptoms or *dis*-eases you experience associated with this food. *Then* make your decision.

You may decide to eat it anyway. We all do from time to time. But at least you have made a *conscious* decision. That's the most important thing to start. The more you practice this, the more you will increase the chances of making wiser decisions and the easier it will become. Don't get too serious about doing this, have fun with it. Think of it as a little game you can play with yourself. But practice it regularly to reap the benefits.

Practicing any new skill or behavior regularly is what leads to mastery. Because it is a lifelong process, not an event, this is especially true when it comes to healthy eating. The key to success is consistent action over time. So, if you fall off the proverbial horse, keep getting back on. Whether you are learning to ride a horse or a bike, or are trying to quit smoking, exercise regularly or eat healthy consistently, if you want to conquer the beast you've got to keep trying and practicing until you get it right.

For example, studies show that it takes 6-7 tries on average before a person is able to quit smoking for good. I believe the same is true for healthy eating. So, if you have tried to adopt and maintain a healthier eating lifestyle a few times already and have

If you don't give your body what it needs, how can it give you what you need?

Debbie Sarfati

failed, that's the good news. It means you're almost there! So, whatever you do, don't give up now. Just think if you had given up the first couple of times you toppled over when first learning to ride a bike because it was too hard. You never would have learned how. Even though it was challenging to start, didn't it get easier each time you fell off and got back on? Eventually it wasn't hard at all and you just cruised right along. That's how *Eating for Health* will become for you if you just keep at it.

Speaking of quitting smoking, there are a lot of similarities between this health-robbing habit and poor eating. Another such similarity that is important for you to be aware or reminded of is the withdrawal phase that often comes along with both. Everyone knows that when trying to quit smoking, many people suffer from acute withdrawal symptoms such as headaches, fatigue, nervousness, irritability and cravings for nicotine. What many people don't know, however, is that when transitioning to a more nutritious diet and letting go of foods that fall below *Level I of Eating for Health*, you may experience similar withdrawal symptoms as the body seeks to rebalance its internal environment. This is especially true if you consume a lot of the extreme foods that we talked about in the second *Eating-for-Health Guideline*, but may be true of other foods as well. It's critical that you understand this and expect it if you decide to go cold turkey on certain foods so that you can arrange your schedule and otherwise prepare yourself.

Don't let the thought of withdrawal scare you off though. You will be so much better off once you get to the other side. Isn't a smoker better off having gone through an acute withdrawal period in order to rid himself of this life extinguishing habit than to have kept smoking? What it comes down to is a matter of a few days of discomfort during the withdrawal process, versus the many years of discomfort that may be experienced from the conditions that can arise from the habit of smoking or poor eating. *Chapter 9 ~ Clear the Way*, will walk you through this transition process step-by-step to make it as easy as possible and minimize whatever withdrawal symptoms you may experience.

Another thing that can be enormously worthwhile in easing some of the difficulties associated with maintaining a balanced eating routine is developing the art of selective perception. To give you an idea of what I mean by selective

> If the pilot of an airplane decides to change its direction by even half a degree the plane will arrive at a completely different destination.
>
> Andreas Moritz

perception, a couple of years ago a former coworker was giving me directions to a function. She told me to go down the main street and turn left at the Burger King on the corner, approximately a mile from my house. Although I had lived in the neighborhood for several years and had driven by there hundreds of times, I had no idea where the Burger King was. When I told her so, she laughed in dismay and then remembered that I was a health food nut.

"Wow, you mean you really don't even notice places like Burger King?" she exclaimed. "I wish I could do that, I'd probably be able to lose that extra 20 pounds!"

I honestly don't notice fast-food places anymore. They're like noise on the side of the road to me. My selective perception filters them out. In the past I could have told you not only where every fast food restaurant was within a 20 mile radius, but I also could have told you everything available on their menus along with their prices.

Today I couldn't tell you the fast-food joints that I drive by every day, but I could tell you where every natural foods store and health food restaurant is this side of the Mississippi and quite a few on the other side too (a slight exaggeration, but close!). The generally unassuming signs of health food havens jump out at me like neon against a black sky. My psychological radar is now wired to seek out places offering pure, healthy foods, and I get a little thrill when I discover them. This selective perception developed naturally over the course of time, as it will for you the more you start to eat better. However, you can accelerate the process by once again practicing and playing a little game with yourself around it, which I highly recommend.

The game can go something like this. You see your favorite fast food or other not-such-a-healthy-choice restaurant and you get a pitter patter of excitement and desire for what they have to offer. Notice that this is what you are thinking and then STOP! and see how fast you can think of other choices that would serve you better health-wise. For example, going to the café down the street that serves fresh salads assembled with chemical-free produce and dressing, or a nearby grocery store where you could pick up a roast chicken or an additive-free, natural brand frozen entrée you could take home. You may still give in and go for the triple-decker cheeseburger with everything and a jumbo milk

Achievement is largely the product of steadily raising one's levels of aspiration . . and expectation.

Jack Niklaus

shake, but once again, at least you made a *conscious* choice. The more you practice playing this game with yourself, the more likely you will be to start making wiser choices.

Similarly, you can also begin to make it a point to set your radar for natural foods stores and restaurants that are available in your immediate surroundings and whenever you are in an unfamiliar area. Doing so helps you to expand your thoughts about what is available to you. This is really important in this day and age, as most people's brains tend to be on automatic pilot, set in the direction of our degenerate popular food culture, which frequently prevents them from even recognizing other possibilities.

Always remember that you are like a target with a big black dot on your forehead for profit-minded restaurants and food manufacturers peddling energy-draining, *dis*-ease-causing, weight-producing primarily fake foods. Peel that big black dot off your forehead and turn the tides. Start thinking for yourself and become a magnet for those food producers that have something better to offer. Just from having read this you will start to notice health-oriented vendors and better food choices more often, watch and see!

All well and fine, you say, if I were on my own. However, most people are immersed in a community that includes immediate and extended family members, friends, colleagues, co-workers, and various other human beings. Co-habitation and social get-togethers with these numerous other humans almost always involves food, which can indeed be a problem. Because it can pose challenges of such great magnitude, the entire next chapter is devoted to dealing with this other-human interaction factor. So we will not go into this topic in detail here. To get started though, start thinking of yourself as an adventuresome pioneer blazing the trail.

It's a jungle out there, a junk-food jungle filled with strategically placed, enticing poor-quality, pseudofood choices everywhere you turn, in addition to a ubiquitous media landscape and native inhabitants that are continuously taunting your taste buds to indulge in this indigenous cornucopia of injurious food. But you, you are a trailblazing pioneer representing a new cultural frontier. Armed with your newly acquired knowledge and understanding, you see beyond the social smoke-screen that's

> Think of yourself as a target.
>
> Restaurants and stores are competing for what the industry calls "share of stomach."
>
> Like any retailer, they'll do everything they can to tempt you to buy more.
>
> Nutrition Action Healthletter 12/01

altering people's perceptions about the foods they eat. When lured by such enticements as the mesmerizing glow of the lights emanating from the little window of the vending machine that lurks at the end of every shadowy hallway, you stop and remind yourself what's really going on...

the impact of cultural influences

The first thing is to get mad.

We've got to view these enticements to eat as an industry wanting us to consume bad products so they can make money.

...They're making it easier and easier to eat a terrible diet.

Kelly Brownell
Yale University

What's really going on is that we as a society are in the midst of what could be described as a manic episode when it comes to our relationship with our bodies and our diets. We are eating lower-quality foods in greater amounts than ever before. And a national health crisis has ensued as a result. We have already discussed much of this topic in *Chapter 1*, primarily on a social level. Now is a good time to think about this issue in the context of this particular chapter. What's happening on a social level has a great deal to do with how you think as an individual, which in turn dictates your actions and choices, often without you being aware of it. Because of this, it is wise to understand and be cognizant of your social conditioning with regard to food, especially when seeking to make a shift in your eating habits. There are a couple of points that are paramount in bringing about greater awareness of this phenomenon at a personal level.

Ninety percent of food budget dollars are spent on popular brand processed, packaged, heavily advertised foods in this country, while a meager estimated 9-12% of the population is eating the government's recommended *5-A-Day* fruits and vegetables. This is no surprise when you consider the gargantuan advertising budgets of the former, which squashes the comparatively meager efforts of the latter. Processed food manufacturers spend a total of $34 billion a year on making sure you are aware of their products. It's staggering to think about how much money is being spent on the promotion of nutritionally bankrupt food — a $10 million annual budget for Altoid mints, $50 million on any nationally advertised candy bar, and $100 million for a nationally advertised soft drink. In one year alone, McDonald's spends $1 billion in advertising, in stark contrast to the *5-A-Day Program*, which spent a mere $2 million in its peak year. To fathom the vast difference, consider the following:

- *1 million seconds = 10.4 days*
- *1 billion seconds = 32 years*

When you consider the magnitude with which we are being deluged with multi-media advertising and marketing campaigns designed by leading psychologists to infiltrate our minds and manipulate our behavior, you can't help but conclude that as a society we are being subjected to a kind of bad food brainwashing. And, as the dramatic changes in our eating habits show, it's working. Remember this whenever you are faced with making decisions about what to eat.

Many people's way of thinking has been radically altered by this insidious assault on their psyches, often to the point of overriding their common sense when it comes to making food choices. For example, I have encountered many people who are afraid to eat eggs, a whole, fresh, natural food that has helped sustain generations, but don't think twice about slurping down one or more sodas per day, loaded with copious amounts of sugar, caffeine, and a host of other *dis*-ease-causing chemical additives. This defies logic, and is a prime example of how extremely imbalanced our popular food culture has become.

Because it has become so skewed, even a small deviation in the direction towards health-producing foods is still frequently a long, long way from what is natural or healthful. It may now be *normal* in our modern Western society to eat 90% processed foods, but it is still completely un*natural*. Even consuming foods at *Level I of Eating for Health* is completely unnatural, as they are still processed foods. I often hear people brag, "I eat better than anyone I know." I hate to burst those people's bubbles, but in light of the present era of extremely imbalanced eating this isn't saying much. Unless someone ranks among the top 5-10% of healthy eaters in this country, they are more than likely still eating in a manner that is out of synch with their natural biological processes.

Like any machine, our body runs best when operated according to its design principles. Unfortunately, most people in our modern world today are running their human machines in complete opposition to the original instruction manual, in much the same fashion as Mr. Whitless was operating his ailing automobile.

Without your knowledge or consent, they control what you eat, when you eat, how much you eat, even the way you think of food.

The food giants have done everything they can to keep you from finding out.

They've warped your food consciousness to make you a willing participant in your own demise.

Paul A. Stitt
Fighting the Food Giants

very cheap

....food is cheaper. In 1950 U.S. families spent 21% of their disposable personal income on food. In 2000 it was 11%. The price of food in stores has fallen and the price of eating out has fallen.

very abundant

The average number of products carried by a typical supermarket has more than tripled since 1980, from 15,000 to 50,000. In 1998 alone, manufacturers introduced more than 11,000 new foods. More than two-thirds of them were condiment, candy and snacks, baked goods, soft drinks, cheese products, and ice cream novelties – much of it loaded with empty calories.

very available

...some gas stations are planning to install touch screens at the pump so you can order food directly from the mini-market while you're filling up.

Nutrition Action Healthletter, 12/01

Another factor contributing to the virtual mania going on with regard to the food we eat has to do with the fact that processed food has become very cheap, very abundant, and very available. According to a recent article in the *Nutrition Action Healthletter,* a monthly periodical put out by the Center for Science in the Public Interest (CSPI), in the last two decades the amount of food produced in the U.S. has increased 500 calories per person per day; the price of food in both stores and restaurants has fallen; and consumers can now choose from an estimated 320,000 different processed, packaged foods. This dramatically influences what comes to the forefront of your mind when deciding what foods to eat, when and how much.

Never before in history have we had so many poor food choices so readily obtainable and so affordable. People used to be limited to the amount of food their livestock could produce and their fruit tree could bear, which was frequently not enough. Today we are inundated with an inordinate amount of low-quality, low-cost, seductive food. We can't get away from it.

The other day I bought a 2-liter bottle of soda for a pseudofood display I was putting together for a talk I was giving. It's been a long time since I have purchased such an item, so I pulled out $3 guessing that would cover it. I was absolutely astounded when the clerk said, "That will be $1.23." Similarly, I have heard that a popular fast-food restaurant is now offering a burger, fries, and a soda for only $3. The thought of these old favorite foods at these low prices was tempting even for me — for just a split second. My well-trained mind immediately reminded me of the high price I would pay in loss of health and energy. But it's no wonder people are buying and eating this stuff *en masse.* (By the way, if you ever see me in line at the store preparing to purchase soda or any other pseudofood item, trust that I am buying it for a bad food display, no need to tackle and launch an intervention!)

To compound the challenging nature of the situation, there is an equally excessive amount of polarized and conflicting nutritional information we receive, both in general and with regard to specific foods. Bookstore shelves are overflowing with books by doctors and researchers with lots of letters after their names denoting high degrees of scientific and academic achievement. Consult ten different books and they'll tell you ten different things. How can this be science? Despite this flood of what can only be considered pseudoscientific or incomplete scientific information at best, on a cultural level the quality of our diets and subsequent state of health is not getting better, it's getting worse. Clearly, this route is not the answer.

The real road to attaining a sustainable diet and resultant better state of health lies in the nutritional knowledge and understanding that has stood the test of time, coupled with following the innate guidance of your body and mind. In order to do so, remember that we are in a cultural era of *extreme* poor eating and shed unwanted social conditioning as much as possible. Then begin to develop a new relationship with food, one that acknowledges nature, timeless nutritional wisdom, and the messages of your body as the ultimate resources for guidance.

the proof is in the pudding

"Do you have any clinical study that you could provide to back up your claim that regular caffeine consumption can compromise your health?" someone asked after a lecture one evening.

"I'm sure I could come up with something, and probably an equal amount of research that said otherwise. So, why play that game?" I responded. "Go off caffeine for six months and see how *you feel*," I further advised. "Let that be the study that influences your decision whether to consume caffeine or not."

Too often people let pseudoscientific input cloud their thinking and decision-making. We have a tendency to inflate the value of research and academia in this country, sometimes to our personal detriment. As I always say, the proof is in the pudding! There's nothing like empirical evidence to shift your paradigm and assist you in knowing what is appropriate for your body. I highly encourage people to try something for themselves and see how it works for them. That goes for the concepts presented in this book as well. Don't just take my word for it. Give the guidelines and recommendations here a try, a real try for an appropriate amount of time, and let your own experience decide. It certainly can't hurt and more likely you will be doing yourself a favor. As you have been learning, most of what is advocated here amounts to common sense with which few could argue.

In order to truly put things to the test, however, you must really give them a try. Some people who only make a half-hearted

> Too much theory interferes with practice.
>
> Unknown

attempt, then claim that they tried it, but it didn't work, are doing themselves a great disservice. To reap the benefits of an accurate assessment, you must undertake a sincere initiative for an adequate amount of time. To return to the pudding metaphor once again, you have to be sure you have used the right ingredients, in the right proportions, and allowed them to congeal for the right amount of time before you judge the merit of the recipe. Anything short of meticulously following the recipe renders the experiment irrelevant.

So, what constitutes a sincere effort and an adequate amount of time when it comes to dietary experimental endeavors? A good recipe would be to follow through with recommendations 90-100% of the time for at least 3-6 months. For extreme addictive foods such as caffeine or sugar, it would be wise to stay off them 100% for the same duration. Otherwise, you run the risk of yo-yoing and skewing your results.

As you are putting dietary changes to the test, it is imperative that you keep in mind the withdrawal factor we touched on earlier, especially when it comes to extreme, addictive foods. For example, if you were drinking a fair amount or sometimes even a small amount of coffee or caffeinated soda every day and went off it cold turkey, you might very likely experience some caffeine withdrawal symptoms such as severe headache, constipation, fatigue, or irritability. This is *not* a sign that caffeine is good for you because resuming consumption makes these symptoms abate. On the contrary, it is a clear indication that your body's chemistry is out of balance as a result of consuming caffeine regularly; the worse the symptoms, the greater the imbalance that has been created. Taking a yo-yo approach, whereby you go back and forth having it and not having it, is not advisable, as doing so can cause you even more physical and emotional ups and downs than going through a complete withdrawal. More help with how to go about getting off addictive foods with the least amount of discomfort is coming up in *Chapter 9 ~ Clear the Way*. But for now, just remember to factor in the withdrawal process when experimenting with changes.

People who take me up on this challenge of trying the *Eating-for-Health* recommendations, experience such a dramatic improvement in how they look and feel that they frequently write or tell me later that they never realized the degree to which the

The only research lab that I've found to be proven consistent over a long period of time, however, is nature itself, which has been feeding humanity for thousands of years without the least confusion.

Dr. John Douillard
The 3-Season Diet

food they were eating was affecting both their body and mind. Unfortunately, some others never give it a try because they are caught in an intellectual quagmire of socially accepted, albeit, questionable science.

For example, a dietician who once attended an *Eating-for-Health* program was overweight, fatigued and experiencing some chronic *dis*-eases. It was painful to watch this woman discount information that I'm confident would have tremendously improved the quality of her life and health because it didn't fit with her textbook training. Although her textbooks may have said that it was all right for her to consume 'moderate' amounts of coffee, diet soda, and chemical-laden processed foods, clearly it was not all right with her body. Her body was falling apart like Mr. Whitless' car. I don't know why she thought she was having so many health problems. Like many people, she probably thought it was due to a genetic weakness or some mysterious forces of nature "that just happen."

As stated earlier, the truth is, there isn't any condition in the body that can't be improved by improving your diet. But don't take my word for it, try it for yourself and see. The proof really is in the pudding.

> Many people suffer in poor health not realizing that their unhealthy lifestyle habits are the main cause of their sickness.
>
> Paul Bragg

as you eateth...

Marisa had been experiencing chronic depression and irritability. It had gotten progressively worse over the course of the previous year and she was reluctantly considering going on anti-depressant drugs to get some relief. When I explained to her that depression and other mental disorders were frequently rooted in diet, I could immediately see her internal wheels start to turn. When I asked if there were any foods she consumed regularly that she suspected might be causing or contributing to her chronically depressed and irritable frame of mind, her face lit up like a light bulb.

"Yes, diet soda!" she proclaimed. "I have been having 1-2 diet sodas a day for a little over a year now. I wondered at one point if this might be the problem, but when I asked my doctor he said it couldn't be. So, I discounted my suspicions." She now decided her suspicions were worth investigating and decided to experiment by eliminating her daily dose of diet soda.

A week later Marisa returned and announced that she felt like a new person. The sense of gloom that had dominated her life for so long had lifted. Relations with her spouse and children had greatly improved and she felt more at ease with others as well. She also reported having more physical energy and a renewed interest in things she loved to do that she had lost sight of over the past year.

We have talked much about how foods affect your physical well-being. Marisa's story illustrates how important it is to understand how food affects your mental and emotional well-being as well. In this case: *as you eateth, so too shall you thinketh and feeleth.*

The fact that food has a tremendous influence on how you think and feel is a fact frequently ignored, diminished or not known. Whether it be chronic depression, irritability, anxiety, fear, anger, obsessive thinking, or constant worrying, the *Standard American Diet* is loaded with foods that not only cause physical imbalance and deterioration, but mental and emotional imbalance and deterioration as well. At the same time, the *Standard American Diet* is lacking in the whole, fresh, natural foods loaded with the vital nutrients needed for proper brain function and mental health. Having an awareness and understanding of this can significantly increase your ability to decipher which foods are best for you, and can also significantly increase your chances for successfully changing your eating habits.

As mentioned earlier, there is a lot of discussion about what is referred to as *emotional eating*, which is another aspect of this association between food and mood. The concept of *emotional eating* is most often based on the notion that people become emotionally upset, which then leads them to binge on large quantities of primarily low-quality junk foods as a source of comfort. What is seldom discussed, however, is what triggered the emotional upset and cravings for certain foods in the first place. It begs the age-old question: *which came first, the chicken or the egg?* Or in this case: *which came first, the emotional upset or poor nutrition and junk food binging?*

This is an important distinction. Negative emotions don't just spring out of nowhere. Improper nutrition is a primary *cause* of imbalanced psychological states and frequently triggers emotional upset, which in turn perpetuates the cycle of imbalanced eating and imbalanced emotional states. The only way to loop out of this vicious cycle is to balance the body's internal

---

...your mood (often created by the foods you choose) determines what you eat at your next meal.

Imbalanced eating habits trigger a vicious cycle where you feel worse and worse and turn repeatedly to the wrong foods for a quick fix....

In contrast, when you make the right food choices, you're providing fuel for a healthy body, a good mood, an active mind, and a high energy level.

Elizabeth Somer
Food & Mood

chemistry by providing adequate nutrients and eliminating the offending foods.

With regard to this topic of emotional eating, I have heard Oprah repeatedly proclaim on her world-famous talk show that, "It's *not* about the food." Each time I hear her say this I jump to the edge of the couch and yell at the T.V., "It *is* about the food, Oprah! It *is* about the food!" I then slump back into the couch with frustration, knowing that she can't hear what I'm saying, then send up a prayer that one day this book will find its way into her hands and she will not only hear what I'm saying, but also understand it.

As people begin to eat healthier and develop more body awareness, they are frequently amazed to discover that more often than not, poor eating in general and certain foods in particular trigger emotional upsets that cause them to unconsciously eat more of the offending foods rather than the other way around. And in fact, the healthier and more balanced they eat, the healthier and more balanced their mental and emotional states become. Because normal brain function has been restored, they no longer react to situations as they would have in the past. They find that they are able to maintain this balanced state of mental and emotional well-being as long as they maintain their healthy eating lifestyle.

As you make the change to a healthier eating lifestyle, remember that proper nutrition is as much about the foods you eat as it is about those you don't. Foods to which you are sensitive or allergic, including the common food allergens, processed foods containing chemical additives, such as aspartame and MSG, and stimulating extreme foods such as sugar and caffeine, are all major culprits in creating a psychological environment ripe for emotional fragility and overreacting to situations you might otherwise let slide. Equally problematic are the nutritional deficiencies that can result from the absence of nutrient-rich foods in your diet. In other words, it is as important to identify and eliminate poor quality offensive foods, as it is to be sure you are getting high quality nutritious foods and adequate amounts of the basic nutrients such as green foods and essential fatty acids. Following the *Eating-for-Health Guidelines* and the upcoming *Dietary Basics*, in combination with heeding the messages of your

> The greatest tragedy that comes to man is emotional depression, the dulling of the intellect and the loss of initiative that comes from nutritive failure.
>
> James McLester
> Former A.M.A.
> President

body, will help you determine how best to accomplish this in accordance with your body's particular needs.

Whether someone is emotionally binging or experiencing acute, chronic, or intermittent irritability, depression, anxiety, hypersensitivity, fear, anger, worry or any other disagreeable psychological condition, learning to listen to the body and correctly interpret and respond to the messages it sends is a worthwhile skill for everyone to develop. The best way to do this is to become a body awareness detective. Keeping a written or mental journal of what you're eating and any corresponding physical or psychological symptoms is one way of playing detective with yourself. Another way, and probably the most effective, is to train yourself to investigate situations in the moment, and at the same time take immediate action to remedy the current situation and reflect on how to prevent yourself from repeating the causative behavior in the future.

To do this, take a moment whenever you are feeling out of sorts to stop and ask yourself the following questions:

1. *What exactly am I feeling both emotionally and physically (i.e., headache, fatigue, irritability, emotional sensitivity, anger, spaciness, etc.)?*

2. *When did I start feeling this way?*

3. *What foods or beverages have I had, or not had, today or yesterday that may have caused or contributed to this imbalanced state?*

4. *What foods or beverages do I regularly have or not have that may be causing an overall state of imbalance in my body and mind?*

5. *What actions can I take at this moment to start feeling better and get my body and mind back into a balanced state of well-being?*

6. *What actions can I take to help prevent this from happening in the future?*

For many people, it will take some time to get to know what your body is trying to tell you. Keep implementing this interrogative technique and playing detective with yourself, and it will help accelerate the process. *Chapter 9 ~ Clear the Way,* contains more

...we eat Krispy Kremes even though we know that the results over time and distance spell something far more disastrous than a rash or a headache.

We've got to be smarter than that and send our taste buds to school.

The only way for your health to be permanently better is for you to change and train your taste buds to enjoy foods that will bring you all you want most out of life.

The Brain Garden Food First Program

information and solutions for curbing food cravings that will help you as well. The more aware you become of what precipitates symptoms and reactions, the better you will be able to correct the situation at hand. In addition, as the specific associations between what you're eating and how you feel become clearer, the more motivated you will be to eliminate the foods and habits that are causing the problems in the first place. The desire to feel good will soon override the desire for injurious foods.

If the mere mention of eliminating certain foods to which you may have become attached sparks a twinge of fear and resistance within you, remember that taste is acquired and it can be *un*acquired as well. Because this issue of taste is so emotionally charged for so many people, it is a topic well worth revisiting and briefly expounding on.

try it, you'll like it!

"I hear everything you're saying, but my problem is I can't stand the taste of vegetables," a young woman once confided to me. This is a common complaint I have heard from others as well. In the infamous style of tell-it-like-it-is Dr. Phil McGraw, my response to this complaint in short, is — get over it!

Chances are, there are several things you didn't like at first, but later learned to love. Coffee and alcoholic beverages are a good example. Unless you were one of those rare and rather odd children who liked to sip from Uncle Fred's beer can at family picnics, or grandma's coffee mug at the kitchen table, you probably wrinkled your nose and screwed up your face with disgust the first time you tasted the smallest sip of these pungent adult beverages. But most of you kept on drinking them anyway when you came of age, because you wanted the 'buzz' and the 'cool' status that came along with them. You essentially forced yourself to learn to like these drinks, to the extent that after not too long you actually came to love them.

It's interesting to ponder that as a society we think nothing of training ourselves to acquire tastes for things that are unhealthy, such as coffee and alcohol, yet balk at the notion of training ourselves to acquire tastes for things that are good for us, such as broccoli and Brussels sprouts. Similarly, we don't think twice about eating processed foods saturated with harmful amounts of fat, sodium, sugar and toxic chemical additives. As a

Taste buds are creatures of habit— and habits can be changed.

Yolanda Bergman, Food Cop

society we have become very complacent when it comes to what we put in our mouths. Quite often, people don't have a clue what's in the food they're eating and they don't care either. As long as it tastes good and everyone else is eating it, it's O.K. Would you knowingly eat rat poison just because it tasted good and was the popular thing to do? No, of course not. To do so would defy logic and go against your basic survival instincts. Yet, that's what we've been essentially conditioned to do, albeit on a slightly lesser, but nonetheless damaging scale.

The primary criterion for making food choices should be the quality of the food and its benefits to the body, with taste as the secondary factor. You can have both, to be sure. But to put your taste buds and social acceptance before your health and well-being is a recipe for physical and mental disaster.

If you currently find vegetables and other healthy foods distasteful, chances are your taste buds have acclimated to the unnatural faire of the *Standard American Diet*. Because of their extreme nature, these highly refined foods with their artificial flavorings and excessive amounts of sugar, refined salt and bad fats, literally burn out your taste buds. If this is the case, and it is for most people, don't despair. While you may never develop a taste for Brussels sprouts (I certainly haven't!), you *can* develop tastes for healthier foods and believe it or not, actually come to prefer them. We will be talking more about how to go about making this transition in upcoming chapters. For now, just know that it *can* be done and that with time you will get an even better 'buzz' from eating natural, nutrient-rich foods; a constant buzz in the form of strength, energy, contentment, emotional balance, and overall health and well-being. All this, instead of the highs and lows (which eventually develop into primarily lows) that you get from eating unnatural, nutrient-poor foods, including overly stimulating substances such as caffeine, alcohol, refined salt and sugar.

For me, the former Queen of Junk Food, a taste for healthier foods came about naturally over time. Put that old six-pack, liter of Pepsi, jumbo bag of Doritos, and pack of cigarettes I used to yearn for in front of me today, and I'd cringe with disgust. On the other hand, give me a fresh glass of carrot, apple, beet juice and my face will light up with delight!

Champions are willing to do the things they dislike to create something they do like.

Don't let the things that matter most be at the mercy of the things that matter least.

Dexter Yager

It's like reformed smokers who can't stand the smell of smoke. Not only am I repulsed by the extreme nature of the addictive pseudofoods I used to adore, but my body has become highly sensitized to these *dis*-ease causing foods as well, especially those with toxic chemical additives. My taste buds and body chemistry have now reached a balanced, healthy internal state. On the *very rare* occasions that I happen to encounter one of these fake foods (usually at some unavoidable social gathering coupled with a very weak moment) and lose temporary sight of my sensibilities, my finely-tuned human machine immediately lets me know about it via a headache, brain fog, fatigue, irritability, gas, bloating or other unmistakable warning signal. I thank my body for reminding me why I don't want to run these foods through my system anymore! Which brings me to another issue of concern some people express regarding making the switch to a healthier eating lifestyle.

don't disconnect the oil light

A former co-worker once jibbed that I needed to go to McDonald's and have a Big Mac and a jumbo chocolate shake in order to put some meat on my bones. I laughed and told her I had no desire to do such a thing because it would make me sick.

"That's what happens when you eat so healthy," she responded. "I would love to lose weight, and as you can see I really need to! But I would never want to become so sensitive to the foods that I love that I couldn't eat them because they made me sick."

What she failed to recognize was that these foods *were* making her sick. Ever since I had known her she had had severe digestive problems, allergies, fatigue, recurrent colds and flu that hung on for weeks at a time (i.e., lowered immune function), and was now gaining excessive weight. But as with so many people, with the exception of the weight gain, she did not associate these chronic conditions with the poor quality of her diet.

What she meant of course was that she didn't want to become so sensitive to junk foods that she experienced an immediate reaction such as stomach upset, diarrhea, hives or the like. I have heard this sentiment expressed by others as well. They say they are concerned about adopting healthier eating habits because doing so may reduce their tolerance for the 'bad'

As the organs start working better... (they) tell the person when he or she is making mistakes... What a person can get away with is apparently reduced.

This is a bit of an illusion, as the person didn't really get away with anything before. They just didn't experience any immediate reaction...

In fact, the body did have a bad reaction but didn't have the strength to indicate it. It's these many little accumulated suppressed reactions that eventually add up to "sudden" breakdowns such as heart attacks or cancer...

Jon Matsen, N.D.
Eating Alive

stuff they love. Whether or not this is a legitimate concern or a creative excuse, I think it is worthwhile to reflect on this line of thinking.

To revisit the smoking analogy, when most people smoke their first cigarette or two, their bodies react quickly and dramatically. Watery eyes, coughing, choking, headache and dizziness are all common reactions when someone takes their first few drags. These are healthy reactions, the body's attempt to reject toxic substances and thereby protect itself. They are also loud warning signals, sending clear messages to cease and desist whatever it is that you're doing. If the person ignores these signals and keeps smoking, however, we all know what happens. The body eventually gives up and adjusts to the injurious inhalations. The acute warning signals stop, but the silent internal destruction has just begun. The body's internal chemistry is now dependant on tobacco and the opposite occurs as a result. The person now craves cigarettes and gets irritable, headachy, and starts coughing when they don't have them, as the body once again seeks a state of chemical balance.

A very similar phenomenon happens with food. When people first start eating poor quality foods, usually at a young age, their sensitive, healthy bodies often respond with immediate reject and protect reactions such as vomiting, diarrhea, sinus congestion, etc. Or, because their system is so clear and strong, they are able to move the offending substances right through without an acute reaction at all. In either case, just as with smoking, eventually a healthy body's ability to respond with an acute warning signal will diminish with time as it becomes overloaded and weakened with the continued ingestion of offending foods. The warning lights will stop flashing and as with smoking as well, the person will begin craving these foods and go through withdrawal when they go without them.

So, to return to the original concern, is it really desirable to want to have a body that is so weakened and desensitized to harmful, offending substances that it can no longer respond in a healthy manner? You'll have to make that decision for yourself, but in my opinion, it is not. Maintaining a certain degree of sensitivity, while annoying on occasion, is a good thing in the long run for two important reasons. One, it indicates a clear, healthy system (or a system that is weakened and overloaded and can't

> Man's mind once stretched by a new idea, never regains its original dimensions.
>
> Oliver Wendell Holmes

process anymore!) And two, it is one of the greatest tools your body provides for keeping you away from offensive foods and other substances that will compromise your health. It's a miraculous instinctual feature, a feature designed to keep us safe. Unfortunately, many of our natural desires and built-in safety mechanisms have been extinguished by the overpowering taunting of the food industry and our subsequent modern food culture.

Wanting to disconnect the body's warning signals in order to consume *dis*-ease-causing foods is a bit like someone wanting to disconnect the oil light on a car. There's some degree of logic missing. And yet, that's the line of thinking many people have adopted due to the unnatural relationship we have developed with food as a result of our popular food culture.

If you are someone who is concerned about developing sensitivities to the foods you currently love, I invite you to reflect on what has been said here and let this concern go. What the issue really comes back to is that notion of feeling deprived or missing out on foods you enjoy. Remember what we discussed in the last segment: you will discover and come to love other, healthier foods just as much as those you most enjoy now. More importantly, you will also enjoy the many benefits that eating a quality, nutrient-rich diet will provide. Many of them you may not have even realized were available to you, as we will discuss next.

> Take the pebble out of your shoe, rather than learn to limp.
>
> Chinese Proverb

jaguar or jalopy?

When I was fifteen my father bought an old Dodge Dart. It had manual steering and a clutch that was as difficult to handle as the three-in-the-tree shifting mechanism. Years of Midwestern weather had dulled its finish and rusted the bottom rim. With its rugged appearance and operational challenges, this vehicle resembled more of a slow-moving tank than the flying dart its name implied. "The Dart," as we called it, was the first car I ever drove.

Then one day my friend's older brother pulled up in a shiny new red Corvette. I begged him to let me drive it and was ecstatic when he agreed. Because I was so used to driving the Dart and didn't know any different, once in the driver's seat I wound up my leg, slammed down the clutch, jammed it into first gear, and yanked the power steering wheel so hard we almost landed in the ditch.

"Whoa! — settle down there missy," my friend's brother exclaimed. "This is a finely-tuned machine, not a tank!"

This was my first lesson in the difference between driving a new sports car and an old junker. Once I relaxed into the sensitivity with which this dream machine operated, I couldn't believe that driving could be such an easy and enjoyable experience. Its speedy acceleration sent us cruising down the road with grace and ease. The smooth power steering took barely a touch to redirect our course, and turned corners at a speed the Dart barely reached going straight ahead. After taking this marvel for a little spin, I burst out joyfully, "Wow! — now that's what I call driving! I never knew driving could be so fun!"

I share this story with you now because this is precisely what many people go through with regard to their human vehicles. They are driving through life in a body that is operating at the level of an old Dodge Dart. They could easily trade in their old clunker for maybe not a sleek new sports car, but certainly a smoother running mid-size economy model just by upgrading their nutrient fuel intake. The problem is, many people often don't even realize they are riding around in an old clunker. Just as I became used to driving the Dart and thought that's just how driving was, they have become used to headaches, digestive problems, lack of energy, PMS, sinus problems, joint stiffness and a host of other aches and pains and ailments. They accept these conditions as normal and don't give them a second thought anymore.

For example, a woman once came to a healthy eating program I facilitated with the intention of losing weight. I remember her telling us at the beginning of the program that she didn't have any health issues or concerns, and that she just wanted to lose ten pounds. After learning the *Eating-for-Health Guidelines* during the program, she became so inspired she went home and cleared her cupboards of all denatured, chemical-laden pseudofoods and replaced them with naturally processed foods and whole, fresh, natural foods. I saw her about a month later and asked how she was doing.

"I can't believe it," she began. "Not only did I lose ten pounds, but I also *feel* so much better! I have so much more

The future is just the past catching up with us.

Today is the preview of tomorrow's reality.

In the future we will say one of two things. "I wish I had" or "I'm glad I did," but we make that choice today.

Unknown

energy, my head is so clear, I'm sleeping better, and I also noticed that I didn't get PMS this month. My husband and I are also getting along better."

"What's so funny is that I thought I was fine," she reflected. "I never realized how bad I felt until I started eating better and then feeling better. Who would have thought that just making a few changes in your diet could do so much? It was much easier than I thought, too. Both my husband and I feel so much better. I can't thank you enough for sharing this information."

Just as I had become accustomed to driving the Dart, this woman, and so many others like her, had become accustomed to walking around in a body that was in poor condition and didn't even know it. Having had the experience of feeling better in her body by improving her diet, her thoughts around food and its relationship to her body were forever changed. This is true for everyone who takes the same initiative and is even more pronounced for people with conditions that are causing them discomfort. But what's really great about having this experience is that once someone starts feeling better and having more energy, more often than not they like feeling better so much that the desire to maintain this level of health and vitality drives them to continue with their new found eating habits. They don't want to go back to feeling the way they did before. Would you want to have to go back to driving the old Dart after driving a new Corvette? Not likely.

You can look, feel and operate like a junk-heap, a finely-tuned racing machine or something in between. Jaguar, Jetta, or jalopy. It's your choice.

inner child gone wild

Another factor to consider with regard to your psychological machinations around the issue of food has to do with the relationships between the different parts of your personality. A good example of how these internal relationships can affect your food choices is illustrated by the case of Nancy, a 50-year-old woman who came to me for nutrition and health coaching. She wanted help getting her eating habits "under control," as she put it, lose a substantial amount of weight, lower her high blood pressure and relieve joint pain.

> The greatest trouble with many of us is that our demands upon ourselves are so feeble, the call upon the "great within" so weak and intermittent that we make little impression upon our creative energies; and therefore we fail to access the force that transmutes desire into realities.
>
> Unknown

During her initial consultation Nancy talked about her past experiences and what she wanted to create for her future. She began by telling me that she wanted to accomplish her goals of weight reduction and health improvement in a way that "honored her inner child." When asked what had prevented her from maintaining healthier eating strategies she had adopted in the past, Nancy said that she would be going along doing very well, and then she would have a desire for ice cream or a doughnut, for example, and because she wanted to honor her inner child, she would eat them. From there things would spiral back down to the level of her previous poor eating habits.

As Nancy continued to talk, I couldn't help notice that she mentioned the need to honor her inner child several times. When she finally finished, I had to ask, "Where is your *inner parent* in all of this?"

Nancy responded that she had grown up in a very restrictive, sometimes abusive household. As an adult, she had pursued many avenues of therapy and somewhere along the way implemented the concept of nurturing and honoring what is referred to in psychological circles as her *inner child*. She felt that doing so had contributed greatly to her personal growth and healing.

In an attempt to break free from the traditional, authoritative approach to childrearing so popular in days of old, baby boomers were the first generation to embrace the concept of the inner child and herald its existence. Unfortunately, implementing this concept can sometimes go too far. The inner child goes wild and turns into the inner brat, ultimately wreaking havoc on a person's life. This was clearly what was happening with Nancy. She had, in large part, dismissed her *inner parent* because for her, the term *parent* itself had strong negative connotations associated with it. Her inner child had consequently taken control, at least when it came to the food she ate.

There's nothing wrong with the concept of honoring the inner child. Acknowledging and allowing the inner child to emerge, especially for those who experienced a restricted or difficult childhood, provides many benefits and can often lead to a more authentic, joyful adulthood. It's only when the inner child is left unchecked or put in charge, that problems begin to surface. As

True effectiveness requires balance.

Stephen Covey

the wiser and more mature of the two, the *inner parent* is the best choice for running the show.

Notice I said inner *parent*, not inner *dictator*. You want to establish an inner parent with well-developed and well-intentioned parenting skills, not an inner dictator you come to loathe. As is often the case with adults who struggle with food issues, upon further investigation I learned that Nancy would vacillate between letting her inner child go wild and imposing severe food sanctions on herself, food sanctions that were so severe they could only have been imposed by an *inner dictator*. She would describe herself as "being good" when she adhered to these restrictions and as "being bad" when she ate excessive amounts of the sweets and treats she loved. This is a very common pattern; a very frustrating and unproductive pattern that sets up and perpetuates an inner struggle. Continuously flip-flopping between extremely restrictive eating and boundless junk-food pig-outs ultimately prevents a person from establishing an enjoyable eating lifestyle. Striking a balance is key.

Ideally you want to treat your inner child the way you would treat any other child placed under your care. You wouldn't let a child in your care run wild in the street or in the candy store, indulging any whim she fancied. Nor would you want to be so restrictive that the child grew to reject and despise you. As a responsible adult, you would want to establish a balanced approach to the caretaking of the child by maintaining safe, healthy boundaries and flexibility when appropriate. Your own personal inner child deserves this same attention and respect.

So overthrow any inner dictators, install an even keeled inner parent, teach your inner child some manners, and create something that all parts of yourself can be comfortable with. That's when you're really being good, when you do what works for your *inner everybody*!

> All that a man achieves and all that he fails to achieve is the direct result of his own thoughts.
>
> James Allen

as you thinketh, so too shall you eat

In the late 1800's, James Allen wrote a book entitled *As a Man Thinketh*. After realizing he had neglected the other half of the human race, he later wrote *As a Woman Thinketh*. These tiny little books became classics. I highly recommend them for anyone who wants to grow personally in any area of their life. The essence of these books that "as a man or woman thinketh, so too shall they become," expresses the foundation of this chapter.

Next to thinking and breathing, eating is the thing we do most as humans. For this reason, when it comes to making lasting changes in the way we eat, willpower alone won't do the trick. Re-approaching how you go about it, on the other hand, will. Remember that you *chooseth* what you *thinketh*, and you can choose to think differently. Hopefully this chapter has got you choosing some new and different thoughts that will help you re-approach your relationship to food and eating.

These new and different thoughts, however, may be inspiring you on the one hand and concerning you on the other. They may be concerning you primarily because, although you are enthusiastic about making changes, you are now wondering how you are going to implement and integrate a new *Eating-for-Health lifestyle* in the midst of finicky offspring and significant others, friends, co-workers and every one else you share and enjoy food with, who may not be sharing your same enthusiasm. And that's precisely the topic we will address next.

Do you
believe
everything
you think?

Bumper Sticker

Chapter Five 🍎

children & others

Gaining Support & Helping Them, Too

Unless you're a recluse or a hermit living in a cave, you interact with other humans on a regular basis. A significant amount of that interaction involves food. And therein lies one of the biggest obstacles people encounter when trying to make a break from the current *Standard American Diet* and our popular food culture. For this reason, it is important to muster up as much support as possible when undertaking such an endeavor. In fact, whether or not you are able to get the support you need can mean the difference between success and failure.

Once someone has become aware of our popular food culture and the devastating effects of the *Standard American Diet*, it is only natural for many to want to gain support for themselves in adopting and maintaining healthier ways. In addition, many others also develop the desire to help those around them to do the same. Whether it's the members of your immediate family or strangers you meet in line at the grocery store, you may start to notice a growing desire to impart your newfound knowledge and experiences on others. You will no doubt realize quickly that, while the urge is strong, scrutinizing the grocery cart of the person standing in line in front of you at the grocery store may not be the best approach. Sharing your enthusiasm on the topic of healthier eating with your spouse or the kids may similarly not be

Success depends on the support of other people.

The only hurdle between you and what you want to be is the support of others.

David Joseph Schwartz

welcomed with the same enthusiasm with which it is delivered. This may leave you frustrated with the question of what to do with this growing desire to help others to eat healthier and get well too. This desire is often especially pronounced for those with children and often met with a lack of interest and sometimes, even disdain by those you are trying to help.

In this chapter we will address these concerns and devote much of it to the topic of what the upcoming generation is facing. Whether you are a parent or not, you will still want to read these segments. What is happening with our children today with regard to our popular food culture is a social issue that affects us all. Even those who are not parents themselves come in contact with children or their parents sometime in their lives. Having an understanding of what is going on can help you to bring greater awareness to this issue. You will also glean further insights and reinforcement for your personal quest to eat better from reading these segments. But first, let's get back to the most important person in this equation — *you.*

gaining support

Debbie was a 32-year-old woman referred to me by her medical doctor. She was having severe bouts of diarrhea followed by long periods of constipation that were making her life miserable in a variety of ways. Her mother, who suffered similar symptoms throughout her adult life, eventually died of colon cancer. Debbie was determined to create a different destiny for herself. By the time she came to see me, she already had a pretty clear idea of what foods aggravated her condition and understood the benefits and basics of a whole, fresh, natural foods diet. Her biggest challenge was implementing what she knew.

Debbie worked with her husband, who owned a successful construction company that involved frequent get-togethers with workers and their wives or girlfriends, most of whom were also Debbie and her husband's close friends. These business/social get-togethers entailed a lot of hearty partying. Debbie had been somewhat successful in avoiding most of the party food on these occasions by eating before she went or doing her best with what was available. A few people were curious about the changes in her eating patterns, but nobody seemed to care too much whether or

> Use your willpower and better judgment to select and eat only the foods which are best for you, regardless of the ridicule or gibes of your friends or acquaintances.
>
> Dr. Richard Field

not she was eating, or what she was eating when she did. When it came to drinking alcohol, however, that was a different story.

The pressure for her to join in and drink with the rest of the gang, as she had always done in the past, was so strong that it resulted in some people actually getting angry with her if she didn't, including her husband and two of her closest friends. More often than not in these situations, she would hold out as long as she could, but eventually cave in to their taunting and have a few shots and a beer or two. She would then spend the following two or three days in the bathroom or lying on the couch writhing in pain as a result. Not only would she be physically incapacitated, but she would suffer emotionally as well. She began to feel a growing sense of despair about the situation. Short of leaving her husband and completely disassociating herself from their mutual combined business and social circle, she didn't know what to do.

Debbie's eyes teared as she relayed the details of her plight, the challenging nature of which I had no trouble understanding. When I asked if she had sat down with her husband or her two friends to talk to them about how she felt and what was going on with her health, she said no. She had mentioned bits and pieces of course, but was kind of embarrassed about her condition so never really gave them the whole story or asked for their support. Although Debbie's predicament was a little more extreme than most, the nature of the social and familial challenges she faced were quite common.

As previously mentioned, when it comes to making lasting dietary changes, gaining the support of those around you, especially those closest to you, can make all the difference in the world. It's up to you, however, to initiate, make specific requests for, and maintain the support you desire from them, all the while realizing they may not provide it. Sometimes those you want and expect support from the most, as Debbie was learning, will be the ones who give it to you the least. In which case, you will have to accept this and look for backing elsewhere. There are, however, things you can do to increase the chances of rallying others around you. The simplest, most effective, and often most neglected of which is to clearly identify and communicate your needs to them. And that's exactly what I suggested Debbie do.

There's a simple way of getting payoffs directly – asking.

'Would you please pay attention to me for a few minutes?'

'Could I have some support?'

...Yes, there's risk involved – you might not get it.

But – as you may have discovered – negative behavior doesn't always get it, either.

John-Roger & Peter McWilliams

the talk

Because those closest to you are the ones who have the biggest effect on you and are the most affected *by* you and your decision to make new dietary choices, it is wise to take the time and forethought to engage in a good old-fashioned heart-to-heart with them about what is going on for you. The most obvious people you would want to have this talk with would be immediate family members, significant others and anyone else who lives with you. You may also want to have a modified version of this talk with close friends or co-workers that you dine with regularly (or drink beer with, as the case may be). Either way, there are certain guidelines that are wise to follow and specific points you will want to make in order to get the most out of this conversation. Our relationships with others are very individualized, so you will want to spend some time thinking about what's most appropriate for you and each person you will be talking to. Following is a list of top ten suggestions that can help:

1 ~ set the time and space for the talk

...to demonstrate its importance and ensure you have your listener's undivided attention.

During the commercial break of your spouse's favorite T.V. program or at the breakfast table when the kids are running late for school are obviously not the best time or setting to have your heart-to-heart talk with them. You will either want to set an official date or plan it for when you know you will have uninterrupted time, such as a lengthy car drive. Also be sure to allow enough time to have a leisurely conversation. So often in our high-paced contemporary lives we tell each other things in passing, only to have them forgotten because our attention was somewhere else. By setting a special time and date to have a talk, you are demonstrating the importance of what you have to say and will ensure that you have your listener's full attention. You may even want to make some naturally sweetened cookies or *No-Bake Apple Crisp* (recipes in back of book) for the person you will be talking with to give them a little taste of what you're learning. And of course, providing a little treat is always helpful in the public relations department as well :-)

The educating of one's environment is a constant, natural and eventually effortless process, but it may take a while to reeducate the folks and things in your life on how you now want them to be or provide for you.

And it will take time for you to access the exact language you will need to say what you want to say and to get what you need without having to strain yourself or the other person.

Thomas Leonard

2 ~ include all members of the family
...when you have this talk, even the little ones.

You may want to speak with them separately, but be sure you talk to all members of the family no matter what their age, even infants and toddlers. Little ones understand more than we give them credit for and they appreciate being included. Even though they may not understand your every word, they hear and respond when you speak from your heart. They understand your general intentions and are happy to have been included in whatever is going on.

3 ~ focus on yourself
...use sentences that begin with "I" and speak from your heart.

When we start to make personal changes, especially changes important enough to require help, it can sometimes make those close to us feel a little uncomfortable. Keeping the focus on yourself and using statements beginning with "I" (i.e., I would like some help..., etc.), is not only less threatening, but also helps others to more clearly understand what you are saying, both of which will greatly increase the odds that you will be heard and receive a favorable response. Another effective means of approaching this kind of intimate communication is to put yourself in the other person's shoes and think about how you would want to be addressed and what would help you to be more receptive.

> If your imagination leads you to understand how quickly people grant your requests when those requests appeal to their self-interest, you can have practically anything you go after.
>
> Napoleon Hill

4 ~ tell them what you are doing and why
...with regard to your decision to make changes in your diet and develop a healthier eating lifestyle.

Tell them that you are learning lots of new and interesting things about food and healthier eating that you are trying to integrate in your own life. Share with them specific reasons you want to do this (i.e., lose weight, relieve digestive disturbances, etc.). Also, be sure to include any reasons that may relate to them in particular (i.e., you want to increase your energy so that you can play baseball with them, make mad passionate love to them, etc.). They will be very happy to hear these reasons and will be more likely to lend support. Be honest, however; people can see right through insincerity and you don't want to say anything that could come back to haunt you.

5 ~ invite them to join you

...but let them know that you honor, accept and respect them if they don't.

This fifth suggestion primarily applies to other adults and older teens in your life who are in a position to make decisions for themselves. This is a great opportunity to let them know that because you love and care about them you would love for them to start eating healthier too. Remember to keep using those "I" statements. For example, "I would love for you to join me and start eating healthier, too," versus *"You need* to start eating healthier too." These are two very different approaches and will elicit very different responses. Nobody likes to be told what to do. With younger children in your care, however, you are in a position to be telling them what to do until they are old enough to make decisions for themselves. This would be a good time to let them know that because it is your responsibility to care for and nourish them, you will be helping them to discover new, healthier foods that they will enjoy as well.

6 ~ tell them what to expect

...from you as you are making the transition.

Sometimes when people start making changes to their diet, especially if they are getting off any extreme addictive foods such as sugar or caffeine, they will feel tired, cranky, headachy or otherwise out of sorts temporarily as their bodies adjust. This same kind of withdrawal experience can happen when eliminating some other foods as well, especially any of the common food allergens such as wheat, dairy or soy. This is something you not only want to be aware of and prepare for yourself, but this is also information you will want to share with those closest to you who may be affected by any changes in your mood or behavior. Plan as little as possible for the first critical days in which you are weaning yourself off these foods, including letting others know how you might be feeling and asking them to give you some space to go through it. Also, let them know that there will be certain things you will no longer want or be willing

Most of us talk more than we need to.

Most of us tell people more than they need to know.

Most of us ramble too much, and most of us take too long to say things.

If you accept this, you can begin to clean up your conversation and become someone people want to listen to, instead of someone they feel they *have* to listen to.

Roger Ailes

to do that you may have done together in the past, such as going to certain restaurants or indulging in certain treats. Giving them a heads up now will help avert problems down the road.

7 ~ make specific requests
...as to how they can show their support and help you.

Tell them you would really appreciate their support and make very specific requests as to how they can provide it. You will want to think about this before you sit down to talk so you can make the most of this opportunity to ask for help. Set your listener and yourself up for success by making no more than 1-3 clear, simple requests that can easily be accomplished. For example, "Please don't entice me to go to Dairy Queen and have a double fudge banana split," "Walk the dog after school so I have more time to prepare a nutritious meal," "Give me a dozen roses instead of a box of chocolates for Valentine's Day," or whatever is appropriate for you. You can always make future requests and take things to the next level once the first ones have been integrated, but keep it very simple and doable to start.

> Others can stop you temporarily – you are the only one who can do it permanently.
>
> Zig Ziglar

8 ~ do not advise them
...about their eating habits at this time, this talk is about you.

Do not use this time to nag them about what you think they "should" or "shouldn't" or "need" to be doing. Remember this talk is about *you* and your requests for support. Keep these issues completely separate or you will, no doubt, sabotage your efforts on both fronts. We will talk about how you may be able to help them shortly.

9 ~ be brief and to the point
...to make it easier for them to hear what you are saying and grant your requests.

Think in advance about what you would like to say. You may even like to jot down a few notes if you need to, so that when it comes time for the talk, you can be as brief and to the point as possible. Don't ramble on and on, or get off track on other topics, or you run the risk of losing your listener's attention and possibly their support. The more precise and poignant you can be, the better chance of being heard and receiving a favorable response.

10 ~ politely remind and repeat

...them of points you have made in your talk in the days to come until new routines are established.

Just because you sat down and had this talk doesn't mean that your listeners are going to remember everything you said, and immediately begin fulfilling all your requests. Remember that this issue is important to *you*, not them. Don't get mad when they forget things you have told them. *Expect* that they will forget and that you will have to politely remind them. It will take a little time and repetition before they are able to develop new patterns of behavior. Repeat commitments or requests you have made nicely and often, until they become integrated into your collective lifestyle.

_____

These top ten suggestions will be a tremendous help to you when talking to your dear ones about your intentions to create a healthier eating lifestyle for yourself, and garner their help as well. Do take the time to have this talk with your loved ones even if it feels a little out of your comfort zone. It will pay off in the long run and help you to move in the direction you want to go. If Debbie had had a talk as outlined here with her husband and close girlfriends from the very beginning, she could have spared herself a great deal of physical discomfort and internal turmoil. As for other people in your life who do not fall into this close-quarters category such as friends or extended family members, but who may still be affected by the changes you are making, it is wise to have a modified version of this heart-to-heart talk, as mentioned, or address the topic as it comes up. Whatever fits best for that particular relationship.

Regarding more casual relationships such as co-workers or fellow members of the P.T.A., unless there's a specific reason to do so, there's no need to broadcast the fact that you are undergoing a nutritional transformation. Especially in the beginning, when you haven't quite rooted yourself in this transformation, it is often smart to keep this matter private. Otherwise, you run the risk of

Those things, people, situations and experiences you don't like – avoid them.

Stay away. Walk away. Do something else.

Some might call this cowardly. We call it smart.

The world is brimming with things, people and experiences.

...So why not associate with the ones that naturally please you?

John-Roger & Peter McWilliams

opening yourself up to criticism, teasing and even heated discussions, all of which are better avoided. Of course, whether you say anything or not, people will begin to notice your absence from the buffet table you used to loiter around, or your unwillingness to pick up that box of Krispie Kremes on the way into work, for example. In those instances, if someone inquires, unless you are certain they will be supportive, it is best to keep your response brief and go with a simple one-liner or two. "Double fried chicken wings just don't agree with me anymore," "I'm allergic to dairy products," "Yep, I'm cutting down on the sweets," are all good responses that require no further explanation.

When met with someone you are certain will not be supportive, and who may also be predisposed to teasing or arguing (we all know one or more of these type people), it is best to keep quiet and smile, or give a little giggle to any insulting or aggressive comments and make a gracious exit if possible. No use subjecting yourself to such treatment when you are trying to do something nurturing for yourself. Some people can get really funny about food and beverages. Even though you may be talking about what *you* are doing, if it isn't in agreement with what they're doing or pushes their guilt buttons about what they think inside they should be doing, some people can get testy and take it out on you, as Debbie learned from her experience. As much as possible, especially in the early stages of making changes in your diet and lifestyle, it is best to associate with those who are supportive of your efforts and avoid those who are not.

the company you keep

Many religious groups encourage their patrons to keep in the company of the holy in order to keep their faith and their religious practice strong. While you don't have to become a dogmatic fanatic about the way you eat, there is wisdom in the notion of keeping company with supportive, like-minded people. Doing so is especially helpful when you first start making the transition to a healthier eating lifestyle and the pull in the other direction may still be strong. As I told Debbie, in terms of the relationships in your life, there are basically four general scenarios that will play out as you embark on your dietary and lifestyle transformation.

Who are you around, what have they got you thinking, what have they got you saying, what have they got you doing, where do they have you going?

Jim Rohn

First, your relationships with certain people will gradually fade and these people will fall away. You will experience a natural parting of ways as you go along your new path and they continue along theirs. This may not be forever, however. Don't be surprised if one day one or another of these people shows up in your life again. I have seen this happen many times. As their own health begins to break down, they decide it's time to get off the destructive path they were on and look to those who have gone before them for guidance.

Second, there will be people in your life who will just accept your new ways and the fact that you don't slam shots or frequent fast-food joints anymore. The nature of your relationship may change a little and go through some initial adjustments, but they will endure. This is the most common scenario for immediate and extended family members and others that are very close to you. It's what unconditional love and acceptance is all about.

Next, you may actually be fortunate enough to have one or more people in your life who not only accept your new ways, but actually start moving in the same direction along with you. I am very blessed to have had this particular scenario play out with my oldest and dearest friend I have known since I was 12-years-old. We went from days of smoking, drinking, and binging on massive amounts of the junkiest junk foods in our teens, to practicing yoga, drinking carrot juice, and sharing healthy recipes. This was a parallel transition that evolved organically over time as part of our individual self-discovery and maturation process. It's hard to say who started it. We both began exploring different avenues along the same route and have been a great source of information and inspiration for one another along the way. It's my wish for everyone to have such a friend or partner in their life, whether you already know them or not.

Which leads us to the final category of relationships that can play out in your life: the possibility of meeting new, more self-care conscious people who reflect your desire to create a more nurturing way of living for yourself. This one usually requires some initiative on your part. For many adults making new friends and associates can be a scary proposition. If this is the case for you, make an attempt to go beyond your comfort zone. It will pay off and may not be as uncomfortable as you might think. Fortunately, there are an increasing number of places to turn

Don't join an easy crowd; you won't grow.

Go where the expectations and the demands to perform are high.

Jim Rohn

when it comes to the search for new, more health-minded camaraderie.

Local healthy eating and cooking classes are a great place to meet people with this same interest. The Internet is also a very comfortable, safe way for many people to connect through message boards, forums and chat rooms. I offer healthy eating teleconference programs where people can learn and meet other natural food enthusiasts from around the world. For more information visit: www.FoodFitnessByPhone.com. Local support groups that are familiar with the *Eating-for-Health* philosophy outlined in this book are also springing up. If there isn't one in your area yet, you can always start one! Bear in mind that at the same time you are seeking out new people to connect with, there are others seeking to connect with the likes of you as well. If you look in earnest, it is only a matter of time before you meet up with each other.

Hiring a coach is another fantastic way of putting someone in your corner, not only for education and support, but also for holding you accountable for following through with your commitments. There is a reason all of the best sports teams and individual athletes have coaches — coaching works!

Buddying-up with an old or new friend can be helpful in the same regard, and it doesn't cost a thing. I always encourage people attending my programs to buddy-up with either another person in the program or someone outside the program for the same reasons someone would hire a coach. When you find someone who is interested in being your healthy-eating buddy, if you're not in one already, you can join a healthy eating program or take a cooking class together. Whether you attend an outside class or program or not, you will want to set up some kind of parameters and regular action steps. Arrange to meet once a week, have a brief daily phone or e-mail check in, or whatever works for the both of you. Make it realistic and then hold each other to the commitments you make. It is often helpful, albeit not always possible or desirable, to have your spouse or significant other be your buddy. Whatever you decide to do or with whom, this kind of mutually supportive partnership can be a lifesaver.

Relationships with others may be the single most influential factor in how you conduct any area of your life. They have the power to propel you forward or hold you back, but it is

Building character means taking the actions that challenge you to face your fears.

...It means creating such a strong relationship with yourself that you develop the emotional strength to go against the norm when your beliefs conflict with those around you.

And it means being willing to rock the boat in order to stand by your convictions so you can protect your rights as well as the rights of others.

Cheryl Richardson

you who has the power to determine the nature of the relationships you choose to maintain in your life. If there are relationships in your life that are holding you back, either make some changes or let them go. Regardless of what transpires with old relationships, you need to get validation, acknowledgement, and encouragement from like-minded people who share your desire to restore or maintain your health and well-being through a balanced diet and lifestyle. As mentioned earlier, this is especially true for those who are just beginning to turn away from the accepted, destructive popular food culture and establish a solid nutritional foundation for themselves.

Although there are those who will walk with you for some or much of the journey, and you will encounter many others along the way, this trek through life is ultimately an individual one. Whether you manage to procure an adequate external support system or not, you can never rely on others to do what only you can do for yourself. Throughout your life you must continually turn to that internal support system for help, for therein lies your most reliable and ever-present source.

> Nothing splendid has ever been achieved except by those who dared believe that something inside them was superior to circumstances.
>
> Bruce Barton

it's all about *you*

I once met a woman who taught me some valuable lessons. Her name was Rhonda and I met her while working a temporary job in downtown Los Angeles many years ago. Soon after starting, I noticed that Rhonda disappeared about every 15 minutes, then wafted back in, enveloped by the stench of smoke. She was anxious and on edge most of the time. This, I surmised, was no doubt related to the one can of Coke after another that never seemed to leave her trembling hands. The intermittent candy bars she munched on throughout the day probably weren't helping much either, I thought. Even in my worst days of smoking and junk food binging I was never *that* bad, I further observed. In those first few days of working alongside Rhonda, I found her personality offensive and her behavior aberrant. Then I learned she was a recovering heroine addict, and ate humble pie.

Rhonda told me her story during lunch one day. She had been a successful songwriter who, at her peak, wrote a few top ten hits recorded by a famous female artist. As sometimes happens in the topsy-turvy world of the recording industry, a couple of years and a few failed contracts later, Rhonda found herself broke, homeless, and addicted to heroine. It was when she woke up in a dumpster one morning that she hit bottom and became determined to turn her life around. Kicking the heroine habit was the most obvious and necessary place to start. So, not wanting to deal with the authorities, Rhonda locked herself up in an old friend's apartment who reluctantly went out of town for the occasion.

For four days, Rhonda sweated, vomited, shook uncontrollably, and climbed the proverbial walls as she withdrew from heroine without medical supervision. During the worst of it, she prayed that she would die rather than have to go through it. But go through it she did, and was now on the other side. She described those four days as the most horrific event of her life. Now, with a fresh can of Coke in one hand and an unlit cigarette in the other, Rhonda concluded her dramatic saga.

"Today I wake up every morning grateful to be alive and well and heroine free. Now I'm addicted to cigarettes, Coke and candy bars," she laughed. "Some day I'll deal with those too, because they're not good for me either. But if that's as bad as it ever gets, I can live with that!"

Feeling complete, she then stood proudly and announced she was going out to have a cigarette. The unspoken criticism and judgment I had held up until that moment now faded into respect and admiration for this woman's incredible courage and determination. Instead of the previous silent scorn I gave to this announcement, I sighed relief at the outcome of Rhonda's story and called out, "You go girl!"

I tell you this story now because I believe it offers a number of lessons that we can all draw from. It illustrates the incredible amount of willpower, endurance, and resolve that we are capable of as human beings. It reminds us to focus on ourselves and suspend criticism and judgment of others. It demonstrates the importance of knowing when it's time to employ every bit of willpower and strength to pull ourselves out of the dumpster, and when it's time to give ourselves a break. It helps put things into perspective, and makes the prospect of kicking a sugar addiction seem like a piece of cake!

But more importantly, it speaks to the fact that when it comes to making changes in any area of life, you can make requests and ask for support from others in a myriad of ways, but

The single most important thing we must do to eliminate our physical problems is TO STOP DOING WHAT CREATED THEM!

George Malkmus

in the final hour it all comes down to *you*. No one else can think for you, eat for you, or withdraw from heroine for you. When it comes to the majority of choices you make and actions you take in life, you're on your own. For this reason, the relationship you maintain with yourself is of utmost importance.

Although others unknowing of her situation may have looked on judgmentally, as I did initially, Rhonda was not beating herself up for smoking 2 packs of cigarettes, guzzling a 6-pack of Coke, and eating several candy bars a day. She didn't hide, make excuses, or apologize for these habits. On the contrary, she was quite content to have them. Rhonda judged herself relative to where she had come from and in accordance with where she was headed. As for what others might think, she didn't care. She had reached a place of loving acceptance with herself that overrode anyone's opinion of her, a place worth taking note for us all.

It's not where we stand in the world, but in what direction we are moving.

Unknown

If you have already started, or are in the market to make changes in your diet and lifestyle, you are going to have to develop some internal fortitude to follow through with your convictions in this regard. If you are as yet a little wobbly, as most people are in the beginning, taking a little time out to recreate yourself may be in order. As someone seeking to free herself from the king of all addictions, Rhonda understood the importance of this. Whereas you may not have to go to the extreme of locking yourself up in an empty apartment, temporarily removing yourself from temptation while you practice and integrate new eating habits and rebalance your biochemistry, is the wisest course of action to take.

So many people put themselves in the face of the very foods they are trying to pull away from and then wonder why it is such a struggle for them. Give yourself a leg up by taking a little reprieve from social activities and eating out for a few days or a few weeks or whatever it takes for you to strengthen your foothold. This is one of the best ways there is to support yourself during this time of transition. Once you have gained some strength, confidence and know-how with what you are doing, as you venture back out into the world other people and situations will have less influence over the choices you make. In some cases, you may even inadvertently begin to influence them.

helping them, too

As mentioned before, one of the most frequent questions people ask me once they embark on the journey to healthier eating is how to help others to do the same, especially their loved ones. Which brings to mind the most valuable lesson Rhonda's story has to offer. It was the dramatic turnaround that she was able to make in her own life that is most inspiring to others. Her personal story is a testament to what is possible and makes others want to do better in their own lives. This kind of inspiration is one of the greatest gifts anyone can impart to another. Just as Rhonda's triumph was inspiring, your testimony will be your greatest tool for helping others to make changes as well. Your personal actions and testimony speak louder than any words you could possibly say. The old saying "you must lead by example" is true.

> The leader is the one who climbs the tallest tree, surveys the entire situation, and yells, "Wrong jungle!"
>
> Stephen Covey

Equally as true, however, is another quote. In his book *The Seven Habits of Highly Effective People,* Stephen Covey writes: "The leader is the one who climbs the tallest tree, surveys the entire situation, and yells, 'Wrong jungle!'" With the information you now possess regarding the pitfalls of our popular food culture will come a calling for many of you to let others know we are rambling around in the wrong jungle and help lead the way out. People are not sheep, however, and those who don't want to will not be led, especially when it comes to the foods to which they may have become ferociously attached. Striking a healthy balance between knowing when to keep quiet and focus on yourself, and when to cry "wrong jungle!" becomes key.

It's important for me personally that people get the information I have to offer. But I remain unattached, as much as possible, as to what they decide to do with it. I hope, of course, that people will use it to improve the quality of their lives, but accept and respect their choice to do otherwise. It is *their* life after all and they have free will in the matter. Information delivered without attachment to the outcome is the easiest for other people to receive. It can also be the hardest to deliver when it concerns those we love. With children who are in our care, the scenario is different, of course, and we *can* impose what we believe to be right and healthy for them as part of our caretaking responsibilities. But for the adults in our lives we cannot.

This doesn't mean we can never broach the subject with them, however, only that we must do so gingerly. Unless you are directly asked for your advise, anything and everything you say that may be *perceived* to be nagging or telling someone else what to do will more than likely be rejected on contact. *Perceived* being the key word here. Your intentions may be good as gold, but what you say may be perceived and received in another way. For this reason, sharing what you are learning, doing, and experiencing in your own life without a hidden agenda can not only be one of the best ways to gain support for yourself, but also holds the possibility of generating interest on the part of others as well.

share & share alike

It is especially important at this juncture for us to share what we know with regard to our prevalent popular food culture and it's relationship to *dis*-ease of the body and mind. There are so many people today who are suffering from chronic *dis*-ease and resorting to toxic drugs, surgery, and other high-risk procedures that will inevitably make their problems worse. Most of them are not aware that the foods they are eating or *not* eating are the root cause of what ails them and, therefore, also provide the only real solution. If they are made aware of this reality, at least then people can make informed choices about which path they choose, rather than feeling as if there are no other alternatives. One of the ways to do this, in addition to giving a brief synopsis during your heart-to-heart conversation with loved ones, is to share information regarding the relationship between diet and *dis*-ease in the course of casual conversations.

Often when I give a presentation I present some of the *Scary Statistics* outlined in the first chapter in the form of a Pop Quiz that I go over with the audience. I have had many people subsequently tell me that they later share this information with family members, friends, and co-workers. They say it makes for interesting conversation and they feel a sort of moral obligation, as I do, to inform others of the severity of the situation in which we now find ourselves.

Similarly I have had many people give copies of this book to others as a gift. I recently received a beautiful thank you note from a woman who received such a gift. She had suffered debilitating migraine headaches for three years, been to several specialists, undergone a plethora of diagnostic tests, taken numerous prescription drugs, and spent thousands of dollars —

There is nothing more difficult to take in hand, more perilous to conduct or more uncertain in its success than to take the lead in the introduction of a new order of things.

Machiavelli
The Prince

with no relief. As mentioned earlier, her sister-in-law then gave her a copy of this book and she immediately began to implement the first *Eating-for-Health Guideline.* In her note, this woman told me her migraines had ceased as a result. Sharing can be a good thing and may even turn out to be a life-changing gesture, as it was in this, and many other similar cases.

Nutritional consultations, coaching, and healthy-eating classes or programs such as the *Food Fitness by Phone* tele-programs also make great gifts. Most businesses offering these programs and services have gift certificates. If they don't, just ask. More than likely they will be happy to whip something up for you. It is always preferable to give such gifts to those who you believe will be the most receptive. For those who are more likely to dismiss such gifts, you may want to get a little more creative. A woman who took one of my healthy eating programs, for example, later told me she was able to inspire her husband to eat better by reading this book to him in bed at night. While this may not be the best approach for everyone, it is a good idea to be creative and to share what you are learning. With some people the exact opposite approach may be more effective — saying nothing at all, thereby generating a natural curiosity. But whatever you decide to do, keep in mind that you are only delivering the information and others have a right to discard it. Don't take yourself too seriously. Keep it light and have fun.

> It's good
> to share.
>
> All Good
> Mothers

Books, articles, statistics, healthy eating programs, nutritional tips and tidbits are all great things to share. But remember, the greatest thing you can offer is your own personal experience and testimony of how changing your diet and lifestyle has improved your overall health, energy and any specific health conditions. The experiences and testimonies of others can be very informational and inspiring to yourself and others as well.

don't tow the party line

There is another critical element to consider when it comes to communicating with people. It has become the socially accepted norm to speak about various issues associated with diet, *dis*-ease, and our popular food culture in a manner that skirts personal responsibility and diminishes, or completely denies the role of nutrition. Refraining from such language in every day conversations is another valuable way of helping both yourself and others to move in a healthier, more honest direction. To do otherwise is to contribute to the spread and perpetuation of the kind of world in which our old friend Mr. Whitless resides (a Whitless world, if you will), which is disempowering and isn't going to help anyone.

For example, how many times have you heard someone say, "So-and-so was perfectly healthy and then they *suddenly* had a heart attack or 'got' cancer, ..." This is not possible. These are chronic degenerative diseases that develop in the body over a number of years, and they are more often than not also preventable, as we discussed earlier. As individuals and as a society, we have to stop kidding ourselves with the words we speak and the actions we take — food matters!

This is especially important when it comes to how we think and speak about the less threatening ailments and *dis*-eases, such as arthritis, asthma, sinusitis, allergies, acid reflux, and other digestive and eliminative problems. These everyday maladies are more often than not falsely believed to be inherited or to have come about as a result of some mysterious, uncontrollable force of nature, and are therefore unavoidable and irreversible. Nothing could be further from the truth. These conditions are all indications of a system that is weakened, congested, and not receiving or absorbing the nutrition it needs. Unfortunately, because the prevalent societal belief structure ignores the root cause of an ailing system as a whole, instead of clearing and strengthening their internal environment, most people take massive amounts of prescription and over-the-counter drugs, which ultimately contributes to their problem of an overburdened, compromised body-mind system.

Betty's story at the beginning of this book is a good example of this phenomenon. Another good example has to do with sinus problems (i.e., sinusitis, allergies, hay fever, etc.). Many people today still believe that these problems result from outside influences. They will make statements such as, "I'm allergic to dust, ragweed, etc." or "I have really bad hay fever this year because there is so much pollen in the air," as if these pernicious airborne substances were the *cause* of their problems. The truth of the matter is that these substances are only *exacerbating* an existing condition. They are the last straw that causes an already weakened, congested and overloaded system to react in an acute

You don't catch diabetes or obesity, you create it.

Brain Garden

manner. Once a person strengthens and clears her system with proper nutrition and cleansing, which is frequently needed as well, more often than not, her sinus troubles go away. The same is true of asthma, skin problems, digestive disturbances, arthritis, recurrent colds, and virtually all conditions and *dis*-eases.

Being aware of the language we use and hear others use is a valuable way to at least begin to align our thoughts, beliefs and words with the truth of the matter. Next time you find yourself or hear someone else perpetuating myths or illusions about the root cause and relationship between diet and *dis*-ease, stop and take notice. You can go a step further by amending what you say when you catch yourself, and in some cases may even want to call someone else on something they have said, too. Be cautious with the latter, however. You may be challenging some deep-seated beliefs and ruffle some feathers. Many people may not understand and some may even want to debate the issue.

the debate team

When I was in college I had a good friend named Danny. He used to joke with others that we got along famously as long as we didn't discuss religion or politics. Today Danny might have added nutrition to that list, as it has become another hotly debated issue often generating the same high level of emotions as the topics of religion and politics. If you find yourself entering into such a potentially confrontational conversation regarding any aspect of diet and nutrition, my advice to you would be to do as my old friend Danny and I attempted to do, and just not go there.

Of course, invariably we did go there and you probably will too. In fact, those conversations were the most fun and lively aspect of Danny's and my friendship. No matter how heated the debate got, however, we would always end by laughing at ourselves and get back to the realm of mutual respect for one another. Keeping your debates in a similar realm of frivolity would be wise, especially if it's with someone close to you. Vow at the beginning, if only in your own mind, to bring the conversation around to a place of neutral feelings towards each other. In the midst of the debate, however, let me provide you with a little fuel for your debating fire, so you can give it all you've got!

Learn to accept the behavior of others that doesn't fit the pattern of your opinions.

Learn to praise the idiosyncrasies, the eccentricities, the quirks and the singularities of others.

It will help you to praise your own.

John-Roger & Peter McWilliams

First of all, stick with bottom line, factual generalities such as the fact that only 9-12% of the population is eating in accordance with the guidelines for a healthy diet as outlined by the government, guidelines that in many natural health care circles are considered to be very conservative and in some cases inadequate. Furthermore, contrary to popular belief, the basic nutritional recommendations that emanate from the legitimate scientific community, and essentially what is put forth in this book, have changed little over the past few decades.

This does not appear to be the case, however, because we are constantly being bombarded with conflicting and flip-flopping nutritional information usually focused on one particular food or nutrient. This is due to the media's appetite for sensationalistic stories, which the food industry eagerly supplies due to its appetite for profits. The media has become entertainment in a race for ratings and a pawn for corporate and other promotional schemes. It is not a viable resource for health and nutritional information. Unfortunately, the mass media has become the average person's exclusive source for nutritional information. People tend to believe without question what they hear and read, not realizing that it is the food industry's savvy marketing teams, not true science that is feeding this information to the media outlets.

For those of you who would like to tap into some big guns for debating this issue in an informed manner, *Food Politics: How the Food Industry Influences Nutrition* is a fabulous resource written by Marion Nestle. Although fascinating and well researched, there was no media firestorm when this book was released because it takes the food industry to task, one of the mass media's biggest sponsors. For those of you who prefer the crib notes, following is a passage from the introduction:

> *Since 1988, in my role as chair of an academic department of nutrition, a member of federal advisory committees, a speaker at public and professional meetings, a frequent commentator on nutrition issues to the press, and (on occasion) a consultant to food companies, I have become increasingly convinced that many of the nutritional problems of Americans – not least of them obesity – can be traced to the food industry's imperative to encourage people to eat more in order to generate sales and*

Reporters highlight unusual findings to grab your attention...

It is...not the latest headlines that should influence food choices...

Uncertain science — especially when mishandled by the media— is often at the core of a seeming flip-flop...

Be cautious of overzealous reporting that flies in the face of conventional wisdom.

Controversial news sells, but don't rely on it for advice.

Adrienne Forman, R.D.

increase income in a highly competitive marketplace. Ambiguous dietary advice is only one result of this imperative. ...the industry also devotes enormous financial and other resources to lobbying Congress and federal agencies, forming partnerships and alliances with professional nutrition organizations, funding research on food and nutrition, publicizing the results of selected research studies favorable to industry, sponsoring professional journals and conferences, and making sure that influential groups — federal officials, researchers, doctors, nurses, school teachers, and the media — are aware of the benefits of their products.

This is a great passage to share with people. Sourced from an academician, it succinctly addresses the issue of how the food industry, through a variety of channels, has been instrumental in creating our popular food culture by manipulating nutritional recommendations and influencing what we eat. Once this is understood, it becomes obvious to most that a nutritional debate based on media supplied information is frequently sketchy and often worthless. Ask a variety of people and they'll give you a variety of answers depending on the derivation and agenda of their source, which is usually based on splashy headlines and sensational sound bites that fill the pages and airtime of corporate sponsored magazines and news shows.

Similarly, what is or isn't being taught in the public schools isn't necessarily accurate either. K-12 curriculums are also influenced by industry propaganda, often lag behind the times, and are slow to change. For example, I had a client who wrote me a frantic e-mail telling me that her daughter's home economics teacher had told the class that enriched white bread was more nutritious than whole wheat bread. She wanted to know a good resource she could provide for this teacher to bring him up-to-date and protect her daughter from this misinformation. I recommended she refer to *Eat, Drink and Be Healthy: The Harvard Medical School Guide to Healthy Eating*, by Dr. Walter Willett, head of Harvard's department of nutrition. This is another great resource to employ in nutritional debates based on up-to-date *real* science, independent of the food industry.

When it comes to discussing and debating dietary issues, whatever you do, don't venture into the realm of scientific

The food processors hire lobbyists to get legislation passed allowing them to call these foods, of all things, *natural*.

Ever wonder how a food that is over 50% *processed* white sugar and dripping with additives can be called natural?

Legislation, m'boy, legislation!

Harvey & Marilyn Diamond
Fit for Life II

information that you don't fully understand and can't articulate. You'll lose, and also run the risk of discrediting other valid points you may have made. Instead, stick with generalities, and also encourage others to do some research on their own by referring them to reliable resources untainted by the mass media and food conglomerates, such as those just cited and others listed in the back of this book.

As for challenging popular beliefs about health conditions and the inclination to deny or diminish the role of diet in creating them, an observation I first heard voiced by Dr. John Lee can be useful. Dr. Lee was a well-known physician and author of several books on women's wellness. In a lecture he gave a few years ago, he said, "When it comes to health issues it takes a generation for us to realize what we're doing wrong, and another generation to fix it." He was speaking about the risks involved with hormone replacement therapy (H.R.T.) during this lecture. We have all watched as the truth of this statement has unfolded with regard to this particular treatment. There are numerous other instances throughout history that support this observation as well. The history of antibiotic use is another good example.

> When it comes to health issues it takes a generation for us to realize what we're doing wrong, and another generation to fix it.
>
> Dr. John Lee

In the generation in which they were first introduced, antibiotics were thought to be a Godsend and the development and usage of this new class of miracle drugs was rampant. Of course, in many cases they *were* miraculous and took healthcare to a whole new level. However, we now know that widespread unbounded use of these drugs can be detrimental. It took a generation to fully discover this and the exact nature of their pitfalls, the development of antibiotic resistant strains of bacteria and viruses being one of the most serious. Today, antibiotics are prescribed more prudently and people are advised to take probiotics to replenish their intestinal flora that may have been destroyed during the course of their treatment, another problem we now know to be associated with antibiotic use. Increasingly, antibiotics are being put in their rightful place by being limited to priority usage.

The observation that it takes a generation for us to figure out what we're doing wrong and yet another generation to reverse the damage would seem to apply not only to health issues, but to a broad spectrum of social issues as well, and could most certainly be said of the current climate surrounding our popular food culture and declining state of health. We are currently in the midst of the first generation to be indulging in widespread unbounded consumption of processed, packaged pseudofoods in unprecedented amounts, much like antibiotics when they first became widely available. With the skyrocketing rates of obesity and chronic degenerative *dis*-ease in this and other industrialized countries, what we're doing wrong is becoming increasingly evident with regard to the down side of this practice as we discussed in *Chapter 1*. Similar to antibiotic use, it is now time to start putting processed, packaged fake food in its rightful place by limiting its consumption, and go about the business of fixing the damage that has been done.

Drawing parallels between what has happened with both H.R.T. and antibiotics and what is now happening with pseudofoods I find to be an effective way of helping people to understand the bigger picture. Using this analogy in combination with the *Scary Statistics* and ammunition provided regarding the food industry will put you in a good sparring position. It is important to remember, however, that in the course of any debate on the topic of diet and *dis*-ease and bringing awareness to the pitfalls of pseudofoods, you are not waging a battle *against* others. On the contrary, there is no *us* or *them* in this situation. Ultimately, when it comes to our health and well-being and that of future generations, we're all on the same human team. And never before in history has there been more of a need to help out the youngest members of our human team, our children.

bull's eye

As we discussed earlier, in recent decades the food industry has aimed their heaviest marketing artillery at the most impressionable and vulnerable segment of our society, with the intention of creating lifelong consumers of their fake-food products. It is now evident that they didn't just hit their target — they got a bull's eye. Our children have been hit and they've been hit hard. The health statistics that are just now starting to emerge as a result of this hit are the scariest of all.

For the first time in history, conditions that were previously associated with aging are now showing up in children at younger and younger ages. *Dis*-eases such as Type 2 diabetes, high cholesterol, high blood pressure, and even heart attacks have

Coincident with the junk-food invasion, which began in the early 1950's and occupied most school lunchrooms by 1960, there (has) been a huge rise in the number of children with brain damage, hyperactivity, or learning disability.

A study at the University of California suggests that the problem has doubled since the 1960's.

Dr. Michael Colgan,
Nutrition Scientist

now reached unprecedented and rapidly increasing numbers among our youth. The *Centers for Disease Control and Prevention (CDC)* predicts that more than one-third of American children born in the year 2000 will become diabetic. For those who are black or Hispanic, the estimate is closer to half. Dr. K.M. Venkat Narayan, a diabetes epidemiologist at the CDC, considers these estimates to be "quite conservative" and further warns that the medical community is not equipped to handle such an onslaught. And this is only the forecast for diabetes.

Allowing these kinds of predictions to come to fruition will make for a sad commentary on this generation in the history books of the future. We are setting a whole generation up for physical, emotional and economic ruin. This is a very serious issue that needs to be addressed and needs to be addressed fast. We are looking at adding to an already overburdened healthcare system the sickest, fattest generation the world has ever seen. Unless this trend is reversed, we will all suffer as a result.

We have a moral obligation as the stewards of this next generation to do everything in our power to turn this trend around and give our children every opportunity to live normal, healthy lives. We are not only robbing them of their childhoods, but the quality of their adulthoods, and possibly their very lives as well. Despite the troubling predictions and burgeoning health crisis that is emerging, an abundant supply of soda, junk food and pseudofood continues to flow into the mouths of our youngsters. One of the most alarming dispensaries of these anti-nutrients is in the very place children should be the safest from manipulative marketing maneuvers — our public schools.

scary predictions

Overall, 39% of the girls who now are healthy 2½-3-year-olds and 33% of the boys are likely to develop diabetes.

For Hispanic children, the odds are closer to one in two: 53% of the girls and 45% of the boys.

The numbers are about 49% and 40% for black girls and boys, and 31% and 27% for white girls and boys.

U.S. Centers for Disease Control

just say 'no' – to soda

Sixty-percent of public schools across the nation have lucrative contracts with soda companies to dispense their products in school hallways. Mega-chain fast-food companies have similarly infiltrated many school cafeterias. That fast food is a major health-compromiser is a no-brainer in the minds of most. However, because the soft drink industry has been so successful in making their products so widely accepted and available for daily — often multiple times a day — consumption, soda is frequently not perceived to be the liquid candy and potential health hazard that it is. This accepted practice of regular and excessive soda consumption concerns me to such a degree that I felt compelled to speak before the Denver Public School Board in the Summer of 2003 urging them *not* to renew their contract with Pepsi. I did so in the context of their monthly public forum as part of the established agenda. In the allotted three minutes each individual was given to voice their opinion on the topic, here is what I said:

We are now the fattest country in the world. The rate of obesity among our children alone has tripled in the last two decades, the same two decades in which soda consumption among children has tripled for boys and doubled for girls.

According to a study recently cited in the Lancet Journal, *drinking one soda or sweetened beverage a day increases the risk for obesity among children by 60%. In addition, soda consumption puts children at risk for learning and behavioral disorders and Type 2 diabetes. Previously known as 'adult onset' diabetes, because it rarely struck those under the age of 50, Type 2 diabetes has reached epidemic proportions among children over the past decade. The same decade in which mass marketing campaigns and mass availability of soft drinks were introduced into the public school systems.*

In response to the frequently voiced argument that students are free to choose whether or not they drink soda, certainly there exist many choices students are free to make and yet are not allowed on school grounds. The question is not whether or not children are free to make the choice to drink soda; the question is does this choice put them at risk?

With the positions you hold as school board members comes the obligation to protect the welfare of the children you serve. The promotion of soda consumption with its inherent health risks is clearly a violation of this obligation.

If you extend the contract with Pepsi, from this day forward the sight of every obese, overweight, diabetic or behaviorally challenged child will weigh heavy on your minds — and if this past decade is any indication of what is to come, there will be many. If instead you forgo the contract, you will look into the eyes of these same children and feel confidant that you have done right by them. I implore you NOT to extend the contract with Pepsi. Do it for the children, do it for yourselves, do it for the future of our nation.

slurp, slurp

A recent study cited in The Lancet *showed that for every soft drink or sweetened beverage a child drinks per day, their obesity risk increases by 60%.*

In the last 20 years, soda consumption has doubled for girls and tripled for boys.

Nearly three-fourths of teenaged boys drink 3 or more sodas per day.

20% of toddlers now drink soda.

Every man, woman, and child in America today drinks an average of 1.6 12-ounce servings of soda per day.

Center for Science in the Public Interest

Two other people came forward to speak to the board on this issue and voiced similar sentiments. One of them was the former superintendent of Denver Public Schools. Members of the board, seven in all, then made comments with regard to their positions. Three members opposed renewal of the contract and similarly voiced grave concerns for the welfare of students and a need to consider future consequences. The remaining four were in favor of renewing the contract, and because they held the majority, the motion to renew the contract was passed.

The comments of these four members in justifying their decisions to vote in favor of renewing the Pepsi contract were both thought provoking and disturbing. They included: diminishing the health risks involved with regular and excessive soda consumption; placing the onus on parents to teach their children not to drink soda (even when it is being made available and, therefore, obviously being endorsed by the schools); the observation that children are purchasing soda anyway, so the schools may as well be reaping some of the profits; claiming that the average student in Denver schools drinks almost ten times less soda than the national average; and of course, the one we would most expect to hear, massive budget cuts which have produced the need for alternative funding.

This final justification would at first seem to be the most legitimate. Admittedly, even I found myself being seduced by this one and sympathized with the board when I first heard it. However, when I later asked what efforts were being made to obtain other sources of funding that didn't involve compromising students' health and well-being, the director of public relations said there were none. In the days soon after this public forum, it became even more difficult for me to swallow this excuse when the local news flashed stories announcing allocations approved for a $6 million dollar park renovation to include a new ice rink and fountain, and a $30 million new state-owned university basketball court to include the latest technology digital score boards. When the news cameras panned across the current premises of each, both looked to be in good order. Yet, a total of $36 million was being spent on these renovations — more than *five times* as much as the $8 million that would be generated through soft drink sales over the five-year life of the Pepsi contract with the Denver Public School District. It became obvious to me that

Soda consumption has increased by over 500% in the last 50 years.

U.S.D.A.

The profit margin on soda is 90%.

the issue at hand was not the unavailability of funds, but about the priorities that determine how available funds are allocated.

Now I realize that the business of budgets at the city and state level are a complex matter. However, the way in which revenue is divvied up in the end provides a clear indication of what we value as a society. Although we like to think otherwise, as this example illustrates, our children and our health have become low priorities. Whether you have children or not, whether you drink soda or not, this is a societal issue that affects us all. Individual values are what ultimately drive social values. I encourage you as an individual to put a higher priority on your health and the health of our children by just saying no to soda pop, especially in the hallowed halls of our public schools!

Although each of the comments made by the Denver Public School Board members in favor of renewing the contract with Pepsi was unsettling, it was a comment made by the final school board member that I found to be the most disturbing of them all. This board member said that while he was greatly concerned about the rising rates of obesity and declining standards of health among our children and the population in general, it was his observation that people seemed to be content to accept this new standard of poor health.

I can assure you that among the many individuals and groups that I have worked with, people are anything but content to accept a fate of poor health. On the contrary, depending on the severity of their condition, most express a sense of desperation not only about their personal condition, but also about the conditions of their children and loved ones as well. In the context of the public forum that night, however, this board member's observation certainly appeared to be accurate. Except for me and the two other gentlemen who spoke, there was not a single teacher, school administrator, parent, or other concerned adult who spoke out in opposition to the renewal of the Pepsi contract. This noticeable absence of any other would-be challengers made the three of us who did speak look like a lone trio of health-food nuts out of synch with popular sentiments. Which led me to ponder why such a seeming lack of interest in preserving our children's health did, in fact, appear to be the case.

One-quarter of elementary school-aged children already have high blood pressure, high cholesterol, or some other risk factor for heart disease.

These are little kids already on their way to a heart attack.

Margo Wootan, CSPI, on ABC News Special 12/8/03

roar, mama roar!

We've all seen the nature show footage: *a mama lion lying with her frolicking cubs; an intruder approaches; the lion's head perks up and she begins a low protective growl; the intruder ignores the beast's polite warning and moves closer; so, mama lion takes to her feet, assumes an offensive posture and lets out a ferocious roar!*

Mama lion's behavior is an instinctual response to imminent danger, a response that we share with her and virtually all other mammals, the natural instinct to protect our young. Unfortunately, in America and much of the industrialized world today, when it comes to the foods we eat, our popular food culture now overrides this primordial instinct. That's what makes the pseudofood weapon of mass destruction the most insidious of all, it is most often not perceived as the imminent danger that it is. It's not that people are "content to accept" a new standard of poor health, or that they don't care, most are just not aware.

Whenever I speak to a group about our pop food culture and spiel off a few *Scary Statistics* as I often do, I watch as people's mouths drop and their heads start to shake in response. People just don't realize the magnitude of what's going on. I believe this is the primary reason that people aren't in an uproar about soda, junk food and other psuedofoods being made readily available to their children at school. This anti-nutrient non-food doesn't look like the boogeyman. On the contrary, it comes cloaked in brightly colored, happy packages, tastes incredibly delicious, and doesn't seem to have any immediately observable ill effects. Besides, grocery store shelves are full of it, and everyone else is eating it and feeding it to their kids, so it must be O.K. (It frequently does, of course, have immediate ill effects, such as hyperactivity, mood swings, crankiness, headaches, fatigue, etc., but people often fail to make this association. Or they make the association to the acute reactions, but fail to recognize the long-term consequences.)

Despite any illusions to the contrary, your children's health and well-being *is* in imminent danger from these fake-food products. Furthermore, whether your child's personal health is directly undermined or not, all children will be affected by the tremendous burden to the healthcare system, and other social, familial, and economic repercussions associated with the masses of those who are.

Nutritional abuse of kids is a form of child abuse...

We don't permit pornographic books in the school libraries, why should we permit pornographic food in school lunchrooms?

Sara Sloan,
School Nutritionist

We don't allow tobacco companies to put their vending machines at the end of school hallways. In fact, even advertising for tobacco products is banned within a certain radius of school grounds. As a society, we have become adamant about sending out a clear message to our youth that smoking cigarettes is hazardous to their health. Why then do we allow the food industry to place their vending machines in school hallways, and in some cases even *serve* their disease-causing, processed junk and fast foods in school cafeterias?

Statistically speaking, these foods cause far greater harm than tobacco. It's unconscionable to be taking advantage of this most precious and vulnerable segment of our society in this way. We should be sending out a clear message to our youth that junk food is hazardous to their health as well. Instead, we are sending out the wrong message or mixed messages by making it readily available in their school environment. Make no mistake about it folks — it's time to take to your feet, pull out your claws, and roar!

Unfortunately, most parents I know, especially single and working mothers, are themselves sick, fat, tired, or exhausted from the foods they're eating and the stressful lifestyles they're living. These overworked, undernourished caretakers barely have enough energy to get through the day, let alone fight city hall or the local school board. Even if they do have the time and energy, most people feel helpless to do anything about this seemingly insurmountable situation. Their family's poor eating habits are firmly established. Just the thought of trying to make changes at the individual and family level can be daunting. Thinking about influencing changes at the level of a school district — well, that can feel downright impossible. After all, we're talking about social change on a mass scale. This can feel so overwhelming that complacency sets in, as people feel powerless to do anything about it. So, they go about living quiet lives of desperation, feeling as though they *have to* accept this situation, but they are certainly not *content* about it.

there's hope

While one finger can rightly be pointed at the food industry for manufacturing and pushing their harmful food products on our children, there are three more fingers pointing back at us the consumers for buying it and feeding it to them. And therein lies

---

Whether or not children eat proper foods, eat regularly, eat carefully, and eat politely has an effect on their health and their personalities.

National Education Association, 1940

When you put faith, hope and love together, you can raise positive kids in a negative world.

Zig Ziglar

our greatest hope for the future. Although many people may feel otherwise, the truth of the matter is that *you* the consumer do have the power to make changes in our popular food culture, and a lot of it. The power is in your pocketbook. Quit buying it, and they'll stop making it. It's that simple.

This is especially true for women who make 8 out of 10 buying decisions. When even a small percentage of women start to change their buying habits in favor of healthier choices for their families and themselves, manufacturers will take notice and respond accordingly. This is already happening on a grand scale as we can see by the proliferation of the natural foods industry in recent years.

And there's more good news on the quest for healthier eating front. When the Denver Public School Board renewed their contract with Pepsi, they amended it, at least somewhat in the right direction, by barring soft drinks from being dispensed in the elementary schools (bottled water and other sugary juice drinks are still allowed). A growing number of major school districts such as Los Angeles and New York City have taken a stand by completely banning the sale of soft drinks in their public schools, setting a bold precedence that will hopefully soon be followed by others. A few private schools have also taken the lead by firing their commercial food services and going with private chefs who make everything from scratch using only whole, fresh, natural ingredients. Not surprisingly, they're finding that this switch to real foods is comparable in price to what they had been paying for the commercial pseudofood service and having a positive impact on the students.

Interestingly enough, in the few weeks that followed the time that I spoke to the Denver Public School Board, I received requests to speak to students and various other groups involved with children, including schools and parent organizations. I am also aware of people coming together to form committees with the intention of reforming school lunch programs. These events are all evidence that there is a growing number of people who are concerned about the poor-eating pit we've fallen into, and they're taking action to pull our children and our country out of it. Everywhere you look there are more and more people jumping on the healthy eating bandwagon.

> Kids are in the process of constructing their reality and they're constructing their reality based on misinformation.
>
> Nirvair K. Khalsa

You can follow in their footsteps by launching your own counter offensive on the home front. You have complete control over what travels across the threshold of your house and makes its way into your cupboards. This is also where you have the most influence. The more you clean up your own diet and restore your own health and energy, the more you will be an energetic dynamo, as well as a role model for helping your children and others. But you don't have to wait. Jump on the bandwagon now and get it rolling!

same guidelines apply

Once adults make the leap onto the healthy-eating-for-children bandwagon, the first thing they want to know is what to feed the young 'uns. Guess what? It's simple. The same *Eating-for-Health Guidelines* apply.

When considering the guidelines as they apply to children, you'll want to magnify their importance ten-fold. Children's smaller, still developing bodies are much more sensitive to low-quality anti-nutrient foods and the many noxious substances they contain, such as MSG, food colorings, preservatives, etc. They are also hypersensitive to stimulants such as sugar and caffeine. Unfortunately, the pseudofoods made especially for the younger age bracket are loaded with all of the above.

Many parents are not aware of, or discount the effects these toxic substances have on their children. I know of one mother, for example, who insists that any juice her children drink be pasteurized, any meat they eat be overly-cooked, and that their hands be washed with antibacterial soap. Yet, she will also insist that they finish their 20-ounce caffeine- and sugar-filled soda before they can leave the dinner table.

As with so many mothers in America today, this mother is afraid of the wrong things. The incidence of illness and death caused by food poisoning and other germs, bacteria, and viruses is miniscule compared to the devastation being caused by soft drinks and fake foods. The slow deterioration of *millions* of children's health over a number of years as the result of regularly consuming processed, packaged pseudofood doesn't make headlines. The dramatic story of *one* child out of millions who dies suddenly of food poisoning does. This is yet another example of

sugar & the brain

Our work also has revealed that there is a direct connection between I.Q. and nutritional status. We tested this in a 1986 study of 1.1 million kids in 803 New York City public schools. We found that there was a fantastic increase in academic performance when the kids' diets were changed to provide more nutrients. Grades in math and English soared. It was the largest documented gain in schools ever in a short period of time.

In addition, the number of learning-disabled kids fell by an astonishing 74,000 in one year...All the schools did was bring in a policy that no food could be served in school cafeterias that contained more than 11% sucrose. Why 11%? Because a lot of fruits and vegetables contain up to 11% sucrose. They decided that if the sucrose is there naturally, that's fine. But out went the sugary sweets.

Stephen Schoenthaler, *Nutrition & Intelligence*

the sensationalistic media shaping people's perceptions of reality and, subsequently, the choices they make.

So many children's delicate bodies and brains aren't able to function properly because they are not getting the nutrients they need. At the same time they are taking in anti-nutrients and stimulants that further interfere with their ability to function normally. There are millions of children today thought to have a host of conditions who are in fact merely lacking proper nutrition. Thousands are being "cured" of hyperactivity, asthma, sinus problems, ADD, ADHD, bed wetting, recurrent colds, flu, upper respiratory conditions, ear infections, skin problems and many other ailments not by a new miracle drug, but by replacing the empty-calorie food items in their diets with real foods full of vital nutrients.

Take any child off processed, packaged pseudofoods, sugar, caffeine and any common food allergens to which they may be sensitive (i.e., follow the *Eating-for-Health Guidelines*), and you will see a significant improvement in their behavior and physical well-being, no matter what conditions they currently may or may not have. Feed them lots of whole, fresh, natural foods as outlined in *Chapter 7 ~ The Basics* and be sure they are getting an adequate amount of essential fatty acids and green foods (the two things most missing from the *Standard American Diet)* and the changes you'll see take place will astound you.

Unless your child is having an acute situation that demands immediate intervention please, please do not subject your children to dangerous, traumatic surgeries, procedures, and toxic drugs until you have explored safe, natural approaches that emphasize nutritional factors. There are thousands of surgeries performed every year on children who have had recurrent ear infections, for example; surgeries that could have been prevented by identifying and eliminating offending foods from the child's diet. As previously mentioned, doctors are not always familiar with, nor have the appropriate diagnostic tools for this task. Either do some research and experimenting on your own (See *Chapter 9 ~ Clear the Way*) or work with a holistic practitioner who is knowledgeable about food intolerances that can help you.

Whether your child is presently experiencing any health challenges or not, you will still want to place a high priority on the foods they eat. The younger children are when they begin to eat

One government study found that only 2% of 2- to 19-year-olds met all five federal recommendations for a healthy diet.

Michael Jacobson, CSPI

harmful foods and miss out on the nourishing foods their body needs, the more likely they are to develop chronic *dis*-ease in the future and at a younger age, whether they currently have symptoms or not. Children's bodies respond quickly to changes in diet one way or the other. Feed them well and they'll thrive. Feed them foolishly and they'll nose dive.

I have a friend who runs a day care facility with a 'nothing-sweeter-than-fruit allowed' policy. For breakfast, lunch and snacks she feeds the children whole, fresh, natural foods and no sweets other than fresh fruit. This is by far the most focused, orderly, relaxed, cooperative group of small children I have ever seen. There are very few squabbles and also very few absences due to illness. These children thrive. They don't feel as though they are missing out on soda or junk food. Some of them aren't even yet aware that it exists. Those who are, are being taught a valuable lesson through this policy. They are being taught to keep junk food and processed pseudofood to a minimum, and to have them only on rare, social occasions rather than as daily faire.

By now I hope you are convinced that helping your children to eat well is essential, and based on the universal *Eating-for-Health Guidelines*, you should have a pretty good idea of *what* to feed them. But I know what many of you are probably thinking now — actually getting them to eat better is another story.

ten things to help kids eat healthier

The best advice for helping children establish well balanced eating habits is to start from the beginning by feeding them primarily whole, fresh, natural foods (80-100%), minimal amounts of naturally processed foods (0-20%), and absolutely no junk foods or pseudofood brands. Keeping kids away from extreme tasting junk and pseudofood is the only sure way to prevent them from developing a taste for it. If it's too late for that, systematically transition them off the undesirable foods and re-educate their wayward palates.

This is not as difficult as people sometimes think. I have seen scores of parents transform their children's dietary habits with little to no trouble. And yes, all of them thought "not my kids!" at first, just as many of you may be thinking now. Although some will fight and kick and scream initially, children learn, make changes, and adapt more easily than adults. Once

If you talk to your children, you can help them to keep their lives together.

If you talk to them skillfully, you can help them to build future dreams.

Jim Rohn

made aware of, and taken off the foods that are overriding their natural sensibilities, kids are often surprisingly more attuned to their instinctual desire for initiating and maintaining a nutritious diet.

Don't rob children of the opportunity to establish good eating habits that will serve them for a lifetime. Developing self-care skills is a critical and sorely neglected part of their education. You must rise to the occasion and make your responsibility bigger than your excuses. Make use of all the information in this book, which can easily be applied to children. Take particular note of the information and techniques discussed in the upcoming chapters *Strategize* and *Clear the Way*, and follow these ten suggestions for helping children eat healthier:

1 ~ have a talk
...focusing on changes that will be taking place.

Once again you will want to take the time to sit down and have a heart-to-heart talk with your kids to let them know there will be some upcoming changes in the household cuisine and why. Use the same recommendations made earlier, only this time keep the focus on them. Let go of any expectations for how you think they might react, however, because you just never know.

I once had a client with three teens who felt they were old enough to make decisions for themselves, and consequently she couldn't 'impose' healthier foods on them. She was afraid they would rebel at the suggestion of eating natural foods, and didn't want to have to deal with the mayhem that would follow. For weeks this client bought and prepared separate food for herself and her testy teens as she transitioned to an *Eating-for-Health lifestyle*. Until one day she couldn't do it anymore. So, she sat down with the brood and told them that knowing what she knows now about the damaging effects of anti-nutrient food, she could no longer in good conscience buy or prepare it for them.

As it turned out they weren't as testy as she predicted. Much to her surprise, no rebellious uprising took place after this announcement. In fact, she reported that her kids merely shrugged their shoulders, mumbled "yeah, O.K., whatever," and went on their way. From that day forward they ate what she made available to them and never heard a word about it.

Role modeling is the most basic responsibility of parents.

Parents are handing life's scripts to their children, scripts that in all likelihood will be acted out for the rest of the children's lives.

Stephen R. Covey

In contrast, a few other clients have reported that their children *did* make a fuss when initially presented with the idea of pending dietary changes (which is often merely a result of poor presentation), only to find that with a little persistence, opposition soon died down and nourishing foods became the norm.

2 ~ be an example
...of what you would like to see them become.

We all know by now that the old saying *do as I say, not as I do* doesn't fly. Let your desire to have your offspring eat healthier motivate you to give to yourself what you want for them, which will ultimately inspire you all. Don't have expectations or uphold standards for them that you are not willing to uphold for yourself. Being an example doesn't mean you have to be perfect, it just means doing *your* best and moving in the direction you want to be going. Find a place that feels comfortable and be willing to raise the bar when the time is right. Use the strategies in the upcoming chapters to help both you and your children make the transition and keep on track. Remember that nourishing your body is a lifelong process, not an event.

> Kids who would never look at a vegetable or a sprout eat them with as much relish as if they were Big Macs – when they grow them themselves.
>
> Sara Sloan

3 ~ educate them
...on the basics of a healthy eating lifestyle.

Educating children on how to properly nourish their bodies is a natural part of parenting that has been lost, to a large degree, in recent decades. Share what you are learning with your children and teach them how to make wise food choices for themselves. Avoid using sweeping statements that can be meaningless to a child, such as this or that food is "bad for you." Instead, appeal to their interests by giving them clear examples of how specific foods affect their bodies both immediately and over time. Most children want to be strong, smart and fast, for example, while many teens are concerned with maintaining clear skin and a normal weight.

Make learning about food a fun adventure. Hands on experience always speaks louder than words, so incorporate it whenever possible. A field trip to a produce farm, sprouting seeds at home, or growing a full-fledged garden are all fascinating to young children and help them to learn about the source of their food. Similarly, a trip to the health food store for choosing and taste testing new foods to find ones that they like is a sure winner. Give them a personal understanding of how taste is acquired by putting the theory that it takes 8 weeks to acquire a new palate to the test in the form of a game. Or ask little ones to take a certain number of bites before they make a decision whether or not they like a new food. To further increase understanding and body awareness, conduct an interesting experiment by having them record how they feel both physically and emotionally before and after eating a large amount of sugar, for example. For more ideas and educational tools, check out the following internet links:

- Bill Moyers program on children and soda: http://www.pbs.org/now/classroom/diet.html

- Interactive children's area on CSPI website: http://www.cspinet.org/smartmouth/index1.html

4 ~ get them involved
      ...with food purchasing and preparation.

One of the best ways to peak youngsters' interest in wholesome foods is to involve them with food preparation as much as possible, at as early an age as possible. The first thought for many of you at the thought of this prospect is nothing short of dread. Yes, initially it can be messy and time consuming. But much like potty training, it will be well worth your efforts in the long run. Invest some of your time to train them now, and it will save you countless hours in the future, as you will have gained a helper or two in the kitchen. More importantly, you will be providing them with practical tools that will serve them throughout their life. There are far too many Generation X'ers and even many Baby Boomers who have been dietetically crippled because they were raised on processed, packaged foods and never learned the skills needed to maintain a real foods diet.

      As soon as they are able to stand, get your offspring in the kitchen learning about foods and food preparation. Get them washing, chopping, cooking, storing, cleaning up or whatever is appropriate for their age. Don't make it a chore, but enjoyable, quality time that you spend together and make part of your daily routine. Don't leave out the boys either. Domestic duties are no longer exclusively female and they will need these important

---

Teaching should be such that what is offered is perceived as a valuable gift and not as a hard duty.

Albert Einstein

skills for themselves when they help with the care of their own families.

5 ~ launch a counter offensive
...to mass advertising and our popular food culture.

You will not only want to educate your children on the principles and practices of a sustainable diet, but you will also want to counteract mass media advertising that preys on their impressionable minds. The food industry spends a great deal of time and money, and hires the top psychologists in the world to get your children to get you to buy their products. And with good reason — it works! Counteracting this programming can be challenging. In order to be effective, take a cue from the food industry: *start young and be aggressive.*

> A study of children ages six through eight found that 70% believed that fast foods were healthier than food from the home.
>
> Kelly Brownell
> Food Fight

One of the best ways to counteract insidious advertising is to limit exposure, especially when the children are very young. Many people mistakenly believe that young children are not taking in information via commercials or television programming because it is beyond their ability to understand. While it is true that the information their still developing brains are receiving may be by-passing their intellectual understanding, the problem is, this information is being downloaded straight into their subconscious, which can have an even greater influence. Savvy food industry psychologists know this, and launch commercial marketing campaigns designed to take advantage of it.

There are a growing number of parents who are aware of this phenomenon as well, and shield their children from mind-altering commercialism by only allowing their children to watch non-commercial public television. Some might consider this extreme, but it's important to remember that the marketing tactics children are being bombarded with are even more extreme. While you may not want to impose such a restriction forever, it is a wise thing to do at least until you have had some time to do some of your own indoctrination, and children are old enough to understand more on an intellectual level. Which leads us to another factor you will want to be sure to include as part of your counter offensive.

In addition to doing whatever you can to limit their exposure to child-oriented advertising and commercials, you will also want to explain to your kids how our popular food culture evolved and the food industry's role in its development. Using age appropriate language, and once again, starting as young as possible, share with your children what you have been learning. Be sure to let them know that they are being preyed upon by the food industry. Encourage them to make their own decisions and not be swayed.

6 ~ equip them with coping strategies
...for dealing with themselves and others.

A lot of
people have
gone farther
than they
thought
they could
because
someone
else thought
they could.

Zig Ziglar

Like you, your children are going to encounter less than supportive people in their lives. Equipping them with strategies for dealing with the inevitable taunting and urgings of these people, as well as their own internal propensity to be pulled into the fray, is another critical part of counteracting our popular food culture and establishing an ongoing *Eating-for-Health lifestyle.* Review the previous chapter as well as the beginning of this one, and share the strategies provided with your children. To generate interest and make it a little more fun, quiz them as to how they can be pro-active and role-play possible dialogues they may encounter in different social situations. In doing so, you will increase your child's preparedness and the likelihood of them implementing what they learn. Keep reminding them of the benefits they will derive from regularly nourishing their bodies with safe, wholesome foods. Be sure to teach them how to incorporate planned indulgences (more on this in the upcoming chapter) so they won't feel deprived.

7 ~ make healthy choices available
...and keep junk foods out of the house.

One of the best things you can do to help your children (and yourself) in the endeavor to maintain a balanced way of eating is to always keep healthy choices on hand, and keep junk food and pseudofood out of the house. That way if anyone is going to have it, they'll at least have to go out to get it. This is *the best* strategy there is for greatly reducing the percentage of time you or members of your family indulge in poor-quality foods. And don't try to hide it. If it's there, they'll know it, find it and eat it. Instead, keep plenty of nutritious snacks readily available. Giving children choices and telling them what they *can* have is important.

Quick and easy alternatives to packaged junk foods include almond butter with fresh apple slices, raw veggies with additive-free ranch dip, homemade granola and organic yogurt, fresh fruit or fruit salad, homemade popcorn or any of the recipes from the *Sweets & Treats* recipe section such as *Frozen Banana Cream Treat* or *Almond-Date No-Bake Apple Crisp.* Engaging children in the art of creating their own medley of trail mix, which will introduce them to a variety of nuts, seeds and the natural sweetness of dried fruits such as dates, figs, apricots and cherries (sulfite-free, of course!), is another delicious snack idea that gets them involved and learning as well.

Think ahead when venturing out of the house by packing a bag with natural foods. That way you can stop at a park with a playground for a little activity, fresh air, sunshine, and good food, which is a much better choice than having to resort to stopping at a fast-food restaurant. If the weather is bad, sit in the mall near the fountain. As soon as children are old enough, let them pack their own lunch and snacks, and yours too!

> Setting boundaries is a nurturing act.
>
> Laurel Mellin

8 ~ set clear boundaries
...remembering to include planned indulgences.

Don't be afraid to set and hold firm boundaries with your children when it comes to what they eat — it's your job! They may not like you for it initially, but they will respect and appreciate you for it, and possibly even brag about you later. People are constantly bragging to me about how their parents were really good about not letting them have the 'bad stuff' when they were growing up.

On the other hand, many other adults have confided that their parents allowed the free-flow of junk food, and they have had to struggle with addictions to these non-foods throughout their life as a result. Many are resentful of their parents for not imposing restrictions

Set boundaries for what your children can eat, how much, and how frequently. Be fair and be consistent in the implementation of whatever boundaries you set, however. Also be willing to negotiate on occasion without compromising the integrity of your overall intentions. If you are too restrictive it can backfire on you when they get older. Also, let kids take part in some aspect of whatever boundaries are established, allowing them to choose what they will have and when they will have it when it comes to a special weekly treat, for example. Establishing boundaries around food is a very tangible way of teaching and putting into practice the concept of delayed, versus immediate gratification, a valuable lesson that will serve your children in other areas of their life as well.

9 ~ speak up on their behalf
...in school, sports, family and other social situations.

Our lives begin to end the day we become silent about things that matter.

M.L. King Jr.

When dealing with other adults, it is not only *not* your business or responsibility to advise them on the state of their eating habits, as discussed earlier, it is usually not in your best interest either. When it comes to the health and well-being of your children, on the other hand, it *is* your responsibility and no time to be timid. Never before has it been so vitally important for grown-ups to speak out on behalf of our youth with regard to what foods are being made available to them. It makes your job easier at home when you have the support of other caring adults in both academic and recreational situations, and gives your children a much needed reprieve from the constant bombardment of junk food enticement they must endure.

Encourage, and even insist, that other parents, coaches, teachers, school administrators, family members and friends make healthier choices available at all youth-oriented functions, and limit the availability of junk and pseudofoods. As the interest in helping children eat well grows, making such requests will become the norm. In the meantime, be a trendsetter and know that other concerned parents will follow your lead. Offer suggestions and even consider bringing your own food to events, plus a little extra to share with others.

As mentioned earlier, one of the Denver Public School Board members shockingly stated that he felt it was incumbent upon the parents to teach students not to buy soda from school vending machines. Schools should be supporting such efforts on the part of parents, not sabotaging them by making it readily available to children throughout their day. And no one should be capitalizing on the innocence of children, least of all the schools. The notion of taking advantage of those students whose parents may not have the best parenting skills, as this statement implies, is deplorable. Speak out and demand that other adults live up to their responsibility to all of our children, especially school officials who have an obligation to do so.

10 ~ be persistent and consistent
…with your actions and your words.

Be persistent and consistent over time with your words, your actions, and everything you implement to help your children eat healthier foods on a regular basis. Once again, you will want to politely remind and repeat often, until new routines are integrated as habit. Transitioning to a healthier eating lifestyle is a process that won't happen overnight. Like any new skill, it takes practice. One of the biggest mistakes people make is giving up too soon. Don't ever give up. Anything worth having is worth working for. Isn't your family's well-being worth having?

Failure is
the line
of least
persistence.

Zig Ziglar

　　As time goes by, if the only thing you find yourself being consistent about is being inconsistent, modify what you're doing. Bring it into the realm of doable, then forge ahead in digestible increments. *Strategizing* as outlined in the next chapter will help.

shift happens
"People never change," is a very popular sentiment that most of us have heard voiced throughout our lives. It is a damaging statement that puts the brakes on even trying. The fact is, nothing could be further from the truth. People and the world around us are changing all the time. Change is an inevitable part of our human experience. It is our beliefs, intentions and subsequent actions that determine the nature of the changes that occur. We must believe that the inevitable change that will occur with regard to our popular food culture will be change for the better. I hope that this chapter has given you some inspiration and ideas as to how this can happen for you and others in your immediate surroundings. And instead of falling into the popular pit of despair wallowing in the belief that people never change, you will believe in yourself, believe in your children, believe in each other and believe in our society at large.

the talk ~ quick reference

1 ~ set the time and space for the talk
...to demonstrate its importance and ensure you have your listener's undivided attention.

2 ~ include all members of the family
...when you have this talk, even the little ones.

3 ~ focus on yourself
...use sentences that begin with "I" and speak from your heart.

4 ~ tell them what you are doing and why
...with regard to your decision to make changes in your diet and develop a healthier eating lifestyle.

5 ~ invite them to join you
...but let them know that you honor, accept and respect them if they don't.

6 ~ tell them what to expect
...from you as you are making the transition.

7 ~ make specific requests
...as to how they can show their support and help you.

8 ~ do not advise them
...about their eating habits at this time – this talk is about you.

9 ~ be brief and to the point
...to make it easier for them to hear what you are saying and grant your requests.

10 ~ politely remind and repeat
...them of points you have made in your talk in the days to come until new routines are established.

ten things to help children eat healthier ~
quick reference

1 ~ have a talk
...focusing on changes that will be taking place.

2 ~ be an example
...of what you would like to see them become.

3 ~ educate them
...on the basics of a healthy eating lifestyle.

4 ~ get them involved
...with food purchasing and preparation.

5 ~ launch a counter offensive
...to mass advertising and our popular food culture.

6 ~ equip them with coping strategies
...for dealing with themselves and others.

7 ~ make healthy choices available
...and keep junk foods out of the house.

8 ~ set clear boundaries
...remembering to include planned indulgences.

9 ~ speak up on their behalf
...in school, sports, family and other social situations.

10 ~ be persistent and consistent
...with your actions and your words.

strategize!

A Fun, Effective Way to Create Lasting Changes in Diet & Lifestyle

Most people's attempts to transform dietary habits that are health robbing into those that are health promoting either fall short of their intended goal or fail altogether. This happens for three general reasons. Either they never muster up the motivation and get around to it; they jump in feet first, find themselves dog paddling and dispense with their efforts; or they successfully accomplish a short-term goal, only to have the old, unwanted behaviors re-emerge over time. It is rare for people to steadfastly revamp their eating habits and associated lifestyle. Rare, but not impossible, and learning how to *Strategize!* the process can significantly increase your chances for success and expedite the process.

Those who have been successful at adopting and maintaining a relatively healthy eating lifestyle usually did so in stages over a period of time, a period of time in which they let go of the unhealthy foods in gradual increments, rather than all at once. At the same time they start developing tastes for, and the habit of preparing and enjoying more nutritious foods. Progressing in gradual increments is key for establishing new routines.

That's one reason why 30-day, 8-week or other such programs frequently don't work. People make too many changes too fast, which greatly decreases the chances of being able to maintain them. As humans we eat food every day of our lives, not just for the thirty days or eight weeks of a program. Consequently, it is common for people to migrate back to their old ways once they have finished with a particular program. Sometimes they even sink below where they were before, having overexerted their willpower and feeling deprived as a result. In any case, they never integrated what they were doing in the program as routine. This is not surprising. It's challenging to implement a lifetime plan, especially with regard to something that you do every day, multiple times a day, and often have no control over (i.e., social or business situations that involve food).

On the other hand, that's one reason why programs often *do* work, at least for the short time a person commits to them. They outline the do's, don'ts, why's, when's and how's. In other words, they have a clear plan for people to follow. And this is one of the primary reasons people who set out to make changes on their own fail. They don't make specific, concrete commitments. They have no plan to follow. Instead, many well-meaning people say things such as, "I'm going to start eating better." Such statements are nebulous and rarely lead to motivation or action.

The more committed and specific you are about what actions you are going to take, the more likely you'll be to take them. You must have a plan and follow it, a plan that is specific to your personal needs. There is no one size fits all here. It's your life. You must decide how to live it. You must devise a plan that will work for you now, and modify as you go along. This is exactly what the *Strategizing* process outlined next will help you to do. It will help you to successfully transmute old habits into new ones.

You can combine this 10-step process with the information and exercises contained in previous and upcoming chapters, and whatever ideas you may come up with on your own. Remember this really is all about *you*. Before we get to the detailed descriptions of the steps to follow, here is a brief overview of what *Strategizing* will help you do:

- *Set action goals with power numbers used throughout the ages.*
- *Incorporate planned indulgences and natural vacillations to minimize setbacks.*
- *Get back on track when you do suffer setbacks.*
- *Take three steps forward and two steps back to guarantee always being one step ahead.*
- *Identify and circumvent potential pitfalls before you begin.*
- *Move forward at a pace that is comfortable for you and still get results.*
- *Follow up with endurance goals to ensure ongoing progress and desired outcomes.*

By following the 10-steps for *Strategizing an Individualized Program* you can devise a dynamic plan that covers all bases, and keeps you moving in the direction you want to go. When you focus on the action steps, the results will follow. Read through the entire ten steps before you begin. Knowing where you are going will make it easier when you get to each step. Keep in mind that you will be returning to this process over and over in order to make incremental changes over the next few weeks, months or even a couple of years.

In addition, you can use this strategic process throughout your life whenever the need arises. While you are reading through the steps, you will want to think about what is most appropriate for you to do at this time. Take note of the thoughts that first come to mind. With a little refinement, they are usually the winners. Once you have read through the steps, you can either let the process percolate and come back to it later. (Note: *if you are a perpetual procrastinator, don't percolate!*) Or pull out paper and pen, put on your thinking cap and get started.

strategizing an individualized program

1 ~ know your 'big why'
...and identify your primary objective for this particular phase of your program.

When I first began to make conscious changes in my diet, the elimination of foul flatulence was my very clear and immediate objective, as I reluctantly revealed at the beginning of this book. As my overall health declined and began to impinge on my life in more momentous ways, I got in touch with the bigger, more long-term reasons for wanting to mend my ways. This is one of the greatest gifts of compromised health. It forces you to clearly see what's important in life.

Whether or not you have had the gift of compromised health, you will want to consciously identify what your 'big why' is for maintaining a balanced state of well-being. This will help place a value on your health and motivate you to preserve it. Think about things you feel passionate about in life. Some of the 'big whys' that clients have shared with me include building an integrated wellness center, being healthy, energetic, and around long enough to provide day care for their grandchildren, trekking across Nepal, and establishing a charitable foundation for children in North Africa.

Having a purpose bigger than yourself, and reminding yourself of it often greatly increases the likelihood of making lasting changes. If you do not have a passionate purpose in life, you may want to embark on a quest to reveal it. Doing so will benefit all areas of your life. If you have trouble doing this, keep in mind that your body-mind system may be fogged from lack of adequate nutrients and all the extreme and chemical-laden foods you may have been ingesting over time. For many people their sense of passionate purpose in life has gotten lost in the sauce, so to speak. In which case, clearing your body and *Eating for Health* can help you tremendously in getting clear about what you really want in life.

In addition to your 'big why' you will want to identify what your specific objectives are for this particular phase of your program. Priority objectives that are more immediate will serve as stepping-stones to fulfilling your greater purpose. Increasing energy, losing weight, relieving symptoms, and *dis*-ease are all good examples. Cement your 'big why' and the immediate objectives you have identified by writing them down in the form of a declarative statement or positive affirmation you can refer to often.

2 ~ list *possible* action steps you could take
... exploring several possibilities before you decide.

With your 'big why' and specific objectives in mind, you will now want to brainstorm the action steps that will best assist you. You will not be deciding on any action steps, yet. Simply take out a piece of paper and start jotting down the action steps that come to mind that would be most appropriate for you to take at this time. This is a brainstorming exercise. Do not censor. Try on and consider all possibilities. As you continue to work through the 10-steps, you will discover what fits best.

3 ~ establish appropriate time frame
...for this particular phase of your program.

When someone establishes a goal or makes absolute statements about what they are going to do (i.e., I will *never* eat ice cream, chocolate or potato chips, again), the body and mind tend to retaliate. After all, you trained them to do so. Weeks, months or years of repeating a behavior regularly imprints it in the body and psyche. Therefore it is wise to employ special time intervals or gestation periods for making and integrating changes and creating new habits. It takes goal setting to a whole new level.

What time frame you choose will depend on what you are trying to accomplish. You must consider the specific action steps you choose to take in accordance with the magnitude of your primary objectives, your level of willingness to follow through, and the feasibility factor in order to make a firm decision as to the appropriate time frame (i.e., 7 days, 21 days, 90 days, etc.) for this phase of your program.

Keep in mind that it takes between 21-40 days to change a habit and a year to establish it as a lifestyle routine. You may need to work up to lengthier time commitments in stages. I have found it enormously helpful to use the following commonly used intervals, or power numbers, as a guide:

- 3 or 7 days – perfect amount of time for something particularly challenging such as a cleanse or withdrawal from addictive foods.

- 21 days – commonly used as a time interval for shifting habits and behaviors.

- 40 days – another common gestation period used throughout the ages. For example, Jesus fasted in the desert for 40 days, and Buddha sat under the Bodhi tree meditating for 40 days. This interval is not only helpful in shifting and integrating behaviors, but also helpful for increasing body-mind awareness and gaining new experiences.

- 90, 180, 360 days – are all similar markers for accomplishing the same, increasing clarity, wisdom and integrating at progressively higher levels along the way.

- 1,000 days – in ancient yogic teachings, this is considered to be the length of time it takes to attain mastery of an issue, as it requires great discipline and determination. Do something consistently for 1,000 days and your life can't help but change!

4 ~ check your calendar
...and consider what's ahead.

Now that you are starting to get an idea of what you might like to commit to doing, you will want to make sure it is feasible for you to do it. Always set yourself up for success by checking your calendar for any social or business obligations that may pose an obstacle to your efforts (i.e., wedding, holiday, business trip, overtime, etc.). A two-week vacation staying with relatives is not the time to go on an elimination diet, for example. Similarly, two days before Valentine's Day is not the time for a chocolate addict to swear off melt-in-your-mouth morsels.

On the other hand, be careful not to fall into the 'but first' syndrome (i.e., I'm going to eat healthier, *but first* I'm going to finish off this bag of cheese puffs, etc.). There are always going to be temptations and occasions in life that have the potential to get in the way. If you wait for the coast to be clear, you'll never get to shore.

5 ~ decide how to deal with obstacles
...and plan indulgences to solidify follow through.

You'll want to anticipate obstacles that could pop up during the course of your program and decide in advance, as much as possible, how you will deal with them. Sometimes you will want to avoid or go around them. Other times you will want to meet them head on by putting them right into the plan. Planned indulgences are a wise and healthy part of any ongoing lifestyle program, and are often the key to success. Incorporating planned indulgences is an especially smart maneuver when undertaking lengthier commitments. "I will have ice cream and cake on my upcoming birthday" is a good example. You must be reasonable and judicious when you plan indulgences, however, so as not to compromise the overall integrity of your plan. Also do your best to raise the bar on the quality of the treats you do eat, even if they are planned. "I will have organic ice cream and carrot cake sweetened with honey and Stevia (see *Recipes*)" is a good example of how you might accomplish this.

Planned indulgences are one way of dealing with potential obstacles in advance and are particularly helpful for special occasions. You will also want to think about other more common, every day kinds of obstacles, and how you will deal with them before you commit to or begin your program. Remember, you want to cover all bases with your plan. Take into consideration invitations and temptations that may come about during the course of an average day or week.

For example, if you always get pseudo-cheese covered nachos and a jumbo-sized soft drink when you go out to the movies every Saturday night, decide in advance how you are going to handle this situation. Will you completely abstain, sneak in your own healthier alternative, modify your usual order or designate this a weekly planned indulgence? Similarly, what will you do in the face of open dishes of candy for the taking that you may encounter at the teller window or your co-worker's cubicle? Whatever you do, avoid putting yourself in a position of having to decide in the moment. If you do, the chances of that turning into a weak moment are great. Practice dictating the circumstances rather than letting the circumstances dictate your actions.

Not having the foods, equipment, or support you need can present major obstacles as well. Be sure you have everything you'll need before you commit to a plan. *Step 8* can help with this.

6 ~ identify the top 3 *realistic* action steps
...that are most appropriate for you at this time.

By now you should be starting to get a pretty good idea of what you want to do. In this step, you will be identifying the top three actions steps you will commit to taking during an established time frame of your choice. Unless you are doing a short term cleanse, in order to set yourself up to succeed for the long haul, plan on taking three steps forward and two steps back so you will be one step ahead. Do this by choosing one step that will be relatively challenging but still doable, another step that will be moderately challenging and a third step that's relatively easy that you can continue after the program. At the end of the program, you will re-evaluate the more challenging steps and decide then whether or not to continue with them.

When deciding on your three action steps, you may choose to follow the guidelines outlined in *Levels I, II* or *III* from *Chapter 3,* or determine your own individual actions such as going off a common food allergen or stimulant you know or suspect may be causing you problems.

If it's too uncomfortable to think about eliminating things in your diet, start by adding things in. I call this the "crowd it out" method. Instead of focusing on what you *can't* have, start focusing on things you *can* have and may be depriving yourself of. I remember when I first started to eat healthier I rarely thought of things I didn't want to eat anymore. Instead I was always exploring new healthier possibilities. This made making changes a fun and easy adventure. I started by adding more fruits, vegetables, and whole grains to my diet. I'll never forget eating fruit, some of which I had never had before, and thinking what a delight it was and how I had been missing out on these delicacies of nature for all these years. Adding in more nutritious foods may be a great place for you to start as well.

7 ~ commit to your program
...by writing down your plan and marking your calendar.

In this step you will bring everything together and finalize your plan of action. Start by writing down the three realistic action steps you have chosen, the duration of the program, and any planned indulgences.

Now, before you mark your calendar, look over the plan you have written and the commitment you are getting ready to make. Close your eyes for a moment and check in with your physical body and your inner everybody. Consider all the variables in your life at present, and then ask yourself, "Am I really going to be able to follow through with this plan? Does this plan feel right to all parts of myself?" If the answer is a flat out no, or even a wobbly no, amend your commitments. Don't set yourself up to fail. Amend your commitments until you get a confidant feeling of, "Yes, this is it. This is what I *want* to do. And I *can* and *will* do it."

The idea is not to wear out your willpower and risk snapping back to old ways. The idea is to develop *want*power by gradually integrating changes over time that will elicit results and inspire you to continue. Better to make small changes and integrate them over time than try to make big changes you may not be able to follow through with, or may put a damper on future endeavors.

When you have come up with the perfect plan for this time in your life, write down the specifics on a clean sheet of paper. Then mark your calendar as a final declaration of your commitment. Intend to follow through with this commitment *no matter what*!

8 ~ prepare for your program
...by gathering the tools and support you will need.

Now that you have made a firm commitment to your individualized plan, give some time and attention to adequately preparing yourself for what's ahead. From a practical standpoint, make sure you have the kitchen equipment you will need (steamer, food storage containers, etc.), and do appropriate food shopping and menu planning. You may also want to look ahead to the chapters *Be Prepared* and *Recipes.*

From a support standpoint, inform those closest to you what you are doing and ask for support. You may want to call upon a close friend or family member to hold you accountable to your commitment as well. Use what you learned in the previous chapter to help you with these family and other social situations. Review the previous chapter if needed.

Finally, prepare yourself mentally by reflecting on your 'big why,' what we discussed in *Chapter 4 ~ Thinketh,* and most importantly, how setting yourself on this track toward a healthier eating lifestyle is going to improve your life in so many ways. Think about how good it is going to feel to have vital energy and a body you feel good about being in, in every way!

9 ~ Just DO IT!
...doing something is always better than planning on doing something.

This is the most important step of them all. You can do all the thinking and planning and preparing you want, but what good will it do if you never take action? It is now time to take the action steps you have made a commitment to doing. Review your 'big why' and immediate objectives. Then combine your willpower, *want*power, and self-discipline to pave the way for attaining these results and the lifestyle integration that will arrive in due course. There's no such thing as trying. Either you do something or you don't. In this case, you have committed to designing and implementing a plan that you can follow through with — *no matter what!*

The road to you-know-where is paved with good intentions, however, and even the best laid plans and intentions can take a wrong turn. If you find yourself not doing what you committed to, you may need to re-evaluate your plan. A well-*strategized* plan is one you will *want* to do and find yourself easily following. If this is not the case, perhaps you bit off more than you could chew (so to speak!) and can't keep up, or you got off the wagon and things fell apart from there. Whatever it is, don't despair. Just go through the 10-steps to help you identify what went wrong. Revise accordingly and get back on track.

Or, if you have entered into a lengthy program and mess up along the way, consider employing a little creative trickery so as not to lose momentum or become discouraged. For instance, if you have started a forty day commitment, and ten days into it you violate an element of that commitment, consider either starting over if you are not too far along or simply adding on a day or two or however many days you were not compliant (within reason, of course) to your established program and keep going. Keep it light and fun. Make your commitment a game to play with yourself, rather than an obligation you dread.

In many cases it is wise to start with some cleansing and clearing of your system. This will help get you over the withdrawal and craving hurdle that so many people experience. We will discuss this further in *Chapter 9*.

10 ~ reward, review, and recommit
...bringing closure to this phase and devising the next.

This is a critical step as well, and the one most often forgotten or neglected. Some programs have no definite ending, as if you are going to go on with them forever, which is highly unlikely. Others do provide a definite time line such as seven days or eight weeks, then leave you dangling. And dangling is a precarious position to be in. It is wise to avoid dangling whenever possible, as any momentum you have built up is sure to fizzle. In order to prevent dangling and fizzling, you must follow through with this all-important final step, which is really not final at all, but rather a launching pad to the next phase of your ongoing personalized program.

Remember, in the beginning this personalized program will span the course of a few months or weeks, and can be revisited over the course of your lifetime. It is designed to be flexible, vacillate and change just as your life does. This step is what precipitates the ongoing nature of this process. Simply follow these three easy-to-recall 'r' words when you reach the end of each phase:

reward ~ give yourself a big pat on the back, a new outfit, tickets to a ball game or whatever you may fancy. Acknowledge your efforts and accomplishments, including the mere fact that you did anything at all!

review ~ think over what you did and how things went for you. Take note of things that worked, and the results or benefits you derived. This is important. Taking note of the benefits will motivate you to continue by building confidence in both the process and your ability to make use of it. Also, take note of things that didn't work. Avoid beating yourself up by focusing on the strategies implemented, not yourself. Consider that the strategies didn't work, not that you are a loser. Then reconsider your strategies. Contemplate what you could do differently next time to make things more winning. There's no room for failure here, only revision. Learn from any failed attempts, rather than letting them discourage you.

recommit ~ begin the cycle again and keep moving forward by recommitting to the next phase of your ongoing, individualized program. Either continue with what you were doing, revise it to better suit your current needs, or dispense with it altogether and start anew. Whatever you decide to do, don't blindly or half-heartedly recommit, go through all 10-steps and draw up a fresh plan of action. If you adopted the three steps forward two steps back plan, this will come easily. Be sure you have integrated major changes and they have become routine before taking on more.

A couple of days or so before you reach the end of a plan you have strategized is the best time to begin this final step, and start thinking about what you will do next. That way, you can recommit and move right into the next phase. Thinking and planning ahead is the best way to keep yourself from dangling or falling off the cliff.

sample strategies

You can strategize any plan you like. This is your personalized program, after all. Here are a few ideas to get you started:

- Eat two large bowls of fresh vegetables a day.
- Eat 1-2 servings of whole grains per day.
- Eliminate one or more foods to which you suspect you have a problem (wheat, dairy, sugar, coffee, etc.).
- Follow the elimination diet as outlined in *Chapter 9.*
- Eat nothing sweeter than fruit.
- Follow *Level I of Eating for Health* by eliminating all pseudofoods.

Just remember not to make it too difficult. Going from 0-60 miles per hour in thirty seconds is a great feature for a sports car, but not for adopting long-term lifestyle changes. The exception would be if you are in a serious state of *dis*-ease, in which case taking the lickety-split approach to making overall changes and cleansing would be wise. Another exception is if you are going cold turkey on a stimulant such as caffeine or sugar. In most cases, however, slow and steady wins the race. You may like to experiment with different ideas and see how you do before you make a firm commitment to a plan. Play around, have fun!

gaining experience

"So how are you doing since we last talked?" I asked a client with whom I had been working for a few months at the start of her session.

"Oh my gosh, you're not going to believe this. I'm so excited!" she replied. "For the last two weeks I totally went off the wagon and felt like absolute crap," she continued.

"Hmmmm, that's an interesting thing to be excited about?" I remarked puzzled.

"No, I'm serious. I felt like absolute crap, the way I used to feel all the time," she explained. "The difference was that this time I knew what to do about it. For the first time in my life I knew what to do to make myself feel better. As soon as I realized how terrible I felt and acknowledged that it was because I had not been eating healthfully, I started getting back to my healthy foods and drinking my green drink every day and within a very short time I started feeling better again. That's what's so exciting!"

This story illustrates one of the greatest benefits of implementing a strategic plan for making changes and sticking to it. You will start to develop keen body awareness regarding the foods you consume. When you see and feel results, it gives you a reason and motivation to continue practicing new habits and taking them to higher levels. Or in this case, to get back on track when you falter.

This story also illustrates the human vacillation factor. It is a fact — you will vacillate. Expect it, it's natural. You are not bad if you get off track, you are normal. The good news is that like this client, you are accumulating tools, skills and knowledge that will help you get back on track, the most important of which is gaining the experience of feeling better. You will also begin to more accurately interpret the messages of your body. For example, recognizing that a headache isn't your body's request for over-the-counter painkillers, but rather, as one classic song so aptly put it, "It's nature's way of telling you something's wrong." What exactly is wrong will become clearer and clearer as you eat healthier and feel better, and begin to learn what foods and lifestyle habits are causing you to have a headache or any other symptoms or *dis*-ease in the first place.

By developing increased body awareness, you are training your mind to work for you, not against you. As with this client and so many other *Eating-for-Health* advocates, including myself, you will eventually reach the point where you will no longer be willing to feel badly anymore. You will choose feeling well over something that tastes good, but makes you feel bad, any day. And during those times when the human vacillation factor does come into play and you make the opposite choice, you will be motivated and know what to do to pull yourself out of any downward reaching spiral. One of the best ways to ensure that things never spiral down too far is to set a limit of some kind, beyond which you will not allow yourself to go; not letting yourself gain more than five pounds, or have symptoms for more than three days, for example.

And of course, to really make sure you keep moving in an upward reaching spiral of incremental progression, remember...

practice makes perfect

It's not enough to just know something or do something once, as we discussed earlier. As with learning a new language or how to play an instrument, you must discipline yourself to practice eating healthier in order to master this skill. Practice involves repetition over time. Strive for progress, not perfection.

When you fall out of practice, let this book call to you. Go to it like you would go to an old friend, a friend that's always there when you need 'em and knows just what to say. Swipe off the dust if needed, and just for fun, open it at random. Let it speak to you and help surface what is an appropriate next step for you, one that will move you in the direction that you want to go. Flip through different sections to refresh your memory, or discover something you missed the first time that will inspire you to take action now. Then come back to this strategizing process, using it over and over to help you master the art of eating well.

The most important reason to do this is so that you will stop beating yourself up for not doing what you know you need to do. Anxiety is caused by inactivity. Get active now and reduce your anxiety. You will not only start to feel and look better, but also build self-esteem and confidence. These benefits are well worth your time and commitment. The next section will help you further by getting even more specific about how to properly nourish yourself and your family. But first, a quick reference review of this chapter's *Strategizing* process.

strategizing an individualized program ~
quick reference

1 ~ know your 'big why'
> *...and identify your primary objective for this particular phase of your program.*

2 ~ list *possible* action steps you could take
> *... exploring several possibilities before you decide.*

3 ~ establish appropriate time frame
> *... for this particular phase of your program.*

4 ~ check your calendar
> *...and consider what's ahead..*

5 ~ decide how to deal with obstacles
> *...and plan indulgences to solidify follow through..*

6 ~ identify the top 3 *realistic* action steps
> *...that are most appropriate for you at this time.*

7 ~ commit to your program
> *...by writing down your plan and marking your calendar.*

8 ~ prepare for your program
> *...by gathering the tools and support you will need.*

9 ~ Just DO IT!
> *...doing something is even better than planning on doing something.*

10 ~ reward, review, and recommit
> *...bringing closure to this phase and devising the next.*

Section Three

make it so!

Practical Know-How to Make Eating for Health a Reality

The clearer people are about what is best for them to eat, the more likely they are to eat it. This section will further refine what you have been learning, so you can get even clearer about how to properly nourish yourself and your family. In addition, it will provide more specific and practical information to help you transition to, and maintain a healthier eating lifestyle.

The first chapter of this section, *Chapter 7 ~ The Basics*, presents a general framework for daily food intake, without having to use a scale, calculator, or taking a crash course in nutrition science or biochemistry. This chapter is fashioned after the *Eating-for-Health Guidelines* in *Chapter 2*, and divided into two parts for easy access and assimilation. The first part begins with a simple, age-old method for determining appropriate portion sizes, then outlines *Dietary Basics*, a flexible framework for a sound diet that includes recommendations for both children and adults. Each is presented in the form of an easy-to-remember guiding statement, followed by a detailed explanation and suggestions for adapting it to your individual needs. Keep in mind that this is a general framework. As always, I encourage you to experiment and discover what works best for *you*. The second part of this chapter outlines *Healthy Habits* for a nourishing lifestyle. This is followed by quick reference lists for both.

Because the overwhelming majority of people in America and throughout the Western world today eat processed, packaged foods the overwhelming majority of the time, most people have little or nothing to do with the source of their food other than plucking it from the grocery store shelf. As a result, they frequently don't know enough basic information about whole, fresh, natural foods or how to prepare them. They are literally unequipped to reform their diets. Because of this, after hearing the guidelines for the first time, many people's immediate panicked response is, "What are we supposed to eat?" Have no fear *Chapter 8* is here to alleviate this anxious concern.

First, *Chapter 8* provides an extensive list of *Suggested Foods* that you can refer to again and again, to familiarize yourself with the vast array of nutritious, delicious foods available to you. Each category begins with a brief introduction followed by a list of specific foods and products. Parentheses are used to alert you to common food allergens and foods that may be difficult to digest, reinforcing *Eating-for-Health Guideline #4: account for food allergies & sensitivities.* Detailed lists of *Foods to Limit* and *Things to Avoid*, including explanations as to *why* these things are best avoided, then follow.

In addition to the primarily psychological and social obstacles discussed in *Section Two*, people also face formidable *physical* obstacles when it comes to making healthy revisions in their diets. Many people want to make changes in their diets, but they don't want to be left hanging with an ever-present desire to pull up to the drive thru window and make off with a burger, fries, and a jumbo soda. *Chapter 9 ~ Clear the Way* will help you overcome food cravings and free yourself from stimulants, thereby clearing the way to a better way of eating with grace and ease.

The major element outlined in this chapter for making this happen is *Cleanse & Clear*, a basic elimination diet and process for identifying and clearing food allergies and breaking free of food addictions. This process also serves as a regular cleansing protocol that you can implement seasonally or as needed, in order to maintain optimal health and well-being. Also included are natural remedies and recommendations for withdrawing from offensive foods in general, and certain foods in particular such as caffeine and sugar. The chapter also includes a prescription for a healthy kitchen makeover, because it wouldn't be an effective rehab program without clearing your cupboards of temptation.

After reading and applying what you learn in this section, you will start feeling better and having more energy than ever before. You will emerge empowered with increased body awareness and know-how that will serve you for years to come. Regardless of how many times you have tried in the past, this section will help you make *Eating for Health* a concrete reality rather than a far off dream. So, let's get started and make it so!

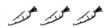

Chapter Seven

the basics

Dietary Basics & Healthy Habits Everyone Should Know

The five basic guidelines for *Eating for Health* are a great place to start in making general food choices. This chapter takes things a step further by building on these universal guidelines. We are all aware that there is much debate over questions regarding portions, frequency of meals, how much protein versus carbohydrates, to eat meat or not to eat meat, etc. The *Dietary Basics* and *Healthy Habits* presented here provide a framework from which to work, while allowing enough flexibility to account for individual needs. For example, amounts are expressed in a range to account for different body weights (i.e., smaller amounts for children, mid-range for teens, larger amounts for adults) and also to allow for varied individual needs (i.e., someone trying to balance blood sugar may need protein 3 times a day, while someone else may only need 1 serving a day, etc.). It is important to find what is right for *your* body at this time in your life.

Regarding servings or portions, this is another area of nutrition that is fraught with confusion. It all starts with the fact that the words *serving* or *portion* are general terms with no universally accepted measurement. For example, I thought I'd found *the* answer to why two-thirds of the population of America is overweight when I first saw the government's former *Food Guide Pyramid* which recommends eating 6 'servings' of grains a day, a seemingly enormous amount. Then I learned that these guidelines define a serving as only ½ cup, which helped to put

The body was designed to run on real foods; a natural foods diet is the ultimate direction in eating for all of us, no matter exactly how we shape it.

Elizabeth Lipski, Digestive Wellness

things in perspective. Others recommend eating a serving size described as a weight, such as 35 grams of lean protein, etc. What exactly does 35 grams look like? No wonder people throw up their hands in surrender when it comes to following these recommendations. You have to be a detective, carry around a scale, or be a scientist just to figure out what size chicken breast you should have for dinner.

To make things easy, the best approach to serving size is in the palm of your hand, literally. Lay out your hand flat with fingers together. There's your serving size for a piece of fish, chicken, steak or other animal protein. Curl your hand into a fist and there's your serving size for grains, a snack or a piece of fruit, give or take a little. Hand sizes vary according to the size of the person. So do appropriate serving sizes. Smaller people have smaller hands and therefore should eat smaller servings. Bigger people have bigger hands and therefore should eat bigger servings. Makes sense, doesn't it?

People who are in sync with their natural biological needs do this instinctively, especially those who eat primarily a whole foods diet. You may already be doing this and just never noticed or thought about it. If you are not, emotions, addictions or food allergies may be overriding your natural inclinations. You may also be eating too many processed foods, which can also interfere, as discussed earlier.

As you read through the *Dietary Basics*, make a mental note of those you are already implementing, and others on which you may be going overboard or missing altogether. Then experiment by following the recommendations and find what works for you within them. Keep in mind as you are experimenting and making changes that discovering what really works for you is a process that can take time. Be conscious that what you may currently consider to be working for you may just be what you're used to and your body has become chemically addicted to, so when first making changes, you may feel worse before you feel better. Given adequate time and effort, however, you will find that adopting a new way of eating works even better for you once you have successfully moved through the initial transition period.

Biochemical imbalances caused by years of eating in a way that did not support and nourish your body may require short-term measures to restore equilibrium. Once equilibrium has been

Fear less,
hope more,
eat less,
chew more,
whine less,
breathe more,
talk less,
say more,
hate less,
love more
and all good
things will be
yours.

Swedish Proverb

restored, a more balanced way of eating may be adopted. For example, if someone has been eating copious amounts of meat for many years, they may do well to not have any meat for a period of time to clear and strengthen the digestive tract. Once their system has cleared, they may then return to eating meat in more moderate amounts. On the other hand, people who have been vegetarians for many years and have become very depleted may do well to introduce some animal protein, then taper off to a more balanced intake once they have regained their strength.

Similarly, those who have been eating way too many sweets and have developed imbalanced blood sugar would be wise to refrain from all sweets, including fruits, until their blood sugar levels are stabilized. The same would be true of fats, and extreme or stimulant foods. Start experimenting within the parameters of the following *Dietary Basics* and you will soon discover what's right for your body-mind system.

Pure water is the best drink for a wise man.

Thoreau

dietary basics

1 ~ follow the eating-for-health guidelines
...*as much as possible.*

The *Eating-for-Health Guidelines* are truly the cornerstone of any health-promoting diet as discussed in detail earlier. As a quick reminder, the five guidelines to *Eating for Health* are:

   1 ~ If it's not food, don't eat it!

   2 ~ Eliminate or relegate stimulants to rare occasions

   3 ~ Eat an abundance of whole, fresh, natural foods

   4 ~ Account for food allergies & sensitivities

   5 ~ Account for ailments

2 ~ drink plenty of pure water daily
...*in accordance with your body's needs.*

Everyone agrees that drinking adequate amounts of pure water is vital for all bodily functions. What exactly constitutes an adequate amount of water is, once again, the topic of some debate. However, because the body expends over a quart of water a day performing its natural functions, it needs at least that much to replace what has been lost and then some. Probably the most well known recommendation is drinking 6-8 eight-ounce glasses of water per day, or a total of 48-64 ounces. Another popular approach advises drinking half your weight in ounces per day. For instance, if you weigh 150 pounds, you would drink 75 ounces.

> The closer food is to its natural, God-created state, the higher its nutritional value.
>
> Dr. Bernard Jensen

With this range as a guide, also take into account that people will have different needs when it comes to water intake, depending on their current health condition, level of activity and dietary habits. For example, people who are eating a whole foods diet rich in high-water content foods, juices, green drinks and herbal teas will have water needs that are generally much less than those who eat a *Standard American Diet* of primarily low water content or concentrated foods, coffee, tea and soda, all of which are dehydrating to the body. Similarly, many people who are ill and have a toxic, weakened system find that they can't seem to get enough water and are always thirsty. Once they start eating an abundance of high-water content foods such as fruits and vegetables, drinking juices and herbal teas, their water needs are satisfied to a degree, and they drink much less water as a result.

The best way to ensure you are getting enough water is to fill a container at the beginning of the day (a liter bottle, for example) and sip it throughout the day so that it is gone by the end of the day. Sipping water throughout the day is preferred, as it is much easier for the kidneys to process than gulping large amounts at once. According to ancient yogic teachings, this is one of the keys to health and longevity. Similarly, it is also best to drink water at room temperature, not chilled or iced. All health experts warn against drinking tap water with its high chlorine and chemical content. Filtered, distilled or ionized micro-filtered water is best. Recent studies have now been finding an array of excreted pharmaceutical drugs in our drinking water, especially antibiotics because of their widespread agricultural use, which is another good reason to drink purified water!

3 ~ eat 2-4 pieces of fresh fruit daily
...preferably organic and in season.

Fruit has been recognized throughout history as truly one of nature's delicacies. The word *fruit* can actually be traced back to the Latin word *fructus*, meaning enjoyment. It is not only our taste buds that enjoy fruit with its sweet intoxicating flavors, but our digestive system undoubtedly enjoys it as well. Eating fruit is very cleansing to the digestive organs and eliminative tract when eaten on an empty stomach in keeping with proper food combining principles. Although fruit is not a great source of balanced nutrition (vegetables are a better source), most fruits do provide fiber, phytochemicals, vitamin C, vitamin A, potassium and also have a high water content, and are thus very hydrating to the body.

Fruit is very sweet and like any food that has a relatively high glycemic index, it can create imbalanced blood sugar levels when eaten in excess and also contribute to the proliferation of *candida* (yeast overgrowth) and other conditions. Consequently, it is wise to keep to the daily 2-4 piece limit. If you already have candida, problems with your blood sugar (i.e., hypoglycemia, diabetes, etc.), or suppressed immune function, it may be smart not to eat fruit at all until your condition is stabilized.

Fruits and vegetables have not escaped the hands of the modern agri-tech industry. In addition to the obvious use of chemical pesticides, herbicides and fertilizers, synthetic growth hormones are also now being used to expedite their growth. After being plucked from the tree or the vine, they are frequently sprayed with chemical fumigants for protection or to accelerate ripening, and chemical colorants and waxes to increase their visual appeal. To avoid ingesting this cornucopia of chemicals, it is wise to consume organic produce whenever possible and wash all produce thoroughly before eating.

Contrary to what many believe, peeling is not a safeguard as sprays and fumigants are able to penetrate the skin and remain in the flesh, and you would also be depriving yourself of the nutrients and fiber contained in the peel and near its surface. All things considered, if you are not able to obtain organic produce it is still better to eat non-organic produce than to not eat fresh produce at all. A piece of fruit is always a better choice for a sweet

> Fruit juices are not OK in unlimited amounts.
>
> There is nothing OK in unlimited amounts except water and vegetables.
>
> Marion Franz, RD

snack than a processed food such as a cookie, pastry, energy bar, or candy.

It is also wise to choose fruit that is in season and locally grown whenever possible to ensure the highest degree of freshness. The fresher the fruit, the more nutrients available and the better the flavor. As with any food, it is best to eat a variety of fruits in order to obtain a broad spectrum of nutrients. This is also helpful for reducing the over-consumption of any pesticides or chemicals that may be common to a particular kind of fruit.

4 ~ eat 3-7 servings of fresh vegetables daily
...preferably raw or lightly steamed.

> Learn to genuinely appreciate vegetables for what they do for you, and your palate will soon follow suit and ensure that you enjoy them.
>
> Mark Percival

While in theory, most everyone agrees that eating an abundance of a variety of fresh vegetables is the best recipe for good health and long life, in practice this food group is the one we eat the least. This is primarily due to the development of our current food culture, which has developed a taste for processed foods and convenience, and lost sight of the importance of nutritional value. The vegetable family, with its many varieties, is one food group to which we have become very disconnected, which has resulted in two specific challenges that many people face when they attempt to incorporate them into their diets.

First, most people today are familiar with only a small group of common vegetables and only limited ways of preparing them, and don't have a clue about the rest. Second, because most people's digestive and eliminative tracts have become so weakened and clogged from years of eating devitalized processed foods, they often have difficulty digesting vegetables when they first introduce them into their diet.

In response to the first challenge, the upcoming *Suggested Foods* and *Recipe* sections will help you start familiarizing yourself with the world of vegetables and how to prepare them. Taking a leisurely, educational stroll through the produce aisle or local farmer's market is also helpful. Take advantage of any knowledgeable grocers or farmers hanging around who are more than happy to give you advice on the best way to choose a particular produce item and the best way to prepare it. You can learn a lot this way.

As for the second challenge, to avert digestive disturbances when beginning to eat more and varied vegetables for the first time, or after a long absence from your diet, begin by lightly steaming those that are easy to digest such as zucchini, yellow squash, carrots, celery, and bok choy. After a couple of weeks of eating the easier to digest variety daily, introduce those that are more difficult to digest one at a time such as broccoli, cauliflower, asparagus, onions, and green peppers. Then begin to introduce raw vegetables gradually in the same way. Raw vegetables contain the most nutrients and enzymes, and also have the highest fiber content, which is why it is wise to start with lightly steamed vegetables, as raw vegetables may be initially the most challenging to digest for those with a weakened digestive system.

Tune into where your body is at in relationship to digesting certain vegetables, but don't banish those you currently have challenges with forever. Instead, come back to them later and see how you do. Remember, that the more vegetables you eat, the clearer, stronger and more energetic your body will become. At the same time, the clearer, stronger and more energetic your body becomes, the more vegetables you will be able to eat!

Dr. Bernard Jensen, a renowned nutritionist, recommends that people eat six different vegetables a day in order to partake of their array of nutrients. This may seem daunting at first, but once you become more familiar with them, you will find it much easier to include more variety and more servings. To demonstrate, consider that if you had a big salad for lunch with a few vegetable toppings (i.e., shredded carrots, beets, celery, sprouts, cucumbers, etc.) it could easily amount to 3-4 servings. And if you then had 1-2 servings of steamed vegetables for dinner, you could easily fulfill both the serving and Dr. Jensen's six vegetable variety quotas. It's most definitely doable and something to aspire to if you are just getting started.

As for those dark green leafy vegetables that everyone is harping about, those are a little less doable for most people (including me!), primarily because many people find them distasteful and therefore have no desire to go about preparing and eating them. By dark green leafy vegetables, I mean kale, chard, mustard greens, collard greens, beet greens, spinach, and the like. Most people enjoy the lettuces and even spinach, but these are not

There isn't any magic daily number or combination of fruits and vegetables for optimal health.

Instead I offer two words of advise: *more* and *different.*

Dr. Walter Willett
Eat, Drink & Be Healthy

enough to fulfill the *variety* quota for dark green leafy vegetables. For this reason, I recommend that people supplement their diets with whole food supplements containing individual greens or a blend of *green foods* to ensure they are getting adequate amounts of the vital nutrients they provide. (More on *green foods* and whole food supplements shortly.) This is especially important today in order to keep up our immune systems, which are being constantly assaulted by all the toxic chemicals, pollutants and stress that come with modern living.

But the most basic weapons in the fight against disease are those most ignored by modern medicine: the numerous nutrients that the cells of our bodies need.

Dr. Roger Williams

5 ~ eat 0-3 servings of protein daily
...animal or vegetable protein, or alternate.

Proteins are the building blocks of the body. They are essential for growth, tissue repair, transporting substances around the body, and they are also used to make hormones, enzymes, antibodies, and neurotransmitters. More than any other macro-nutrient, protein probably elicits the most controversy when it comes to recommendations as to how much and what kind is best to eat. This makes it very challenging for people to know what to do. Because of this tremendous debate, I have tried here to give a lot of room for varying philosophies without going to one extreme or the other. When it comes to specifics, the bottom line is that the question of what is an adequate amount and the right kind of protein for your body at this time presents a great opportunity for you to hone your body awareness and intuitive skills and discover the answer for yourself.

There are many things to consider when experimenting with different kinds of protein in order to discover what works best for you. Notice how you feel after eating it. For instance, some people have trouble digesting the ocean fishes because of the high essential fatty acid content and are best doing without it until their liver and gallbladder are clearer, stronger and thus better able to process it. Turkey has a high tryptophan content and as a result, causes many people to become very tired after eating it, so it is best consumed at the evening meal. Many people rave about the benefits of eating beans and nuts as good sources of protein, but remember that it's not what you eat, it's what you digest. So, if you have a lot of trouble digesting beans and nuts, once again, it would be wise to come back to them when your system can adequately process them. Some say eat protein in the morning, while others say eat protein in the evening or at lunch, while others still say not to eat protein at all. I say eat the kind and amount of protein at the time of day that works best for your body. Once again, experiment and see, and know that this may change over time due to changes in age, activity levels, and health conditions.

We frequently hear that vegetarians are healthier than meat-eaters. Considering that the average American eats excessive amounts of meat, it's not surprising that this is true (although it is not always the case). However, it doesn't mean you have to become a full-blown vegetarian. What it does indicate is that the average American could definitely benefit by cutting down on his meat consumption. Once again, the theme of having a wide variety comes into play. Diversify your protein intake by incorporating as many different kinds of protein into your diet on a rotational basis, while forgoing those that are not in agreement with your system.

6 ~ eat 1-3 servings of complex carbohydrates daily
...either whole grains or starchy vegetables.

Carbohydrates are the main fuel source for the body. There are two main categories of carbohydrates: complex and simple. Simple carbohydrates are *fast releasing*. They include sugar, honey, sweeteners, and refined grains (white refined flour or rice). In addition to causing weight gain, they can wreak havoc on your blood sugar, causing your energy to spike, then drop dramatically, which can lead to a host of other adverse health conditions. Consequently, simple carbohydrates are best kept to a minimum. They are extreme foods that fall into the category of stimulants and *Eating-for-Health Guideline #2: eliminate or relegate stimulants to rare occasions.*

Complex carbohydrates, on the other hand, are *slow-releasing* whole, fresh, natural foods that nourish the body and provide sustained energy. Complex or unrefined carbohydrates include whole grains and starchy vegetables such as yams, sweet potatoes and squash. Many people are shunning starchy vegetables and whole grains these days as a result of the low-carbohydrate craze that has become popular. This is unfortunate

...compared with a diet high in refined carbohydrates, eating intact grain foods is clearly better for sustained good health and offers protection against a variety of chronic diseases.

Dr. Walter Willett
Eat, Drink & Be Healthy

and unnecessary, as complex carbohydrates are a rich, satisfying part of a natural, balanced diet. People aren't overweight in this country because they're eating too many whole grains and starchy vegetables. Most people aren't eating them at all. People are overweight because they are eating too many *refined* and *simple* carbohydrates in the form of white bread, pastries, pasta, processed cereals, soft drinks, sugars, syrups, jams, and jellies. Replace these health robbers with complex carbohydrates and your weight, energy and overall health will come into balance.

7 ~ consume essential fatty acids (EFA's) daily
...either 1-3 tablespoons extra virgin olive oil, coconut oil, ground seeds or other healthy fat, or an EFA supplement.

Fats are an essential part of a healthy diet. However, it is important to distinguish between the beneficial fats and those that are harmful to the body. In a nutshell, essential fatty acids (EFA's) are the most beneficial to the body and as such, are often referred to as "fats that heal." They play an important role in the proper functioning of the brain, the immune system, the cells, the hormones, the skin, the nervous system, and more. A deficiency in EFA's can be associated with a host of adverse conditions in the body, including PMS and menopausal symptoms, ADHD and other brain and behavioral disorders, celiac disease, irritable bowel syndrome, candida, allergies, cardiovascular disease, arteriosclerosis, hypertension, cystic fibrosis, cancer, and more.

Essential fatty acids are called *essential* because the body is unable to produce them on its own and, consequently, they must be obtained through the diet. There are many sources of essential fatty acids, which can be added to the diet in the form of oils, ground seeds, supplements (usually gel-caps), or by eating fish rich in omega-3 fatty acids. As with foods themselves, I believe it is wise to vary the essential fatty acids you consume to allow for a wide spectrum of nutrients and benefits. And also be mindful of what works for your body and in what amounts. Many people have a weakened and toxic liver/gallbladder and may have trouble processing fats of any kind. If this is the case, it is wise to introduce them slowly, in small amounts until your system is healthier.

...there is a desperate need for the medical profession in general to devote far more attention than it ever has to the prevention, and not simply the cure, of disease.

It is upon health, not upon ill-health, that our sight should be fixed.

Dr. Roger Williams

One of the most commonly recommended oils for meeting all-around essential fatty acid needs is flaxseed oil, which contains both omega-3 and omega-6 fatty acids, the two most lacking in our diets. Some people react to flaxseed oil, however, and there is also some debate about whether or not it is a smart choice for regular consumption because of its estrogenic properties. If you are concerned about excess estrogen, avoid flaxseed altogether. Otherwise, test to see if it agrees with your system. You will find flaxseed oil in the refrigerated section of the health food store in black, lightproof containers. Keep it refrigerated and observe the label's expiration date to avoid oil that may have turned rancid. *Do not cook* flaxseed oil or you will destroy the beneficial fatty acids. Instead, add it to your morning smoothie or drizzle over salads or steamed veggies after they are cooked. Some people like to down EFA oils by the spoonful, which is better than not getting them in your diet at all, but can sometimes tax the digestive system. The general recommendation for adults is 1-3 tablespoons a day.

Virgin coconut oil is another fabulous source of medium chain essential fatty acids. After an undeserved and much publicized bad rap a few years ago, coconut oil and coconut milk are returning to their rightful stature as healthy fats that offer an array of therapeutic benefits. They are also quite delicious.

Another great way to incorporate essential fatty acids, as well as a little fiber into your diet, is to consume 1-3 tablespoons of ground seeds a day. Use a coffee grinder to reduce raw flax, pumpkin, sesame or sunflower seeds to a fine meal, which can then be added to salads, smoothies, hot cereals and other recipes. To preserve nutrient content and the integrity of the essential fatty acids contained in the ground seeds, be sure to add them *after* the hot cereal or other recipe has been cooked. Left over ground seeds are best stored in a glass jar in the refrigerator or freezer for no more than a few days to a couple of weeks in order to avoid rancidity.

There are also a number of essential fatty acids available in supplement form such as Evening Primrose oil, black currant seed oil, borage oil and fish oils. They usually come in gel-cap form and are located in the supplement aisles along with the vitamins and herbs. It's best to follow the dosage recommendations given on the label, as potencies will vary with each brand. These are

> The cells of our bodies can become unwell and malfunctioning for two general reasons: First, they may be poisoned; second, they may lack a good supply of nourishing food.
>
> Dr. Roger Williams

especially helpful for people that find the taste of oils offensive or want more convenience.

It is important to clarify that you want to consume a *total* of 1-3 tablespoons essential fatty acids daily by having either a single EFA or a combination of different EFA's. As with all foods, incorporating a variety of healthy fats into your diet is best. Variety may be obtained by either rotating the type of essential fatty acid on a daily basis or alternating them every few weeks or so (i.e., have flaxseed oil one day, ground seeds the next, etc.).

In contrast to beneficial EFA's, we are all aware that there is another group of fats that are harmful to the body. These are often referred to as "fats that kill." These would include highly refined oils, fried foods, and hydrogenated fats and oils found in processed foods. For more information, see *Things to Avoid* in the next chapter.

8 ~ eat a variety of different foods

> *...from meal to meal and day to day, for a wide spectrum of nutrients and to reduce sensitivities.*

After first presenting this concept to a class one evening, a rather strapping young man raised his hand and with a bit of a smirk said, "Now let me make sure I have this straight. You mean if I have a *Bud Light* one night, then I should have a microbrew the next?"

"No, actually you would have a *Bud Light* one night and a shot of whiskey the next," I responded in kind.

Obviously this was a tongue in cheek exchange and not a recommendation that would fall under the category of *Eating for Health*, however, it did serve to make an important distinction. A distinction that is made in the careful wording of this recommendation, "Eat a *variety* of *different* foods..." This may at first seem redundant. On closer examination, however, it makes clear the distinction between eating a variety of the *same* food in different forms, which is what most people do today, as opposed to eating a variety of completely *different* foods. For example, on a daily basis most people will eat a variety of the same food or foods with the same primary ingredient, such as pasta, bread, bagels, and cookies, all of which are made from wheat. Or as another example, they will eat milk, cheese, yogurt, and creamy

---

the spice of life

Every organ of our body needs one chemical element more than others to keep healthy... The best way to take care of this is to have variety in vitamins. The best way to take care of this is to have variety in our foods.

Foods, in a way, are matched to our body organs in that each food is usually highest in one or two minerals and vitamins... Each color has its own activity in the body, because each color carries a chemical element particular to that color.

All red foods are stimulating foods. All yellow are of a laxative nature in the natural food routine. All green foods repair, rebuild and are high in iron and potassium... This is one of the greatest laws to follow.

Dr. Bernard Jensen

dressing, all of which are made from milk. Doing so, as mentioned, can lead to the development of food intolerances and also displaces the nutrients that would otherwise be gained by eating a wide variety of different foods.

One easy way to be sure you are eating a variety of different foods is to regularly eat an array of different *colored* foods — red, green, yellow, brown, purple, etc. Think for a moment about how you would accomplish this and you will come to the obvious conclusion that it can most easily be done by eating an assortment of vibrantly colored fruits and vegetables. Sorry, gummy bears and other artificially colored foods don't count! But that is one of the reasons manufacturers add artificial coloring. It makes them not only more aesthetically appealing, but also triggers our natural inclination to eat a wide variety of brightly colored foods, which in a natural setting would be primarily fruits and vegetables, of course. In addition, you would want to vary the grains and kinds of protein you eat. See *Suggested Foods* for a cornucopia of foods to choose from.

This concludes our outline of the *Dietary Basics* and suggestions for specific daily food intake. We will now delve into recommendations for healthy eating and associated lifestyle habits.

healthy habits

1 ~ eat only when hungry
...and under optimal conditions.

The goal here is to keep your digestive fire burning. Put too many logs on the fire, or food in your stomach as the case may be, and you will stomp out your digestive processes. Good digestion is a key ingredient to optimal health, high energy levels, and normal weight. To help your system operate fully, allow at least 2-3 hours between meals or snacks, more if needed, and don't eat for at least 2-3 hours before going to bed.

Similarly, it is wise to eat only under optimal conditions, not when hurried, stressed, or excessively fatigued, all of which will inhibit your body's ability to process food adequately and with ease.

There is slower digestion because the food gets bogged down in the stomach, and there is less complete digestion.

These two factors are the root causes of the smothering of the healing process, and thus the beginning of disease.

When the digestion is quickened and made more complete, the body immediately reactivates its healing powers.

Jon Matsen, N.D.
Eating Alive

2 ~ don't drink beverages with food
...thereby diluting the digestive juices.

This seems almost un-American given that as a culture we automatically order a beverage with our meals. Knowing that our current cultural food climate does not always take our health into consideration should make letting go of the habit of drinking with meals at least a little easier. The best recommendation is to drink beverages at least 15-30 minutes before meals or snacks on an empty stomach and not for at least a ½-1 hour after eating. This will ensure that digestive juices such as saliva, enzymes and hydrochloric acid are not diluted, which can impede proper digestion.

3 ~ chew, chew, chew
...to ensure adequate mastication and saliva secretion.

It is important to remember that the first step of digestion occurs in the mouth through chewing and the secretion and subsequent mixture of saliva with the food. As a chiropractor I once knew used to say, "chew your juices and drink your food." He would go on to explain that whenever you are drinking juice, bear in mind that it is food and should therefore be held in the mouth and swished around a bit in order to mix with saliva before swallowing. This not only releases the full nutritional value of the food, but also ensures proper digestion and heads off gas or bloating that may occur otherwise. In other words, "chew your juice." Similarly, food should be masticated to a pulp in order for it to be of the finest consistency before entering the stomach and also, once again, to allow for adequate saliva secretion. Thus accounting for the latter part of the saying, "drink your food."

4 ~ follow food-combining principles
...whenever possible to ensure proper digestion.

It's not what you eat, it's what you digest and proper food combining can assist you greatly on that count. Because different foods require different digestive juices and enzymes to digest them, food combining is a way of supporting this natural biological system of processing and assimilating foods. Food combining is a fantastic way to improve your digestion and elimination, lose weight, and increase your energy. If you watch young children, you will see that they often eat one thing at a time, indicating a natural propensity to combine foods properly.

There are a few different schools of thought and entire volumes written on this topic. We will keep things simple here by introducing just the basic rudiments of this practice:

1. *Eat fruits alone on an empty stomach and wait at least 15 minutes before eating something else.*

2. *Vegetables may be eaten with proteins or starches.*

3. *Proteins and starches are best eaten at separate meals.*

4. *Or, if proteins and starches are eaten at the same meal, layer them by eating the protein first, then vegetables, then the starchy food.*

Keeping your meals simple by having only two or three *different* foods at once is another way of lightening the load on your digestive and eliminative systems.

5 ~ follow the body's natural cycle
...eat light in the morning and don't eat after 6-7:00 p.m. or at least 2-3 hours before bedtime.

There is a natural cycle the body follows in relationship to the ingestion, assimilation and elimination of food. This cycle begins in the morning which is the primary time for the body to eliminate waste, thus accounting for the typical morning bowel movement. The rest of the day into the early evening is the body's optimal time for taking in or ingesting food. At night, when we are sleeping, the body then processes, digests and assimilates the food and nutrients ingested throughout the day. The cycle then continues when we awaken in the morning, by eliminating the by-products of the previous night's processing. Simply put, this natural cycle is as follows:

*   Morning = Elimination time
*   Afternoon/Early Evening = Ingestion time
*   Night = Assimilation time

All the rules of prudence or gifts of experience that life can accumulate will never do as much for human comfort and welfare as would be done by a stricter attention and a wiser science directed to the digestive system.

Thomas DeQuincy

To implement eating and lifestyle habits that work in accordance with this natural cycle, many health advocates believe it is wise to eat light in the morning (i.e., fruit, juices, nuts, etc.) to free up the energy of the body for the elimination process. Eat your biggest meal of the day at noon when your digestive machine is at its peak operation. Eat your evening meal no later than 6-7:00pm. And do not eat for at least 2-3 hours before going to bed so as not to disrupt sleeping patterns. This will also give the body adequate rest and time for the digestion and assimilation process that takes place at night.

> Digestion is the process whereby we absorb and utilize nutrients from the foods we eat; so to enhance this process is to benefit the entire body and all of its systems.
>
> Dr. Vic Shayne
> Illness Isn't Caused by a Drug Deficiency

It is important to understand that this does not mean that you skip breakfast, but rather that you eat light, cleansing foods, juices or smoothies. The exceptions to this would be if you have problems with your blood sugar such as hypoglycemia (which would account for millions of people!), if you are very thin and have a high metabolism, or if you do manual labor and expend a lot of energy in the morning. In these cases it would be wise to have a heartier breakfast within an hour of waking up that includes a serving or two of concentrated foods such as eggs or whole grains. The worst thing you can do, which has unfortunately become a tradition for many Americans, is to have a sugar-loaded processed cereal covered with milk in the morning (or any time of day really!)

6 ~ cleanse regularly
   ...to clear and strengthen your entire body.

After doing a cleanse, drinking only the *Green Drink* and juices for a few days, I woke up one morning with an odd yet distantly familiar taste in my mouth. It was very distinctive, sort of metallic, and I racked my brain throughout the day as it stayed with me to figure out where I had encountered it before. It finally came to me. It was the same taste I had had in my mouth for the duration of the ten days that I took copious amounts of a potent antibiotic when I was in the Peace Corps some 15 years before. I had always heard that people release toxins and drugs that have been stored in the organs and tissues when they fast or cleanse, and had always felt this to be true when I had done a cleanse. But this was the first time I had a directly identifiable experience of this.

It is a long held notion among natural health advocates that toxins and chemicals can be stored in the tissues and organs of the body, wreaking havoc with your health. In recent years scientific evidence has proven this historically held theory to be valid. In a recent PBS program, Bill Moyers took a blood test that revealed he had numerous toxic chemicals in his system, including heavy metals, DDT, and other harmful substances. This blood test only accounted for environmental pollutants, however, and did not even include all the toxic chemicals that are ingested from eating processed pseudofood.

Toxins from your natural metabolic processes can also accumulate in the body if it is so overloaded and weakened that it is rendered incapable of performing its rudimentary detoxification process. This is very common in our culture with its poor eating and lifestyle habits and the added burden of environmental toxins and consumption of large quantities of chemicals in the form of over-the-counter and pharmaceutical drugs. For this reason, it is a wise practice to cleanse and rejuvenate the body on a regular basis, and especially if you want to prevent the onset of, or are already experiencing, any ill health. More on this in *Chapter 9 ~ Clear the Way*.

> The road to good health is paved with good intestines.
>
> Unknown

7 ~ troubleshoot digestion & elimination
...to maintain health and keep things running smooth.

People frequently approach chronic constipation, diarrhea or other elimination problems by resorting to laxatives, colon cleansers or anti-diarrhea medications for assistance, treating these challenges in isolation of the digestive function. While this may be advisable in acute cases as temporary assistance to get things back on track, it is important to remember that elimination is the latter part of the digestive process. Everything you do on a regular basis leading up to the elimination event is what's most important. For this reason, in order to achieve optimal digestive and eliminative function on a regular basis, it is paramount to follow the preceding guidelines for *Healthy Habits*. If, however, you should find yourself in a position of having troubles in this area, it is wise to address them as soon as possible in order to get your system in order.

To do this, go off foods that may be slowing things down (i.e. foods to which you may be sensitive such as dairy, wheat, sugar, fried foods, etc.). If things are really backed up, consider taking some herbal cleansing formulas. My favorites include *Cleanse Smart* or *Ultimate Cleanse,* which are available at health food stores, and the *Cleansing Trio* by Young Living Essential Oils (see *Resources*). Drinking ginger or other herbal teas is helpful as well. You may also consider irrigating the colon by doing an enema or having a colonic. Colon irrigation is a time-honored way of cleansing the body and restoring health to a clogged system. You may also choose to go on an elimination diet, eat minimally, or drink only liquids (broths, *Green Drink,* etc.) until the colon clears. Whatever you do, *don't* allow the waste to continue to back up.

Diarrhea often alternates with being constipated. Essentially both conditions are sending the same message: *what you're eating or doing in your life, especially poor eating and stressful living, are not working for you.* Definitely make use of temporary measures, but ultimately you will want to adopt new habits that will eliminate the cause.

One of my all time favorite books that can help you further with this topic is *Eating Alive: Prevention Thru Good Digestion,* by Jon Matsen, N.D. It is a fabulous book that I believe should be a part of our public school curriculum. It will completely change the way you think about food and how your body works. Everyone who has ever taken my advice and read this humorous, yet informative, book has been glad they did.

8 ~ exercise & de-stress regularly
... to keep all body-mind systems working optimally.

There are so many things you can do in this arena and so many thoughts as to what is best. The important thing is that you get yourself moving, breathing, stretching, and relaxing on a regular basis. These are not luxuries of life. They are necessities. So, indulge often. If you don't have things that you like to do already, explore what's available by taking classes at your local community center or YMCA (remember to bring a bottle of water!). Take advantage of free introductory classes offered at dance, yoga, and martial arts studios as well. And don't forget

---

From physical exercise one gets lightness, a capacity for work, firmness, tolerance of difficulties, elimination of impurities, and stimulation of digestion.

Charaka

about walking, one of the best exercises and de-stressors that's absolutely free. When you find a thing or two you like, stick with it. Enlist a buddy to go with you to increase the likelihood of it actually happening. Get moving, get breathing, follow the *Dietary Basics* and *Healthy Habits* and all areas of your life will improve!

dietary basics ~ quick reference

1 ~ follow the eating-for-health guidelines
  ...as much as possible.

2 ~ drink plenty of pure water daily
  ...in accordance with your body's needs.

3 ~ eat 2-4 pieces of fresh fruit a day
  ...preferably organic and in season.

4 ~ eat 3-7 servings of fresh vegetables a day
  ...preferably raw or lightly steamed.

5 ~ eat 1-3 servings of protein a day
  ...animal or vegetable protein, or alternate.

6 ~ eat 1-3 servings of complex carbohydrates a day
  ...either whole grains or starchy vegetables.

7 ~ consume essential fatty acids daily
  ...either 1-3 tablespoons extra virgin olive oil, coconut oil, ground seeds or an EFA supplement.

8 ~ eat a variety of different foods
  ...for a wide spectrum of nutrients and to reduce sensitivities.

healthy habits ~ quick reference

1 ~ eat only when hungry
   ...and under optimal conditions.

2 ~ don't drink beverages with food
   ...thereby diluting the digestive juices.

3 ~ chew, chew, chew
   ...to ensure adequate mastication and saliva secretion.

4 ~ follow food-combining principles
   ...whenever possible to ensure proper digestion.

5 ~ follow the body's natural cycle
   ...eat light in the morning and don't eat after 6- 7:00 p.m. or at least 2-3 hours before bedtime.

6 ~ cleanse regularly
   ...to clear and strengthen your entire body.

7 ~ trouble shoot digestion & elimination
   ...to maintain health and keep things running smooth.

8 ~ exercise & de-stress regularly
   ... to keep all body-mind systems working optimally.

Chapter Eight

suggested foods

Getting to Know Natural Foods to Enjoy & Things to Avoid

Although we have been culturally lulled into believing that eating healthier limits what we can eat, when truth be told, the list of *Suggested Foods* is actually much longer than the overall list of *Things to Avoid.* As Americans we eat a variety of forms of mostly the same foods (wheat, sugar, dairy, meat) rather than an actual *variety* of foods. When you start on the path of making wiser food choices, it is refreshing to meet up with all those delicious, nutritious foods you have been missing. Following is a relatively comprehensive list of specific whole, fresh, natural foods to familiarize yourself with. This is followed by some pointers on natural brand processed foods, whole food supplements, and things to limit or avoid altogether.

Food is an important part of a balanced diet.

Fran Lebowitz

suggested foods list

Although the following list is all whole, fresh, natural foods, as you have learned, not all of the foods listed are going to be appropriate for everyone. Foods that are in parentheses indicate foods that may be problematic. They are either common food allergens or foods that can be difficult to digest. You will learn how to test for these foods in the upcoming chapter *Clear the Way*. In the meantime, make a mental note of these foods and begin to take notice of any possible reactions you may have to them.

My favorite resource to further assist you in getting to know natural foods is *The New Whole Foods Encyclopedia*, by Rebecca Wood. Entries include information on the origin of the food, its health benefits, uses, and practical tips on buying and storing. This is one book that should be on the shelf of everyone who is serious about eating natural foods. For now, the following list will get you started

fruits

Sweet, succulent, juicy, nectar of God is the best way to describe these marvels of nature. Both fresh and dried fruits are great to keep on hand to liven up a dish or as a stand-alone snack. Check the labels on dried fruit to be sure there are no additives such as sugar, colorings, or preservatives. If you run across dried fruits such as apricots, apples, and raisins that are light in color, they may have been treated with toxic sulfites. Dried fruits that are not treated will be brown and more shriveled by comparison. They may not look as pretty, but they are a much better choice health-wise. See *Things to Avoid* for more on sulfites.

apples	grapefruit	(oranges)
apricots	kiwi	papayas
(bananas)	lemons	peaches
(berries)	limes	pears
cherries	mangoes	pineapple
figs	melons	plums
grapes	nectarines	tangelos

Produce should be fresh whenever possible. Frozen would be the next best choice and good to have on hand for quick smoothies.

Canned foods are devoid of vital life force energy and it is best to use them sparingly or not at all.

non-starchy vegetables

Non-starchy vegetables are the only food that everyone seems to agree we should all be eating in abundance. At the same time they are, ironically, the one food that everyone is eating the least. This is true of Americans anyway. In many traditional cultures, vegetables are the mainstay of their diet, which, in large part, accounts for their comparatively lower incidence of chronic degenerative *dis*-ease. As a culture, our eating habits have, unfortunately, strayed from these vital plant foods and we are paying the price. We must take a cue from traditional cultures and reacquaint ourselves with the regular preparation and consumption of vegetables. Begin by perusing this list. The next section contains recipes, food shopping and preparation tips, and will help you further in making these nutrient-packed foods part of your daily diet.

asparagus	cilantro	peas
(avocado)	collard greens	peppers
beans (green & yellow)	cucumber	radish
beets	(eggplant)	salad greens
beet greens	jicama	sea veggies
bok choy	kale	(spinach)
broccoli	leeks	sprouts
cabbage	lettuce	swiss chard
carrots (raw)	mustard greens	(tomatoes)
cauliflower	mushrooms	watercress
celery	onions	zucchini

starchy vegetables

Starchy vegetables are a hearty, satisfying part of a natural, balanced diet. Because most are root vegetables, they are especially beneficial in the cold months due to their warming properties. They are also versatile. You can cook them whole, chop into bite-sized chunks, or purée for a rich sauce or soup base. Another nice feature is that most starchy vegetables have a relatively long shelf life when stored properly, making them easy and convenient to keep on hand.

artichokes	rutabagas
burdock root (cooked)	squash
carrots (cooked)	sweet potatoes
parsnips	turnips
(potatoes)	yams
pumpkins	

gluten grains

Remember as a child mixing flour and water to make glue? It was the gluten contained in the flour that gave this mixture its sticky, glue-like consistency. Gluten is a mixture of gum-like, water-

The more fruits and vegetables you eat, the less your risk of disease...

Most studies show that even small to moderate amounts of vegetables make a big difference.

Eating certain fresh vegetables twice a day, instead of twice a week, can cut the risk of lung cancer by 75%, even in smokers.

Linda Page, N.D.
Healthy Healing

insoluble plant proteins found in many grains. Great stuff for binding paper maché, not so good for the intestines or any other part of the digestive and eliminative tract.

The following grains all contain various amounts of gluten, with wheat containing the most. This is the primary reason wheat is problematic for so many people. Many people who are allergic or sensitive to wheat have difficulty with other gluten grains as well, and are, consequently, better off eating the non-gluten grains that follow. Others do just fine with gluten grains other than wheat, however. Test different grains to see how you do. Spelt and kamut are the two grains closest in taste and texture to wheat. Because of their lower gluten content, however, they are often easier to tolerate.

barley	rye	(whole wheat)
kamut	spelt	
oats	teff	

non-gluten grains

Whether you have a pronounced sensitivity to gluten grains or not, it is wise to regularly partake of the non-gluten grains as well. You don't want to miss out on the nutrients and fiber they offer, and also the opportunity to grant your system a reprieve from having to deal with the thicker, stickier gluten grains.

Brown rice can sometimes be challenging for those who have weakened digestion or elimination. In which case, this otherwise beneficial gain should be avoided, at least temporarily, until you are able to process it adequately. White basmati rice would be a better choice until your system is stronger, as it is much easier to digest. Make sure it is basmati rice and not regular white or instant rice.

amaranth	brown rice	quinoa
buckwheat	(corn)	wild rice
basmati rice (brn/wht)	millet	

animal protein

Many non-vegetarian pioneers of the health food movement, such as Dr. Bernard Jensen, recommend having animal protein 3 times a week. Give or take a serving, this is generally accepted as an

---

Low energy is a very common symptom of gluten intolerance, and it can lead to excessive need for caffeine, nicotine, and other stimulants.

Some of my clients also often complain that they continue to feel hungry even after big meals and just keep on eating.

They never feel full because their gluten-damaged intestines aren't absorbing food very well.

Julia Ross
The Diet Cure

adequate amount to satisfy the body's nutritional needs, while at the same time not too much to run the risk of clogging up your system. As discussed earlier, while you may need to eat more initially to restore balanced blood sugar levels, or less to clear your system, having animal protein three times a week is a ballpark amount to strive for.

Fresh free-range and grass-fed organic animal protein free of additives, hormones, pesticides and antibiotics is always your first choice whenever available. Meat packers that offer these quality standards boldly display this on their tags and labels. If you do not see this information displayed anywhere, you can be sure that one or more of these harmful substances is present in their products and better left alone. When preparing animal protein it is best to cook at lower heats for longer times. In other words, bake, broil, grill, or roast it to preserve the integrity and nutritional value.

beef	fish
bison	lamb
chicken	ostrich
eggs	wild game

(dairy products)

Once again, if you are going to indulge in dairy products, be sure to choose organic products free of preservatives, hormones, pesticides and antibiotics such as Horizon, Alta Dena, or local brands. Fresh from the farm, unpasteurized is best as the pasteurization process uses heat that alters the nature of the milk protein and renders it harmful to the body. Also check labels to be sure you are getting *real* cheese, butter, and yogurt that do not contain additives, artificial sweeteners or refined sugars. Pseudofood dairy products that boast being 'lite' often contain a list of suspicious substances.

Keep in mind that dairy foods are at the top of the list of common food allergens and, as a result, must be completely eliminated from or included only on a rotational basis in many people's diets. Even if you do not have a known or pronounced problem with dairy, it is a food to limit in your diet for reasons that will be explained shortly. Furthermore, when you get to the instructions for the *Cleanse & Clear* process in the next chapter, you will be referring back to this list of *Suggested Foods*. To be clear, dairy products are *not* included in the elimination diet. They are, in fact, one of the food categories you will be eliminating. Dairy products are among the most common food allergens (notice the parentheses) and are one of the foods you will most definitely want to eliminate, then test yourself for sensitivity. More on how to test for sensitivities and intolerances is coming up in the next chapter.

(milk)   (cheese)   (butter)
(yogurt)

beans & vegetable protein

Raw almond butter is a great substitute for peanut butter, very tasty and much easier to digest. Try spreading some on apple slices for a delicious healthy treat. Don't overdo it, however, nuts and nut butters are best eaten in small amounts.

Nuts may be soaked overnight for easier digestion.

Beans are a nutrient-dense food savored throughout the world for their economical, life-sustaining properties. Beans are a great food to include in your regular menu planning, especially if you are looking to cut down on the amount of animal protein in your diet and save money at the same time. Cook up a batch of spicy or seasoned beans and rice, add a side of mixed veggies, and you've got a satisfying meal for pennies.

As we are all aware, however, beans are the musical fruit. Which means, they can be difficult for many people to digest. If this is the case, you should limit them to 1-2 servings a week, or leave them alone completely until your system is stronger and better able to tolerate them. Remember, any food is only highly beneficial to you if YOU can digest it and it agrees with YOUR system. Soaking beans over night will reduce their cooking time and reduce the flatulence production factor as well. Adding a piece of kombu seaweed to the pot while cooking can also reduce gas production, as it helps to break down the hard outer shell of the bean and, consequently, increases digestibility. Some beans are easier to digest than others. Experiment to discover which are best for you.

adzuki beans	lentils	(tempeh -soy)
beans & bean sprouts	(miso)	(tofu - soy)
kidney beans	mung beans	white beans

nuts & seeds

Avoid roasted, salted nuts and seeds. Instead, choose raw, unsalted nuts and seeds in their natural state, as they provide a good source of healthy fats. Limit daily consumption of nuts and seeds to 1-2 small handfuls per day (approximately ⅛-¼ cup). Any more than this can be challenging to digest. If you have known, or suspected problems with your liver/gallbladder or just a generally weakened digestive system, do not eat any nuts or seeds initially. Later, when your digestion is stronger, you can introduce them, starting with a few almonds and see how you do.

Contrary to popular belief, cashews are beans and peanuts are legumes. Both are common allergens and it is therefore wise to test for any sensitivity to them. When it comes to nut butters, almond butter is a much better all around choice than peanut butter. It contains less fat, is much easier to digest, and tastes delicious. Tahini, or sesame seed butter, is another good choice.

almonds & almond butter
(cashews)
flax seeds (ground)
(peanuts & peanut butter)
pecans
pumpkin seeds
sesame seeds & tahini (sesame seed butter)
sunflower seeds
walnuts

oils

The low-fat fad has steered many people away from fats and oils. This is unfortunate, as they are an essential part of a well-balanced diet and highly beneficial to the body — the *good* fats and oils, that is. Look for oils that are unrefined, cold-pressed, and virgin or extra virgin whenever possible. Heat alters the nature of oils and renders them harmful to the body. Cold pressing oils prevents damage to the essential fats caused by the heat process, thereby maintaining the beneficial nature of the oil. Virgin and extra-virgin is the highest quality oil, as it has been extracted from the best produce of the harvest from the first pressing.

Contrary to what we have been told the last couple of decades, coconut oil is the best all-around oil to keep on hand. It is the only oil that maintains its integrity when heated and offers a long list of healthful benefits. To top it off, it is incredibly delicious! Choose from virgin coconut oil, which has a full-bodied coconut taste that adds a satisfying richness to everything you

Polynesian islanders, who get most of their fat calories from coconut oil have an exceedingly low rate of heart disease.

Coconut oil is less likely than other oils to cause obesity, because the body easily converts it into energy rather than depositing its calories as body fat.

Linda Page, N.D.
Healthy Healing

make with it. Or the expeller pressed, which is much milder tasting and, consequently, a better choice for those dishes you'd rather not have taste like coconut. There are a couple decent brands available at health food stores, but *Tropical Traditions*, available by mail order (see *Resources*) is the brand I most recommend. They offer organic, virgin coconut oil that you can buy in bulk and save. Because coconut oil is so stable, you don't have to worry about it going rancid, so buying in bulk is the most cost effective way to go. For more on the health benefits, *The Coconut Oil Miracle*, by Bruce Fife, is a great read and also explains the politics behind why this highly beneficial oil was falsely vilified in recent years.

Extra virgin olive oil is another great all-around oil to keep around and is especially nice for salads and dipping. Butter is also a nice condiment and, in addition to coconut oil, is the best choice for baking. Unrefined sesame oil maintains its integrity at medium temperatures and, consequently, is a good choice for low-heat stir-frying. When sautéing vegetables or meats, use a small amount of coconut, olive or sesame oil with a little bit of water and keep temperature below 350°.

Margarine is not recommended for any use as it contains hydrogenated oils. There are also a few spreads on the market today made from a blend of oils and ingredients. Most of these are highly processed, loaded with additives, and are therefore also not recommended. Following are a list of your best choices.

(butter) or ghee (clarified butter)
coconut oil
olive oil (extra virgin)
(flaxseed oil) - do not heat!
sesame seed oil
sunflower oil

herbs & spices

Travel around the world and you will have dishes placed before you brimming with both common and exotic herbs and spices. Scout around most American kitchens, however, and you will be hard-pressed to find anything other than the classic salt and pepper shaker strategically placed on the dining table. If you do find a spice rack, it was most likely acquired as a Christmas gift, and is now collecting dust or never been opened. This is a shame

If they would
drink nettles
in March and
eat mugwort
in May,
so many fine
maidens
wouldn't go to
the clay.

Old Proverb

because these marvelous gifts of nature don't just add flavor, but are packed with nutrients and offer a wide variety of therapeutic properties as well.

In addition to a host of individual qualities, all are powerful immune boosters that keep the body healthy and strong. Probably the most important feature that almost all herbs and spices offer is that they help with the digestion and elimination of food. When you deprive yourself of herbs and spices, you are also depriving yourself of the therapeutic benefits they have to offer. So, next time you're cooking, see if you can't spice things up a bit. Adding herbs and spices into your diet in cooked foods, fresh salads, or drinking herbal teas is a really easy and enjoyable way to upgrade the quality of your diet. It is particularly smart to add in those that are known to aid any symptoms or *dis*-eases you may be experiencing. Following is just a partial list of the wide variety of herbs and spices available.

> The Chinese do not draw any distinction between food and medicine.
>
> Lin Yutang

anise	dill	pepper
basil	fennel	peppermint
bay leaf	garlic	rosemary
cardamom	ginger	saffron
cayenne	lemongrass	sage
cinnamon	marjoram	spearmint
clove	oregano	tarragon
coriander	nutmeg	thyme
cumin	parsley	turmeric

condiments & dressings

Similarly, when it comes to dressings and condiments most American kitchens are equipped with the standard ketchup, mustard, bottled dressings, and little else. My kitchen is stocked with these cultural standards as well; the natural, additive-free varieties, of course! Following are some other natural, ready-made popular favorites you may want to add to your repertoire.

(Bragg's Liquid Aminos)
(Tamari Sauce)
Herbamare
Tocomere
Mrs. Dash
Spike
Gomasio

Unrefined sea salt
Bottled dressings (such as Seeds of Change, and Annie's)

These are all store bought brands. However, you can also easily make up your own blend of herbs and spices, or homemade dressings. A few recipes for homemade dressings are included in the recipe section. You can also drizzle a combination of olive or flax oil and lemon or balsamic vinegar over steamed vegetables or a fresh salad (remember not to heat flax oil). Or marinate chopped vegetables in olive oil and lemon or balsamic vinegar before roasting or grilling. Use approximately 1 part acid to 2 parts oil for marinating. Keeping these items on hand makes flavoring foods simple and healthy.

natural sweeteners

A woman once came to me because every winter she would get recurrent colds and upper respiratory infections that would linger on for weeks at a time. She was puzzled and frustrated as to why this was happening because relative to the average American, she maintained a pretty wholesome diet, eating fruits and vegetables and all organic foods regularly. When I looked at her food diary, however, her problem became clear. She ate a substantial amount of sweets with almost reckless abandon. Because they were homemade with natural sweeteners such as maple syrup and honey, she mistakenly thought it wasn't a problem. As soon as she reduced the amount of sweets she was eating, her health and energy improved.

Like this client, people often mistakenly believe that natural sweeteners are 'good' for you and don't have any ill effects when, in fact, while natural sweeteners such as those listed below are a better choice than refined sugars, they are still extreme foods that have a stimulating effect and with regular or over consumption can cause the same problems as refined sugars.

As with other foods, there is a wide spectrum of sweeteners. At one end of the spectrum would be white refined sugar and high fructose corn syrup, probably the two that cause the most harm to the body. On the other end of the spectrum is *Stevia*, which is actually beneficial to the body and has little to no effect on the blood sugar. Concentrated sweeteners of any kind, natural or otherwise, are best kept to a minimum. Consider foods

---

I am fond of telling people that if something tastes sweet you probably should spit it out as it is not likely to be too good for you.

This of course, is a humorous exaggeration, but for most people who struggle with chronic illness, it is likely to be a helpful guide.

Dr. Joseph Mercola

made with them as special treats rather than daily events. When you do indulge, the natural sweeteners that follow are your best choice. On a regular basis, keep them to a minimum in accordance with your tolerance level. And cut them out completely if you are experiencing any *dis*-ease, especially lowered immune function or lack of energy.

agave	date sugar	stevia
barley malt	honey	rapadura
brown rice syrup	maple syrup	xylitol
fruit juice, jam	molasses	

natural brand processed foods

Since approximately 90% of Americans today are eating processed foods approximately 90% of the time, it is unrealistic to think that everyone is suddenly going to flip the scales and start eating whole, fresh, natural foods 90% of the time. While processed foods of any kind are not the wisest choice you could be making, natural brand processed foods are certainly a better choice than pseudofood brands that contain toxic chemical additives, as you have learned. They are also a great alternative to fast food or eating out frequently. Refer to the side bar for a partial list of popular natural food brands that you may like to try.

If you raise the bar on what is acceptable to put in your body by making chemical-laden pseudofoods unacceptable and natural brand processed foods the worst you ever eat, you will be significantly raising the bar on your health and energy levels as well. This is a very easy transition to make, as there are now a wide variety of additive-free, natural brand processed foods available, including cookies, snack foods, frozen entrees, soups, pasta, sauces, breads, and more. Give your taste buds time to acclimate and try different brands to find those that suit your palate. Keep the *Dietary Basics* and *Eating-for-Health Guidelines* in mind when making selections. Choose organic whenever possible, and check ingredients labels to know exactly what you're getting.

Sadly, as the popularity of natural brands has risen, some of their quality standards have fallen. Mega-food manufacturers have bought out some of the original mom-and-pop type health food brand companies and have also started up some of their own brands. Some of these companies pay more attention to their profits than purity. Because the natural foods industry is one of

natural food brands

Some popular natural food brands include, but are not limited to:

Alta Dena

Amy's

Annie's Naturals

Arrowhead mills

Barbara's Bakery

Bearito's

Bob's Red Mill

Breadshop

Cascadian Farms

Eden Foods

Fantastic Foods

Garden of Eatin'

Hain

Health Valley

Horizons

Imagine Foods

Kettle Chips

Knudsen's

Lundberg Farms

Newman's Own

Pamela's

Seeds of Change

Shari's Organic

Shelton's

Spectrum Naturals

Westbrae

the fastest growing segments of the economy today, there are many scrambling to cash in on this trend. Consequently, I have noticed examples of this phenomenon showing up more and more as I did on a recent trip to the market.

I live just outside of Boulder, Colorado, which is probably the greatest health food Mecca in the world. As a result, a few regular grocery stores, including one right near my house, stock a good amount of natural food brands as well. I love shopping at this supermarket because it carries most everything I can get at the health food store, in addition to all the most popular pseudofood brands. That way I can keep up with what's being made available on both fronts.

For example, I was recently drawn to investigate a box of frozen fruit pops because it was a brand I would normally never recommend, and yet it boasted 100% Natural on the front of the box. There are many large food brands that are, at least ostensibly, making an effort to improve the quality and nutritional value of their foods. So, I thought I'd check the ingredients and see if this particular product would qualify as food, or if it was just a deceptive labeling ploy to make it look that way. Sure enough, when I checked the ingredients list on the back I was astounded to find aspartame and artificial colorings!

The moral of the story is to stick with long-established, reputable health food brands that maintain quality standards, the *real* natural food brands, such as those listed. Check labels whenever trying a new food product, and eat whole, fresh, natural foods that don't don labels as much as possible. Familiarizing yourself with the upcoming list of *Things to Avoid* will also be of tremendous help.

No nutrient is an island, entire of itself; every nutrient is a piece of the continent, a part of the main.

John Donne

whole food supplements

Because people are eating mostly processed foods and because the few whole, fresh, natural foods they do eat are often depleted of enzymes and nutrients due to modern farming and distribution practices, in addition to the aforementioned suggested foods I also highly recommend augmenting your diet with whole food supplements.

Whole food supplements, as the name implies, are made of concentrated foods with all of their synergistic nutrients intact according to nature's original design. Quality whole food supplements are bio-available, nourish the cells, and do not cause nutritional imbalance or toxicity. They are available in convenient powders, capsules, and tablet form to suit individual needs.

How do you know if a product is a whole food supplement? Read the ingredients label. It will read like a grocery list (i.e., carrots, beets, spinach, kelp, broccoli, barley grass, etc.) rather than a list of isolated vitamins that have been extracted from food and isolated from their companion nutrients (i.e., Vitamin A, B, C, and so on). For those who are interested in learning more, *Man Cannot Live on Vitamins Alone*, by Dr. Vic Shayne is a great resource.

There is no substitute for eating a healthy diet. However, whole food supplements can lend a helping hand when it comes to restoring and maintaining vital health and energy, as well as preventing future *dis*-ease.

There are a variety of whole food supplements available. For broad-spectrum, foundational supplementation that everyone can benefit from, my favorites are the *Juice Plus+® Orchard, Garden* and *Vineyard Blend*s available through independent distributors. The reason I love Juice Plus+® products is because, unlike most supplements, they are scientifically proven to be effective and non-toxic. They are also very affordable, come in easy capsule, chewable or gummie form and they have a fabulous program called the *Juice Plus+® Children's Health Study* that allows children who qualify to get their whole food supplements for free. They are an awesome company and group of people who are dedicated to helping people improve their health through *real* nutrition. (See *Resources*.)

Some of my favorite liquid whole food supplements include *Berry Young* or *Ningxia Red Juice* by Young Living, *Noni Juice* by Tahitian Noni, *Body Balance* by Life Force International and *FrequenSea* by Forever Green. Keep in mind that as with any food, not every whole food supplement is going to be right for every body. When choosing what I call "specialty" whole food supplements such as those just listed, you must take into account *Eating-for-Health Guideline #5: Account for ailments when making wise food choices*. Research and experiment to find what's best for you.

Whole food supplements are especially helpful when it comes to meeting our daily quota of critically important dark green vegetables. In fact, if there is any one whole food

We have created a bizarre situation in which our food is fragmented and sold to us in bits and pieces so that we are forced with the impossible task of trying to reassemble what amounts to a biochemical Humpty-dumpty.

Rudolph Ballentine

supplement everyone should be taking regularly, it is a green food supplement.

green foods

Everyone agrees that consuming fresh green vegetables regularly is paramount to optimal health. But how many of us actually do it? Whole food supplements derived from the fresh juices of wheat grass, barley, kamut, alfalfa, etc., or *green foods* as I call them, are a convenient, palatable way to incorporate these nutrient-packed foods into your diet. They are a necessity for anyone who wants to boost their energy and improve their health. Don't let a day go by without 2-3 healthy doses of fresh green vegetables and *green food* supplements for increased energy and decreased *dis*-ease.

Like whole food supplements in general, there are a variety of green food supplements available in both health food stores and through independent distributors. They are available as individual green foods, such as alfalfa or wheat grass, and also available in green food blends. My favorite single green food supplements are *Just Barley* and *Green Kamut* by Organic by Nature. My favorite green food blend, and the only one I recommend for everybody, is the *Juice Plus+ Garden Blend®* or their children's version that comes in gummies or chewable.

Generally speaking, it is best to consume a green food blend regularly in order to provide the body with a wide selection of nutrients. Take half the recommended dosage on the label when first starting on green foods. They are very detoxifying to the body and, as a result, some people may initially experience classic detoxification symptoms such as fatigue, headache, runny nose, congestion, diarrhea, etc. This reaction is part of the body's natural cleansing process. If this does occur, cut back on the amount you are taking and gradually increase the dosage over a couple of weeks. Soon you will feel even better than before.

Green foods are great to have on hand as a quick remedy for almost anything, especially headaches, stomach upset, fatigue, imbalanced blood sugar, and more. Instead of reaching for Advil, Tums, Maalox or other over-the-counter drugs that may have long-term toxic effects, reach for a dose of green foods and feel better naturally. When you're feeling depleted, doubling up on your regular dosage is a great way to head *dis*-ease off at the pass.

Greens are our most important foods because they provide us with all of the essential components of health.

They are our foods, as well as our medicines.

Where green plants cannot grow, we cannot live.

Udo Erasmus

benefits of green foods:

- *increase your energy and endurance*
- *improve digestion and eliminate constipation*
- *increase mental focus and clarity*
- *balance hormones reducing headaches, cramping, hot flashes, etc.*
- *help clear acne and other skin problems*
- *prevent and help reverse cancer, arthritis, asthma, and other degenerative dis-eases*
- *balance blood sugar - great for diabetes, hyper- or hypoglycemia*
- *eliminate body odor and bad breath*
- *boost the immune system - reducing colds, flu, allergies, hay fever, sinusitis, etc*
- *strengthen nails and hair*
- *reduce food cravings and sensitivities*
- *acts as a natural sunscreen when consumed regularly*
- *high in bio-available calcium to help prevent and reverse osteoporosis*
- *Great for keeping children and pets healthy too!*

Wellness, like life, is always a question of balance.

Wellness Workbook

Now that you have familiarized yourself with the many suggested foods, natural brand processed foods and whole food supplements that are available, it's time to turn your attention to specific foods and non-foods you will want to limit or avoid altogether.

foods to limit

Each of the following foods has been mentioned earlier, sometimes for more than one reason. Here they are presented in the context of an easy-to-remember list of *Foods to Limit,* along with the specific reasons why. While each *may* be considered a food (some are arguably not), unlike the upcoming list of non-foods to avoid, they are problematic foods that are not supportive to the body when eaten regularly, and especially when eaten excessively, which is frequently the case today. Consequently, it is wise to keep these foods to a minimum in accordance with your personal tolerance level. For most people whose bodies are in a relatively balanced state of well-being, this would be somewhere between 1-3 times per week, in contrast to the current cultural trend that has most people eating them 1-3 times *a day*, or more.

Although consuming these food items to this degree may have become the norm here in America and much of the industrialized world, doing so is excessive and unnatural, and one of the primary reasons so many people are experiencing so much chronic *dis*-ease. For those who are experiencing any kind of *dis*-ease, it would be best not to have these troublesome foods at all until your system is stronger. In brief, the list of *Foods to Limit* includes, but is not limited to:

- wheat
- dairy
- soy
- stimulants: sugars, salt, caffeine, chocolate, alcohol

Volumes have been written and could be said about each of these substances, and there is a substantial amount of debate associated with each as well. As with the meat eating issue, I tend to take a position somewhere in the middle. Although you may consider it extreme to advocate having these foods only 1-3 times a week, you must remember that eating these foods to the degree that we are eating them, often in place of other foods that are necessary for proper nutrition, is *way* out of balance. There are many natural healthcare practitioners who recommend not having foods on this list at all, ever. I think this is unrealistic, and although I agree it is wise to take these foods out of your diet if you are having any health conditions, once your body is stronger and back in balance, I think it is possible for many people to include these foods in their diet on a limited basis without compromising their health.

As you read through each of the following you will have a better understanding as to why I recommended curtailing consumption of these foods. We will also discuss how to rotate or eliminate them from your diet and let your body tell you how it feels about them in the next chapter.

Nature's garden provides a great variety of foods, and we need this variety to meet the nutrient needs of the many specialized cells, tissues and organs of the body.

Without variety we can't be healthy, we can't meet the chemical needs of the body.

Dr. Bernard Jensen

wheat

Regardless of whether or not you have a known or suspected allergy, sensitivity, or intolerance to wheat, it is wise for *everyone* to limit this staple grain for several reasons. First, we eat *way* too much wheat in this country. For many it is the only grain they ever eat. This is problematic because it means missing out on the many nutrients that other grains have to offer. In addition, eating the same foods over and over, as we learned earlier, can tax the system, deplete specific enzyme stores, and lead to the development of food intolerances.

Furthermore, unless you are the very rare person who cooks up bowls of wheat berries, which is its whole grain form, *all* of the wheat being served up in this country is processed — the overwhelming majority of which is *highly* processed into white refined flour. This devitalized anti-nutrient is such an aberration from its natural state that it is included in the upcoming list of *Things to Avoid*. Unfortunately, even many of the products labeled 'whole wheat' are themselves highly processed and also frequently contain white refined flour and refined sugars as well. Check the ingredients label to know for sure what you are getting.

In addition, wheat in any form, processed or not, is challenging to digest and eliminate due to its high gluten content mentioned earlier. Of course, this is why we like it so much, too. All that gluten is what makes breads and pastries so fluffy, doughy, and delicious. Wheat is the most ideal grain for making baked goods and pastas. The problem is, while all that gluten may make it easy to create a variety of lovely processed foods, it is not at all easy for the human body to process and the result is anything but lovely.

Because it is so difficult to digest and eliminate, wheat is a notorious mucous-producer and inflammatory agent. In addition to causing and contributing to a host of *dis*-eases including arthritis, sinusitis, constipation, diarrhea, irritable bowel syndrome, Celiac and Chron's disease, fatigue, candida, liver and gallbladder congestion, mental disorders, insomnia, and suppressed immune function, in Chinese medicine wheat is also considered to be one of the primary causes of depression. Regardless of whether or not you are suffering from these or any other symptoms, everyone can benefit from limiting wheat in their diets or going completely wheat-free. Try it and see!

Population studies show that arthritis is most common in countries where wheat is the staple food.

Wheat is possibly the most common arthritis aggravating allergen and definitely near the top of the most allergenic food list.

Scientists have discovered that many people, including some who have never had arthritis before experience arthritis symptoms in a relatively short time when an extract of wheat is placed under the tongue.

Lauri Aesoph, N.D.

Years ago it was very difficult to adopt a wheat-free diet. When I was first diagnosed as being sensitive to wheat and went in search of wheat-free products to replace my daily bread, I mail ordered fresh baked goods (this was before the convenience of online internet shopping) from a company in California who would send their pricey products packed in dry ice. Today, however, it is easier than ever before to go wheat-free or at least to rotate or limit its intake. In addition to a variety of whole grains and whole grain flours now widely available, there is an abundant array of wheat and also gluten-free pastas and baked goods now on the market as well. These products are readily available at all health food stores today, and also increasingly found at regular supermarkets.

When you enjoy these whole grain alternatives, you will not only be giving your system a break from wheat and white refined flour, but you will also be giving your body more of the beneficial nutrients and fiber it so desperately needs to function properly. Refer back to the *Suggested Foods* section for a list of both gluten and non-gluten grains to choose from, and look to the *Recipes* section for how to cook them whole.

Eat a wide variety of grains, including non-gluten grains, reduce or eliminate wheat from your diet, and see how quickly your energy, digestion, and elimination improve. You'll feel better and lose weight too!

> ...dairy products shouldn't occupy the prominent place that they do in the USDA Food Pyramid, nor should they be the centerpiece of the national strategy to prevent osteoporosis.
>
> Dr. Walter Willett

dairy

Like wheat, dairy ranks as one of the most common food allergens and is also eaten *way, way* too much to be healthy in this country. The average per capita consumption of dairy products is 580 pounds per person, per year, which means the actual individual consumption is not quite as much, but an enormous amount nonetheless. There is a reason that wheat, dairy, and soy (which we will discuss next) top the list of the most common food allergens. They are difficult for the body, *any* body, to process. Once again, whether or not you have a known or suspected allergy, sensitivity, or intolerance to dairy it is wise for *everyone* to limit its consumption for several reasons.

Virtually everything that has just been said about wheat can be said about dairy products as well. Like wheat, dairy is also very mucous producing, which clogs the tissues and organs of the body, resulting in congested and inflammatory conditions. Dairy products are most notorious for causing or exacerbating any kind of sinus or respiratory conditions, including sinusitis and asthma, and are best completely avoided whenever someone is suffering from acute respiratory ailments including bronchitis, a cold or the flu. They are also notorious for causing acute and chronic gastrointestinal distress such as gas, bloating, constipation, diarrhea, acid reflux, and liver/gallbladder disorders. Regular or excessive consumption of dairy products can also cause weight gain, weaken the immune system, and cause or contribute to inflammatory conditions such as arthritis and bursitis.

It is important to remember that symptomatic reactions to common food allergens can manifest differently for different people and dairy is no exception. In addition to the preceding list, dairy consumption may be responsible for or contribute to *any* symptom or *dis*-ease you may be experiencing

Compounding the challenge of its allergenic nature, most commercial dairy products on the market today contain synthetic hormones and antibiotics now commonly used as part of dairy and livestock production. Ingestion of these harmful substances carry with them another whole set of problems that we will discuss in the next segment, *Things to Avoid*. Because of the problems associated with hormone and antibiotic ingestion, on those occasions when you do indulge in dairy, be sure the products are organic. The few extra cents you will pay is well worth it.

Also take into consideration that many people, depending on the nature of their sensitivity, do better with some forms of dairy than others. For example, people who are lactose intolerant often cannot have the more liquid forms of dairy such as milk or sour cream, which have a higher lactose content, without immediate and pronounced gastric distress, but have little to no immediate trouble with hard cheeses. Experiment to see what works best for you, all the while keeping in mind that overall limitation of all forms of dairy is your healthiest choice.

I realize that this recommendation may completely contradict what you have been told since you were a small child. "Drink your milk, it's good for you" is indelibly etched upon most of our American minds. For several decades now the dairy industry has done a very good job of leading us to believe that

Contrary to advertising, dairy products are not even a desirable source of calcium.

Absorbability is poor because of pasteurizing, processing, high fat content, and an unbalanced relationship with phosphorus.

Hormone residues and additives from cattle-raising practices also mean that calcium and other minerals are incompletely absorbed.

In cattle tests, calves given their own mother's milk that had first been pasteurized, didn't live six weeks!

Linda Page, N.D.
Healthy Healing

milk and other dairy products are a staple food that we can't live without. Through relentless advertising and marketing campaigns disguised as educational in nature, they have been successful in creating a cultural climate that upholds milk and dairy products as nourishing wonder foods that if excluded from the diet will result in physical calamity. However, this simply is not true.

Consult with the top experts on nutrition who base their knowledge on sound information and research, rather than parroting marketing ploys, and you will find few who disagree with the notion of limiting the amount of dairy, including milk, in one's diet. For example, Dr. Walter Willett, a trained physician and current head of Harvard's Department of Nutrition, states in his recent book, *Eat, Drink, and Be Healthy*, "...there are more reasons *not* to drink milk in large amounts than there are to drink it. I don't recommend it as a beverage for adults and believe you should think of milk as an optional food..."

With regard to the issue of adequate calcium intake, once again I refer to Dr. Walter Willett's book, *Eat, Drink, and Be Healthy*, which contains an entire chapter on this topic entitled *Calcium: No Emergency*. This informative chapter debunks the myth that we are a country suffering from an acute lack of calcium resulting in high rates of osteoporosis. Dr. Willett points to the *National Dairy Council* advertising campaigns as the source of this myth, which has subsequently been expounded upon by the supplement industry pushing the latest and greatest source of calcium in convenient pill form.

"For starters, there isn't a calcium emergency. When it comes to calcium in the diet, the United States is near the top of the list of per capita calcium intake, second only to some Scandinavian Countries and parts of Latin America...," Dr. Willett states in this chapter. "Unfortunately, there's little proof that just boosting your calcium intake to the high levels that are currently recommended will prevent fractures. And all the high-profile attention given to calcium is distracting us from strategies that really work....Curiously, countries with the highest average calcium intake tend to have higher, not lower, hip fracture rates," he goes on to say.

We don't have to look far to see proof of this. Many cultures eat little to no dairy and yet have very low rates of osteoporosis. Asian cultures are a good example.

Cute milk-mustache ads aside, worldwide research increasingly indicates that milk consumption, especially in childhood, can lead to very serious problems: diabetes, heart disease, infant anemia, Crohn's disease, M.S., infertility, and asthma.

There are several good reasons for all of us to minimize the use of milk products whether we can "stomach" them or not.

Julia Ross
The Diet Cure

If you are not convinced and are still concerned about getting enough calcium, there are many other foods that provide even more calcium than dairy products, and in a much more bioavailable form. Green foods and sea vegetables are two such foods. They can be included in your meals and also taken as whole food supplements.

As far as what to put on your cereal in the morning, one of the best alternatives is oat milk. Among the dairy alternatives, to many people it has a taste and texture that is most like cow's milk. Some people can't even tell the difference. Almond or rice are two other recommended choices. I do not recommend soy milk, however, for reasons we will discuss shortly.

Keep in mind that most of these milk substitutes are highly processed and not always the best or most nourishing choice for the body. Water, tea, fruit and vegetable juices are your best choice for beverages. Cold, dry, sugary sweet cereal with cow's milk or even milk substitute is one of the worst choices for starting the day anyway. Use these alternatives as transition foods or once-in-awhile treats, and gradually move onto even healthier choices. When you do buy these milk substitutes, be sure to check the label and always buy the brand with the best overall ingredients and the least amount of added sweeteners. The original or plain variety is usually your best bet where sugar content is concerned.

Goat's milk and goat cheese is another alternative for some people. It is generally easier to digest and less taxing to the body than cow's milk, but still wise to keep to a minimum. Coconut milk is another fabulous alternative that is at the top of my list along with coconut oil. In Thailand people drink coconut milk with the same frequency that we drink cow's milk in this country, and have comparatively low rates of obesity, heart disease, and osteoporosis. They're obviously doing something right and we could take some pointers.

As for other cheese substitutes, I haven't found any good choices. There are a variety of substitutes now on the market usually made from either soy, almonds, rice, or oats. But quite frankly, none of them comes anywhere near the taste or texture of the real stuff and I'm not convinced that they are any better for your insides than the cheese you are trying to avoid. With the exception of soy cheese, which I don't recommend at all, try a couple different cheese alternatives and see if they do anything for

Foods that may look familiar have in fact been completely reformulated.

What we eat has changed more in the last forty years than in the previous forty thousand..

Eric Schlosser
Fast Food Nation

you, once again being mindful that they are processed foods and best kept to a minimum.

Or consider doing what I do, which is to do without the substitutes and enjoy a bit of organic cheese 1-3 times a week in keeping with this notion of having dairy on a limited basis. For some people it may be wise to have it even less or not at all. Experiment to find what's best for you, and know that whatever you discover may change in the future as your body changes. But whatever you do, keep your dairy consumption well below the culturally popular 580 pounds per capita consumption per year if you want to restore or maintain your health, energy, and natural weight.

soy

Like dairy, soy has enjoyed a media and marketing blitz that has become prevalent and enduring. People frequently ask me about soy, expecting that I will respond with a simple "it's good" or "it's bad" for you. It's like asking if potatoes are good for you and if I say yes, surmising from there that potatoes in any form from French fries to potato chips to Pringles are, therefore, good for you. Because this is not the case, instead I reply with a sigh, and then say "soy — oh, boy!" because the answer is a little more complicated than it's good or bad for you. To simplify and separate fact from fiction, following are some things to consider about soy.

Soy is one of the most common food allergens because it contains a protein enzyme (trypsin) inhibitor that prevents it and other nutrients from being properly digested. People with compromised digestive, eliminative, and immune function are especially susceptible. Symptoms range from digestive disturbances such as gas and bloating to severe depression and anxiety, and every other conceivable symptom that may be associated with food allergies or sensitivities. Regardless of any health benefits you may have heard associated with soy, if you have an allergy or intolerance to soy and can't digest it properly (and most Westerners can't!) it won't do you any good and may, in fact, be causing you harm.

It has become a popular trend for people to switch from dairy products to soy milk and other soy products thinking they are doing themselves a favor when, more often than not, they are

---

Today, an alarming 60% of the food on America's supermarket shelves contain soy derivatives (i.e., soy flour, textured vegetable protein, partially hydrogenated soy bean oil, soy protein isolate).

Gerson Institute Newsletter Volume 14 #3

simply trading in one set of symptoms for another (or experiencing the same symptoms, just trading in the cause). Unfortunately, when this happens, people often do not recognize soy as the culprit because they have been led to believe that soy is *so* good for you.

To compound the problem, more than two-thirds of America's soy is genetically engineered. Data published by Monsanto in the *Journal of Nutrition*, March 1996, shows that relative to conventional soy meal, Roundup Ready soy meal contains 27% more trypsin inhibitor, meaning it has even greater potential for setting off allergic reactions and digestive disturbance. In 1999, the York Nutritional Lab in the U.K. attributed a 50% increase in soy allergies to the fact that British consumers had started eating large amounts of imported genetically engineered (GE) soybeans the previous year.

To offset its allergenic nature, soy is best consumed in a fermented form such as miso, tempeh, natto and soy or tamari sauce. Fermentation reduces soybean's enzyme inhibitors to some degree, making it easier to digest and less likely to cause reactions. There are also fermented soy protein powders now available at health food stores. Sprouted soy is also easier to digest and assimilate, and therefore a better choice as well. Tofu, which is known to block mineral absorption, is best eaten warm with a little fish or other animal protein to offset this effect and increase digestibility.

Unfermented soy products, which is what people are primarily eating in this country today, are highly allergenic and best eaten only on a rotational basis—and not at all by those who are sensitive to soy or have weakened digestion and elimination. Similarly, products such as soy flour, soy powders (other than the fermented or sprouted variety), soy grits, soy flakes, soy nuts, and soy nut butter are also best avoided by those who are intolerant or have compromised digestion as they have not had the trypsin inhibitor removed and are, consequently, allergenic. Soy cheeses and soy milks are highly processed food items that often contain poor-quality oils and refined sweeteners. As a result, they are best avoided as well. Milks made from oats, rice, almonds and coconut milk are a better choice for dairy alternatives, especially if you make them at home.

Evidence is mounting that soy allergies are on the rise because of genetic engineering.

The York Nutritional Laboratories in England – one of Europe's leading laboratories specializing in food sensitivity - found a 50% increase in soy allergies in 1998, the very year in which genetically engineered beans were introduced to the world market.

Kaayla T. Daniel, The Whole Soy Story

There are literally billions of dollars of influence in the edible oil industry that is promoting soy's use in natural medical circles so it's use can then be promoted in the general medical public.

They are even able to fool otherwise knowledgeable natural medical physicians.

Dr. Joseph Mercola

In addition to the allergenic nature of soy, there is the issue of its estrogenic properties, which has fostered much debate. Asian women have very low rates of menopausal complaints, heart disease, breast cancer and osteoporosis. The soy industry, with sketchy evidence to support their claims, attributes this to soy foods being a regular part of the Asian diet. These claims, which have subsequently become widely known and accepted due to massive ad and media campaigns, disregard extensive research that shows otherwise. They also disregard other dietary and lifestyle factors at work in Asian cultures.

First of all, there are many Asian populations that do not eat soy as a regular part of their diet, yet still enjoy low rates of the *dis*-eases mentioned above. Among those who do eat soy regularly, fermented soy products such as those mentioned are what is primarily consumed. Traditional Asian populations aren't downing quarts of overly sweetened, highly processed soy milk or popping supplements containing concentrated soy isoflavones, as is becoming popular in this country. Even more important to note, the traditional Asian diet primarily consists of whole, fresh, natural foods, including sea vegetables, which are packed with vital nutrients and one of the richest sources of absorbable calcium. They also eat a lot of fish, small amounts of meat, and little to no dairy products or processed foods. This diet is in stark contrast to the *Standard American Diet*, which primarily consists of processed foods high in sugar, fat, sodium, and exorbitant amounts of meat and dairy products frequently produced with synthetic hormones and antibiotics and, of course, *zero* sea vegetables.

Unfortunately, the media and advertising blitz that has taken place touting the health benefits of soy has been so pervasive that the other side of the debate, including research linking soy to a host of adverse health conditions such as breast cancer and memory loss, is rarely heard or considered.

For more on this topic, once again I refer to Dr. Willett's book, *Eat, Drink & Be Healthy: The Harvard Medical School Guide to Healthy Eating,* which devotes an entire segment to the effects of soy, including an overview of studies that have been done. Dr. Willett's final words on the topic pretty much sum it up: "I'm still a bit cautious about soy, specifically about eating a lot of it....treat concentrated soy supplements or isoflavone pills with the same caution as you would a totally untested new drug...given how little we know about its effect on breast cancer and memory loss, it's wise not to go overboard eating soy products."

Dr. Willett's thoughts on soy, dairy products, and calcium, not only shed light on these specific topics, but also point to larger issues. Namely, something's wrong in paradise when the intentionally misleading and manipulative voice of food industry advertising and media sound bytes has become so loud it drowns out the voice of recommendations put forth by Harvard, one of the world's most respected institutions.

Most of the recent hoopla about the benefits of soy is not based on sound nutritional research, but rather on the interests of a booming industry that is making a gold mine on a cheap, versatile, highly profitable commodity. Don't fall prey to the soy industry's antics. As with any of the most common food allergens (wheat, dairy, soy, corn, sugar), if you are going to include soy in your diet, do so on a rotational basis, consuming it no more than once every 4-5 days (never daily!) in the most natural, bioavailable forms described above. This will allow the body adequate processing time and reduce the likelihood of developing or exacerbating sensitivities and other problems.

stimulants (i.e., sugars, salt, caffeine, chocolate, alcohol)

We have already gone over the detriments of regular and habitual consumption of stimulants in *Eating-for-Health Guideline #2: eliminate or relegate stimulants to rare occasions.* I would be remiss, however, if these extreme foods were not included in this list of *Foods to Limit.* So just a little reminder and reinforcement to keep these items to a minimum or eliminate them completely in order to maintain a balanced, energetic body-mind system, and reverse or prevent *dis*-ease.

Also, remember to distinguish between those stimulants that may be considered foods and those that are not. On those occasions when you do indulge, stick with those that are of the whole, fresh, natural foods variety such as honey or maple syrup, rather than white refined sugar, for example. And of course, absolutely avoid those stimulants that cannot be considered food at all, some of which are listed among the *Things to Avoid,* which we will discuss next.

Alcohol, which is a chemical cousin of sugar, also upsets blood sugar levels.

So do stimulants such as tea, coffee, cola drinks, and cigarettes.

These substances, like stress itself, stimulate the release of adrenalin and other hormones that initiate the "fight or flight" response, preparing the body for action by releasing sugar stores and raisng blood sugar levels...

Patrick Holford
Optimum Nutrition Bible

things to avoid

...like the plague! Following is a partial list of some of the most health compromising substances found in processed foods today. These are all substances that you would be wise to avoid putting in your body at all costs. While the previous list of *Things to Limit* are in fact foods, the following list of *Things to Avoid* are not. Unfortunately, popular brand pseudofoods are filled with them. Eating only natural brand processed foods available at natural foods stores and also increasingly found at conventional grocery stores will greatly reduce the chances of running into these health robbers. However, check labels carefully to ferret out fake health food brands as we discussed earlier. These substances are not food, don't eat them!

In brief, the list of *Things to Avoid* includes but is not limited to the following:

- refined sugars
- white refined flour
- refined salt
- the bad fats
- nitrates & nitrites
- sulfites
- monosodium glutamate (msg)
- artificial sweeteners
- artificial colorings, flavorings & preservatives
- pesticides, herbicides, hormones & antibiotics
- genetically modified organisms (GMO's)

Although we have already discussed the detrimental effects of anti-nutrient pseudofoods in general, it is worthwhile to familiarize yourself with the following specific list of substances regularly contained in these non-foods to gain an even greater understanding, and further increase your awareness and ability to make wise food choices.

refined sugars

It is said that if white refined sugar were put before the FDA today it would not be approved. Unfortunately, white refined sugar and other refined sugars are a multi-billion dollar industry that isn't going away any time soon. Refined sugars are found in just about every processed food today.

Although we rarely, if ever, hear about this in the news media, the fact is that toxins are causing more health problems than most of us realize.

Toxins are chemicals that disrupt biochemical, cellular function and include artificial ingredients, heavy metals, chemical compounds and byproducts of industry.

They include dioxins, fluoride, chlorine, mercury, PCBs, poisonous gasses, formaldehyde, food chemicals (stabilizers, preservatives, etc.) and lead, to name but a few of thousands.

Dr. Vic Shayne

As simple carbohydrates lacking in fiber and nutrients, refined sugars are anti-nutrients that deplete the body of vitamins, minerals, and enzymes. They also cause a dramatic rise and rapid fall in blood sugar levels. Eating these simple carbohydrates is like driving a car with a stuck accelerator: you speed around for a short time, then run out of gas. Regularly fueling your body with quick-burning refined sugars is associated with numerous health conditions, including major diseases such as Type 2 diabetes, obesity, heart disease, cancer, and osteoporosis as well as lesser *dis*-eases such as fatigue, allergies, PMS/menopausal complaints, digestive and eliminative problems, arthritis, asthma, insomnia, depression, hyperactivity, learning disorders, and more.

Check ingredient labels for sugar and its equivalents, including sucrose, high-fructose corn syrup, corn syrup, dextrose, glucose, fructose, and maltose. And don't be fooled by processed foods you find at the natural foods store that are sweetened with refined sugars such as brown sugar, cane juice (evaporated, dried, raw, or milled), muscovado sugar, Turbinado sugar, Sucanat, or Demerara sugar. Their names may convey a healthier image, but these are all still refined sugars and should be avoided. When you do indulge in sweets, stick with the natural sweeteners listed earlier in the list of *Suggested Foods*, keeping these to a minimum as well.

> Refined sugar is 99.4 to 99.7 percent pure calories – no vitamins, minerals, or proteins, just simple carbohydrates.
>
> Nancy Appleton
> Lick the Sugar Habit

white refined flour

Similar to refined sugars, white refined flour is a simple carbohydrate that quickly breaks down into sugar when consumed. Remember the experiment you did as a kid in elementary science class where you took a bite of Saltine cracker, and held it in your mouth to see what would happen? What happened was the taste went from a salty cracker to sweet as sugar within a matter of seconds; the lesson being to demonstrate how quickly white refined flour and refined grains break down into sugar. This happens because the refining process has broken down and stripped the once whole wheat grain, a nutritious complex carbohydrate that is slowly metabolized by the body, into a simple, refined carbohydrate that is now an anti-nutrient. As such, it will not only deplete the body of vitamins and minerals, but will also raise blood sugar as it is quickly metabolized.

Many food items made with white refined flour also have refined sugar added to the mix, especially breads and other baked goods. In addition, white refined flour is processed with toxic substances such as bleach (how do you think it gets white?) and has a high gluten content as discussed earlier. You made paste out of white refined flour, not whole wheat flour, for a reason. With its fiber removed and gluten remaining, white refined flour is the perfect ingredient for making a sticky paste that is great for childhood art projects, but not so great for trying to process through your body. For all these reasons, white refined flour and other refined grains are included in the stimulant category, as well as this list of *Things to Avoid.*

> If the label doesn't say "100%" whole wheat, chances are the bread has more white than whole-grain flour.
>
> Nutrition Action Healthletter, 10/2001

As you start to move away from food products made from white refined flour, be aware that because it is a simple carbohydrate, much like sugar, white refined flour can be addictive in nature. You may need to clear it from your system in order to eliminate cravings, as we will discuss in the next chapter. Also be aware that many pseudofood products sport misleading verbiage on the front label, such as "rich in whole grain" or "made with natural whole grain." A closer look at the ingredients label on the back, however, may reveal another story. Many will list as the first ingredient either "white refined flour," "unbleached flour," or "enriched wheat flour," all of which are refined flour and are best avoided.

refined salt

Many people have cravings for refined table salt as well, because it is another unnatural substance that acts as an addictive stimulant in the body. Refined salt has been processed at very high temperatures and had all the naturally occurring trace minerals removed except for sodium and chloride. Refined table salt is comprised of 99% sodium chloride, plus toxic additives. Sodium chloride causes electrolyte imbalance and prevents nutrients from being transported to the cells of the body, which can cause water retention and inflammation.

Natural unrefined sea salt (*real* salt) on the other hand, contains over 84 essential minerals, including naturally occurring iodine. It helps nutrients to reach the cell interior and does not cause water retention, inflammation, or cravings. Look for fine or coarsely ground natural sea salt available in shakers or in bulk at health food stores. Substitute it for refined table salt in cooking and to flavor foods and you will also be substituting health consequences for health benefits.

the bad fats

In contrast to the essential fatty acids that are beneficial 'fats that heal,' there is another group of harmful 'fats that kill.' This group includes *saturated fats* such as those contained in meat and dairy products, which may be harmful when consumed in excess; and *trans fatty acids* or *hydrogenated* fats, which are created when manufacturers heat liquid oils at high temperatures or otherwise alter them to extend their shelf life. These man-made fats are found in most processed foods (another good reason to avoid processed foods!) such as margarine, commercial vegetable oils, peanut butter, roasted nuts, potato and tortilla chips, cookies, crackers, pastries, frosting, salad dressings, and more. Even natural brand processed foods often contain these health-robbing fats. Fried foods would also be considered *fats that kill,* as frying foods damages otherwise healthful oils creating free radicals that are harmful to the body.

Poor quality fats have been associated with a host of *dis-eases* in the body including cardiovascular disease, obesity, impaired immunity, increased free radical production, increased cholesterol levels, infertility, diabetes, and cancer. In addition, they also inhibit the body's ability to make use of the beneficial fats or essential fatty acids and are a major cause of digestive disturbance. For this reason it is smart to avoid these "bad" fats and consume only the good fats such as the essential fatty acids and healthful oils listed in the *Suggested Foods* and *Dietary Basics* sections.

nitrates & nitrites

These nasty little toxins are primarily used as color fixatives for processed meats such as bacon, sausage, hot dogs, cold cuts, meat spreads, deviled and cured ham, and smoke-cured tuna and salmon. High levels of nitrates can also be found in vegetables that have been grown in soil heavily fertilized with nitrate fertilizers. The biggest problem associated with nitrates and nitrites is that when they combine with stomach saliva and food substances, they create nitrosamines, which are powerful cancer-

If you are a fat addict, your real problem probably isn't that you are eating too much fat, it's that you aren't eating enough of the right type.

You are probably so deficient in certain essential, healthful fats that your body continually calls for oily, creamy foods, hoping that you will eventually swallow the particular kind of fat that it really needs.

Julia Ross
The Diet Cure

causing agents. In addition, many people experience acute reactions to these carcinogens, often in the form of headaches, irritability, or fatigue. Because of their carcinogenic nature, food manufacturers voluntarily removed nitrates and nitrites from baby foods in the 1970's. However, the FDA's efforts to ban them completely in 1980 were thwarted by the manufacturer's claims that there are no adequate substitutes. An interesting claim when you consider that there are numerous brands of processed meats readily available at health food stores that do not contain them. These are your best choice when it comes to processed meats, and fresh, organic meats are even better!

sulfites

Sulfites are added to foods as both a color fixative and preservative. The Food and Drug Administration estimates that one out of every hundred people is sulfite-sensitive. Asthmatics are particularly at risk. Reactions range from severe to mild, and may include acute asthma attack, loss of consciousness, anaphylactic shock, diarrhea, nausea, brain fog, muscle aches, headaches, and extreme fatigue. In addition, seventeen fatalities occurred as a result of sulfite ingestion before the FDA finally banned the most dangerous uses of sulfites, and set strict limits on other uses in 1986.

Sulfites are still found in a variety of cooked and processed foods, including baked goods, condiments, dried and glacéed fruit, jam, gravy, dehydrated or pre-cut or peeled fresh potatoes (often used to make French fries or hash browns), molasses, shrimp, and soup mixes and also in beverages, such as beer, wine, hard cider, and even some fruit and vegetable juices. Although there have been no sulfite-related deaths reported since 1990 and the reports of severe reactions has declined significantly, many people experience mild to moderate reactions to sulfites contained in processed foods, often without realizing the cause. It is believed that sulfites accumulate in your system over time and, consequently, some people develop reactions to them later in life.

Because of their extreme allergenic nature, it is now required by law to list them on the ingredients label of packaged foods. They may show up as sulfites, sulfur dioxide, sodium bisulfate, or sodium and potassium metabisulfite. Dried apricots present the most obvious visual clue as to whether or not they

Researchers at Michael Reese Medical Center linked infinitesimal amounts of nitrite to cancer in young laboratory mice, especially in the liver and lungs...

Nitrosamines also produce cancer in hamsters similar to pancreatic cancers in humans.

Ruth Winter
Consumer's Dictionary of Food Additives

contain sulfites. Check the label of dried apricots that are bright orange in color and you are sure to find sulfites listed, in contrast to dried apricots that do not contain sulfites, which are a dark brown and a little more shriveled. Red wine is another favorite that also frequently contains sulfites, and is often the reason people experience an intensified hangover after drinking it. Natural brand processed foods, wines, and dried fruits that do not contain sulfites are available at health food stores.

Sulfites should be avoided by everyone, and should especially be avoided by asthmatics and children. Unfortunately, the FDA has yet to require restaurants to disclose which of their foods contain sulfites, which is yet another reason to patron restaurants that provide whole, fresh, natural foods whenever possible.

monosodium glutamate (msg)

We have discussed MSG in previous chapters. The following will provide even further insight into this menacing neurotoxin, as well as some effective natural antidotes to MSG reactions.

Since writing this book and otherwise educating people about the problems associated with MSG, I have received numerous testimonies and thank you notes from people who have benefited from eliminating processed foods that contain this chemical flavor enhancer. Although relief from migraines and other headaches are reported the most, many others have reported getting relief from everything from PMS to brain fog to depression by taking this one simple action.

Other symptoms that can be associated with MSG include burning sensation, numbness, tingling, chest pain or tightness, rapid heartbeat, drowsiness, foggy thinking, weakness, irritability and angry outbursts, pressure around eyes, blurred vision, runny nose, sneezing, shortness of breath, asthma attacks, frequent urination, swelling of the prostate or vagina, depression, dizziness, anxiety and panic attacks, hyperactivity, behavioral problems, ADD, lethargy, insomnia, seizures, chills and shakes, muscle and joint pain/stiffness, bloating, nausea, vomiting, and stomach or intestinal cramps.

MSG is now estimated to be added to over two-thirds of pseudofood brands. It is primarily found in soups, broths, bouillon, salad dressings, sauces, frozen meals, candy, seasonings,

hidden sources of MSG

Be aware that MSG (monosodium glutamate) in addition to being listed outright, may also be found in any foods that contain the following, which is all the more reason to avoid all foods with chemical additives:

autolyzed yeast

broths or bouillion

calcium caseinate

carrageen

enzyme modified flavoring

artificial flavoring

natural flavoring

gelatin

hydrolyzed oat flour, vegetable or protein

malt extract

malto-dextrin

plant protein extract

potassium glutamate

sodium caseinate

soy sauce

textured protein

yeast extract

seasonings

any foods that are fermented, protein fortified or ultra pasteurized ice cream and candy. Eating whole, fresh, natural foods and purchasing only natural brand processed foods is the best way to avoid MSG. Do check labels in the health food stores, however. Unfortunately, I have run across it in a few natural brand processed foods as well, usually listed as "autolyzed yeast extract," or "yeast extract." Although some people may have no reaction to MSG in these forms, those of us who are very sensitive to it may.

Especially if you are sensitive to this toxic flavor enhancer, you will want to familiarize yourself with the many names under which MSG may be hidden listed on the side bar. It is also important to understand that MSG accumulates in your tissues. So if you know or suspect you have a sensitivity to it, it would be wise to take measures to cleanse it from your system to help reduce your sensitivity. If you are not currently sensitive to MSG, also understand that because it accumulates in your system, there is a good chance that you may become sensitive to it down the road.

For acute reactions to MSG, also known as MSG syndrome, there are two remedies that I have found to be very effective antidotes. One is to drink spearmint tea and/or take a bath in spearmint tea. And the other is to take 50mg of vitamin B6 three times a day for a couple of days until symptoms subside. Although I don't normally recommend taking isolated nutrients, this is certainly a much better choice than taking over-the-counter medications, which usually don't give you relief anyway. There is also a homeopathic remedy for detoxifying MSG available online. This is helpful for flushing out accumulated MSG from your system and reducing overall sensitivity.

Everyone can benefit from increasing awareness about the problems associated with MSG and ways to avoid it; if not for themselves, then certainly for a loved one or someone else they may encounter. For this reason, I have included several references on this topic in the *Resources* section, including books and websites. People who know or suspect that they are sensitive to or having a problem with MSG will find these resources especially helpful.

> MSG toxicity is cumulative, so even if you don't react to it immediately, it could still be causing you problems that you're not aware of and won't be aware of for years to come.
>
> Marilu Henner

artificial sweeteners

When it comes to nourishing our bodies, it is not possible at this stage of our evolution to improve on what Mother Nature has provided for us to eat. While scientists have been successful in creating artificial sweeteners that may have little to no calories or little to no effect on blood sugar, they have not been successful in doing so without creating a multitude of harmful side effects at the same time.

For this reason, when it comes to artificial sweeteners — you name it, I don't recommend it. Whether it's Saccharin (*Sweet'n Low*), aspartame (*Equal, Nutrasweet, Spoonful*), sucralose (*Splenda*), Acesulfame K (*Sunette, Sweet One*), each of them is shrouded in controversy and reports of adverse reactions ranging from seizures to headaches to asthma attacks, to liver and kidney damage, and even weight gain. I have personally worked with a number of people who have been relieved of both depression and anxiety by going off diet soda that contains aspartame. None of these are food, they are all synthetic chemicals that have no business in your body.

There are volumes of information available on each of these artificial sweeteners. Do your own research and chances are, you will end up with more suspicions than confidance in these substances. Once again *when in doubt, do without*. There are so many natural sweeteners that we know for sure are safe, why take the chance?

When you get the urge for something sweet, have a piece of fruit. It's loaded with vitamins and minerals, packed with fiber, and naturally sweet and delicious. For baked goods or to sweeten your tea, use whole food sweetners such as those listed earlier including honey, maple syrup, and agave. If you are looking for a natural noncaloric sweetener that has little to no effect on blood sugar, go with Stevia or xylitol (birch sugar).

artificial colorings, flavorings & preservatives

Food additives of all kinds have long been suspected, and frequently proven to cause adverse health conditions including cancer, hyperactivity, ADHD, and allergic reactions. All pseudofood products, and many other products such as vitamins, pharmaceutical and over-the-counter drugs, including cold and cough syrups, toothpaste, and even skin care products (60% of

Do additional approved sweetening agents truly contribute to good health?

Do they really meet special dietary needs?

Or, do they merely further encourage poor dietary choices?

...There is no clear-cut evidence that sugar substitutes are useful in weight reduction.

On the contrary, there is some evidence that these substances may stimulate appetite.

Consumers' Research Magazine

which are absorbed through the skin), contain chemical additives that have been linked to numerous health problems. Children are especially at risk due to the smaller, more sensitive nature of their developing bodies, and the fact that most processed and junk foods geared to the younger set are loaded with artificial colorings, flavorings, and preservatives.

In the early 1970's, Dr. Benjamin Feingold, who was Chief Emeritus of the Department of Allergy at the Kaiser Foundation Hospital and Permanente Medical Group in San Francisco, was one of the first medical professionals to report diminished symptoms of hyperactivity and ADHD in children who eliminated additive-containing foods from their diet, especially artificial colorings. The Feingold Association was soon established as a non-profit organization to help children and adults apply proven dietary techniques for better behavior, learning and health. Their website, www.feingold.org, is a fabulous resource.

As we have seen, behavior problems aren't the only health risk associated with food additives, and children aren't the only ones who suffer from their effects. Because of the many health risks posed and general anti-nutrient status, adults and even family pets can certainly benefit from their elimination as well.

pesticides, herbicides, hormones & antibiotics

Although you won't find these listed on an ingredients label, the practice of using pesticides, herbicides, hormones, and antibiotics in agricultural production has become widespread in this country. Unfortunately, it is a practice that is having serious consequences we are only just beginning to realize and understand. Some of these consequences extend far beyond the mere individuals who are consuming the foods produced with these harmful substances, consequences that are upsetting the natural balance of our precious ecosystems and will affect generations to come.

Many plastics, household chemicals, personal care products, and environmental toxins, pesticides, herbicides, hormones, antibiotics and other synthetic drugs, send manmade hormone-disrupting chemicals into our bodies and the natural environment. Although the extent to which this exposure affects human health is unknown, there is growing evidence that suggests it may be responsible for recent worldwide increases in health problems, including precocious puberty, breast and

Yellow 5 dye causes asthma, hives, and a runny nose.

A natural red coloring, cochineal (and its close relative carmine), causes life-threatening reactions.

Dyes can cause hyperactivity in sensitive children.

Michael Jacobson
CSPI

prostate cancer, infertility, low sperm counts, auto-immune diseases, and even osteoporosis. They are also linked to a host of lesser symptoms and *dis*-eases such as allergies, food intolerances, candida, learning disabilities, PMS and menopausal conditions. In addition, the food industry's excessive use of antibiotics for both therapeutic and livestock growth purposes is contributing greatly to the problem of antibiotic-resistant bacteria and viruses. Toxic chemical pesticides are similarly creating pesticide-resistant bugs.

It's unnerving to think that less than 100 years ago it took 4-5 years to bring cattle to slaughter. And now, with the help of enormous amounts of corn, protein supplements, and drugs, including growth hormones and antibiotics, it only takes 14 months. When you consider what these aberrant practices are doing to the animals who are subjected to them, it isn't too difficult to imagine the impact these practices could be having on our own bodies and our surrounding environment.

Whether it's animal products or produce, the best way to avoid toxic pesticides, herbicides, hormones, and antibiotics is to eat certified organic foods and those that state clearly on their labels that they do not use or contain these substances. For more information on this very serious topic, *Our Stolen Future: Are We Threatening Our Fertility, Intelligence, and Survival?*, by Theo Colburn is a well-documented book that presents an eye-opening overview. In addition, there are several other resources listed at the end of this book.

genetically modified organisms (GMO's)

You won't find these listed on food product labels either, despite the fact that over 90% of Americans say the FDA should require labeling of genetically modified organisms (GMO's), also known as genetically engineered (GE). Not surprisingly, strong lobbying on the part of the food industry has managed to prohibit such a requirement.

GMO's are a topic of much debate, a topic that looms over us like a dark cloud of uncertainty. The biggest problem — that we know of, thus far — associated with genetically modified foods in terms of the immediate effect on human health is a dramatic increase in their allergenic potential. In terms of environmental concerns, genetically engineered organisms cross-pollinate with other non-GMO crops and the subsequent

Hormone disrupters, like silent saboteurs, have invaded the highly sensitive endocrine systems of our children.

Whether from chemical exposure in the environment or from the hormone-laden meats and dairy products, or chemically laced personal care and household products, exposure to dangerous chemicals has now reached the highest level of exposure in the entire history of human civilization.

Is there any wonder why precocious puberty is a worldwide epidemic.

Sherrill Sellman

transmutation is irreversible. This is most alarming when you consider that the long-term consequences for both humans and the environment are, as yet, not fully known. What is eminently clear, however, is that there are problems (potentially catastrophic problems) associated with these Frankenfoods, as opponents often call them, and further testing and regulation are needed.

When in doubt, do without, is clearly not the motto of the biotech industry, the formulators of genetically modified organisms, as they are moving forward full steam ahead. This is a greedy, shortsighted move on their part. It is also unfortunate when you consider the damage that may be done is irreversible and has the potential to affect every living creature on the planet.

In addition to the health hazards, the biotech industry is undermining the livelihoods of farmers the world over, forcing them to purchase their patented seeds year after year, and suing them for exorbitant amounts if they don't. The practice of planting saved seed is a practice as old as farming itself; a practice that is a necessity for many farmers, especially those in underdeveloped nations who cannot afford to purchase new seed every year.

To avoid contributing to the unscrupulous endeavors of the biotech industry, and keep your family and the environment safe, once again, consume foods that are certified organic and clearly state that they use non-GMO ingredients. For the most up-to-date information on the biotech and organic foods industries, visit: www.OrganicConsumers.com. I also highly recommend *The Future of Food*, a fabulous documentary on this topic available at: www.TheFutureOfFood.com.

> Because of vested commercial interests, greed, convenience, apathy, and *gross* misinformation, far too many people have been lulled into believing that anything they can get down their throats is okay to put there.
>
> It's not.
>
> Harvey &
> Marilyn Diamond
> Fit for Life II

onward & upward

So as not to leave this chapter on a sour note, think back for a moment to all those luscious whole, fresh, natural foods we talked about at the beginning in the *Suggested Foods* section. Then move on to the next chapter, *Clear the Way*, and start clearing food cravings, sensitivities, and addictions, so you can more easily transition to eating more of these delicious, nutritious foods and live a healthier, happier, more vibrant life.

Chapter Nine

clear the way

Transitioning to Healthier Foods, Clearing Food Addictions, Cravings & Sensitivities

In addition to the primarily *mental* obstacles discussed earlier, people also face formidable *physical* obstacles when it comes to making healthy revisions in their diet. Food cravings and chemical dependencies to stimulants can bind people to bad foods like drug addicts are bound to their drug of choice, literally. This chapter lays out general tips and a step-by-step process for breaking these bonds and setting you free to make the transition to a healthier eating lifestyle with greater ease.

Everything you need to succeed, is now within your reach.

Unknown

First, we will talk about clearing your kitchen to create surroundings that will best support you. Then we will turn our attention inward to address probably the most formidable obstacle that anyone faces when it comes to changing their eating habits: food cravings and addictions. Next, you will learn how to cleanse and clear your system by following a basic elimination diet, which can also be used to identify and clear food intolerances, which often go hand-in-hand with cravings and addictions.

As you begin to implement what you learn in this chapter you will simultaneously begin to feel better and have more energy. Even more importantly, you will develop and empower yourself with an increased awareness and understanding of what is happening in your body in relation to the foods you eat. This new body awareness and know-how will become a powerful ally that will serve you for a lifetime. Dealing with the mental and social obstacles that often go along with making changes in your diet will become much, much easier when you have a handle on your internal physicality which is, in many cases, a prerequisite. How can you expect to deal with external obstacles over which you often have no control when you have not yet learned how to deal with internal obstacles, which are usually the only ones over which you do have control?

As you read through this chapter, remember that making lifestyle changes is a dynamic process that takes place over time. It is not recommended, or even possible, to do everything suggested here right away. Start with the things that call to you and use the *strategizing* process you learned earlier to devise a plan of action for what is right for you do at this time. The elimination diet in particular is something that most people have to work up to doing properly. Do, however, read through and familiarize yourself with everything offered here now, and return to it later when you are ready to take the next step.

Implementing the concepts presented in this chapter have been instrumental in my success and the success of countless others in being able to make dramatic and lasting dietary changes and creating a healthier way of life. Ultimately it's up to you to decide where to start, but if there were any one place I would most recommend you begin to clear the way to make this transition for yourself, it would be in your kitchen.

clear your kitchen

The single most powerful step you can take to transition to a healthier eating lifestyle is to clear your kitchen of all pseudofoods. There are basically two ways to go about this. Each has its own set of benefits and drawbacks. You must decide which is best for you.

The first and most effective approach is what I call making a clean sweep. You will need to schedule a block of time for this project, a good part of 1 or 2 days on the weekend is perfect, and collect a few sturdy boxes before you get started. Then you will literally make a clean sweep of all pseudofoods in your kitchen, removing them from all the nooks and crannies of your cupboards, pantry, refrigerator and anywhere else they may be

May you fully enjoy the benefits of your new knowledge and the resultant growth as you study and apply these materials, and may you enjoy the rewards to be found in sharing this information with those who you genuinely care for and who share a similar desire to enrich their lives.

Mark Percival

lurking, placing them in the boxes for removal as you go along. What you decide to do with this fake food after you have removed it is up to you. Donating it to a homeless shelter or local soup kitchen is a good idea. Although, I have had several people tell me that knowing what they know now about this weapon of mass destruction disguised as food, they couldn't bring themselves to give it away and inflict it on others. Consequently, they chose to discard it instead. While I completely understand their position, I am more of the mindset that if people are in a desperate situation, pseudofood is better than no food at all. Either way, the dilemma that this scenario presents is food for thought. The next step of the clean sweep process is, of course, to go to a natural foods store and replace these pseudofood items with their natural brand equivalent and some whole, fresh, natural foods.

The payoffs for making a clean sweep of your kitchen are big and immediate. You will see and feel a difference right away as your surroundings go from something that was detrimental to your health and well-being, to something that will support you. You will be setting the stage for a fresh start and exponentially increase your chances for success, just by taking this one simple step.

More importantly, over the next few days and weeks, now that you are no longer regularly consuming anti-nutrient, fake foods and are instead nourishing your body with more real foods, you will start to notice a dramatic difference in your internal environment as well. You're energy will increase and your body will start to feel better in many ways. I don't know anyone who has done a clean sweep of their kitchen (and I know many who have) that has ever regretted it or gone back to their old ways. In fact, the most enthusiastic testimonials I receive come from people who put in the time and money it takes to make a clean sweep of their kitchen.

This initial investment of both the time and money it takes to get the job done are, of course, the two biggest challenges associated with taking the clean sweep approach. Depending on the size of your family and how much food will need to be replaced, it can cost up to several hundred dollars and take the better part of 1 or 2 days, as mentioned.

Working up to a clean sweep and getting creative about obtaining the resources you may need is the way to go if time or

If you're like most people, 70% of the contents of your kitchen right now is unhealthy and has got to go.

But the good news is that there are healthy and tasty alternatives to *everything*!

The transition is easier than you think.

Marilu Henner
Healthy Life Kitchen

money are an issue. For example, asking for gift certificates to your local health food store in place of presents for Christmas or your birthday is one way to offset this cost. Or engage in a little strategic planning, as one client did, by scheduling a clean sweep after a group of relatives were scheduled to visit. She planned in advance to feed as much of the pseudofood that now occupied her kitchen to the visiting relatives, then replace it with natural brand foods after they left. This woman confessed that she didn't feel the least bit guilty about this plan because that is what they would have been eating anyway. As for the time factor involved, you can always hire someone to do a clean sweep for you if the cost is not an issue or enroll other household members to help. Whatever you can come up with to get the job done will be worth every minute and penny you spend.

Speaking of other household members, they can sometimes pose a challenge to the clean sweep strategy as well. The best way around this is to refer back to *Chapter 5 ~ Children & Others*, have a talk with them, and try to get them on board and involved with the process as much as possible. Or for those who are really brave, try just doing it and see if they even notice!

The second strategy for clearing your kitchen of unwanted pseudofoods and making the transition to healthier cuisine is a little less dramatic and, consequently, also produces less dramatic results. This next approach basically entails replacing non-food items with natural brand processed foods one-by-one as you run out. Obviously this will take some time. In addition to missing out on the fresh start psychological boost you derive from the clean sweep method, you won't get the quick and unmistakable improvements in your health and energy, as these changes will occur more gradually. The risk you take with this approach is that enthusiasm can wane, and there is an increased likelihood that you will abandon it before you ever get to experience the benefits. The benefits, of course, are that you won't have to invest an initial chunk of time and money as you do with the first strategy.

Doing a partial clean sweep of salty snack foods and sugary treats is another option. I don't know what the philosophers would say, but I believe that it is a universal law of human nature that if there is something in your cupboard or refrigerator that you like to eat, you're going to eat it! Or at the very least, it will be silently calling your name until it is eaten. For

Most people assume that healthy meals are more difficult and require more time to prepare than junk food.

The truth is that preparing healthy food doesn't have to be more burdensome or time consuming.

The trick is to design your kitchen so that healthy eating becomes simple and convenient.

Marilu Henner
Healthy Life Kitchen

this reason, the very least that you can do in terms of clearing your kitchen to make way for a more nutritious lifestyle is to keep snacks and treats you love, but know aren't good for you, out of the house. You don't have to swear off them completely, just have them when you go out or only bring in one cookie at a time, for example, rather than an entire box. Having them around is too much a temptation for most people, and constantly indulging in them is what perpetuates food cravings and addictions more than any other single factor.

clear your food cravings & addictions

There are many factors that can contribute to or cause food cravings and addictions. However, whether they arise from imbalanced blood sugar, which is often the case with sweets, food intolerances, nutritional deficiency, or in reaction to stimulants, such as caffeine, or neurotoxic additives such as MSG or aspartame, with rare exception, all food cravings and addictions stem from improper nutrition. Even what is labeled emotional eating, as we have already discussed, is most often caused by emotional imbalance, which was caused by biochemical imbalance, which was caused by improper nutrition. It *is* about the food. Understanding this is the first step toward freeing yourself from sometimes irrepressible desires for specific foods and even food in general.

Food cravings are your body's way of speaking to you. And although you are hearing these messages loud and clear, you must learn to *accurately* interpret them. Once again, while each message may relate to a specific factor, the bottom line is that food cravings are your body's way of begging you to feed it properly, and it won't stop begging until you do. It's that simple.

Processed foods of one kind or another are eaten excessively in this country, and in some cases, exclusively. This habit more than anything will cause your body to beg the loudest. You may interpret these messages as a desire for more of these foods, but in fact, your body is screaming for more *nutrients*, not more bad foods. The most poignant and concise explanation for how anti-nutrient, fake foods affect our appetite and create an insatiable desire for them is explained in the book *Fit for Life II*. In this sequel to the classic and highly recommended book *Fit for Life*, authors Harvey and Marilyn Diamond explain:

Eating unnatural substances brings about unnatural appetites that can never be satisfied.

Grace Purusha
The Five Essential Laws of Eating

The appestat is an organ located in the base of the brain. It is something like a thermostat. The appestat is responsible for your appetite. It constantly monitors the bloodstream for nutrients. When they are not present in the necessary amounts, you feel hungry. So what do you think happens when you eat food that has had its nutrient content destroyed? You fill up, but because the food is "empty" the appestat registers that you need still <u>more</u> food. You keep eating and eating but the appestat just doesn't turn off. The result is that familiar complaint, "I eat all the time but I'm still hungry." The body is tricked into thinking it needs more food when it's actually crying out for nutrients. Sadly, there is a beneficiary of this tragic situation — the people making and selling you the empty foods! Your apparently insatiable appetite is a result of the most detestable kind of manipulation of your body chemistry imaginable, and it's all done to increase profits while diminishing your health.

In the now famous documentary *Super Size Me*, viewers see this phenomenon unfold before their eyes as Morgan Spurlock develops strong cravings for the McDonald's pseudofood he has committed to eating exclusively for thirty days. This is a fantastic film that is both informative and entertaining. It is a must-see for everyone, especially those who have an affinity for fast food. Go to: www.SuperSizeMe.com for more information.

Most people who are having problems with food tend to spiral down into thinking something is wrong with them. As you begin to understand the internal machinations taking place in your body such as those just described, you will also begin to understand, as I did, that there is nothing wrong with you. There is something wrong with the food you're eating.

Having this understanding will help you to become a third-party observer to the powerful, seemingly uncontrollable forces of food cravings and addictions. Which is another issue around which you can play a little game with yourself. A little game that could go something like this: first notice that you are feeling like you could strangle somebody for a piece of chocolate (soda, cup of coffee, etc.); or find yourself frantically rifling through the cupboard where you are praying you will find a forgotten candy bar or bag of cheese puffs. Then STOP! Take a

---

So many of our mistakes come from misinterpreting what our body is trying to tell us...

Even if you are not willing to do what you know your body is asking of you, tell yourself the truth anyway.

This is the beginning of gaining skill.

Awareness is the key to change.

Grace Purusha
The Five Essential Laws of Eating

deep breath, center yourself and say, "Gee, isn't it interesting that I could strangle somebody for a little ol' piece of chocolate (soda, cup of coffee, etc.). " Or "Gee, isn't it interesting that I am rifling through the cupboard like a maniac looking for anything I can get my hands on that will suppress this unrelenting desire I am experiencing." Then ask yourself, "What is my body *really* trying to tell me?"

Playing this little game with yourself will help you to stop operating on automatic pilot, and if you're lucky, will also at times stop you from nose diving into injurious foods with reckless abandon. But the most important thing you can do to help overcome irrepressible food desires is to start nourishing your body properly. Giving your body adequate amounts of the nutrients it requires and eliminating problematic foods is paramount to reducing and clearing unnatural food cravings and addictions. To make sure you are getting all the nutrients your body needs, review *Chapter 7 ~ The Basics* to see what foods you might not be getting enough of, or may be missing altogether.

You may also want to review *Eating-for-Health Guidelines #2 and #4* regarding stimulants and common food allergens, as these are the most notorious culprits when it comes to food cravings and addictions. We will be talking about how to identify and clear food intolerances and sensitivities and any associated cravings from them shortly. As for stimulants, in addition to the problems they present that you have already learned, consuming these substances can set up an imbalanced body chemistry that makes you crave other stimulants. For example, eating sweets can lead to cravings for salt as the body seeks balance, and vice versa. So staying away from these extreme foods in general is wise. Staying away from pseudofoods in general, especially those containing MSG and aspartame in particular, is also wise. These neurotoxins are known to induce cravings not only for more of the foods that contain them, but for other poor quality foods as well.

As for cravings for specific foods, they can be an indicator of specific nutrient deficiencies. Cravings for fatty foods such as potato chips, milk, cheese, ice cream and the like can be an indication that you are not getting enough essential fatty acids. Because it is so bitter, a craving for chocolate may mean that you need to eat more bitter foods such as green leafy vegetables. A desire for bitter foods or tart foods can also be a signal that the

> Overwhelming food cravings are the culprit behind every obese body, every broken diet, and every dietary-related disease.
>
> If we can stop the food cravings, the unhealthful eating habits will disappear.
>
> Doreen Virtue
> Constant Craving

body needs help with digestion. When it comes to chocolate, there is no doubt that you are also craving the added sugar, and must address this craving as well. A craving for sugar and other sweets can be a cry for overall nourishment. Sugar cravings may also indicate low blood sugar and a need for more protein or complex carbohydraes to stabilize it.

When used in combination with a nutrient-rich diet, certain herbs and whole food supplements can also help remedy food cravings and addictions.

Noni juice and *Berry Young Juice* are two whole food supplements at the top of my list for overall reduction and clearing of food cravings and addictions. Both nourish the body at a cellular level and for many people quiet the body's demand for poor quality foods unlike anything else. Because of their regenerating effect on the liver, they help with addictions of all kinds, including tobacco and alcohol. As with all supplements, some people will need to consume them regularly for some time before they see results while others will notice results right away. In addition to helping suppress food cravings, noni juice and *Berry Young Juice* are also therapeutic remedies for a number of physical complaints. Give them a try and see what works best for you. *Tahitian Noni* is the only brand I recommend because of its quality standards (see *Resources*). While *Berry Young Juice* is only available from the Young Living company (see *Resources*). It's primary ingredient is wolfberry, one of the world's most powerful antioxidants.

Green food supplements, when taken regularly, will also help stave off cravings by contributing to your overall nourishment. Barley grass in particular quells cravings for sweets because it helps balance blood sugar. In fact, it is recommended by the *American Diabetic Association* for just this reason.

In the realm of herbs, oatstraw, cinnamon bark, dandelion, lemon balm, skullcap and bergamot are all helpful for cravings and addictions in general. As for specifics, bergamot is especially helpful for easing caffeine and salt addictions, and anything that balances blood sugar will help clear cravings for sweets such as fennel, coriander and dill. There are also herbal combinations available for sugar cravings, caffeine and tobacco withdrawal.

Herbs are readily available in bulk, capsule and tincture form at all health food stores. However, my favorite way to access

Craving and overeating fatty foods, especially when you are trying not to, is a signal that something is wrong. The solution is not to cut out all fats, but to find the *right* fats.

Julia Ross
The Diet Cure

the benefits of nature's original medicine is in the form of therapeutic grade essential oils. Because they are so powerful and versatile, I keep a small arsenal of different kinds around the house at all times. You can apply them topically, diffuse them in the air, take them internally, and even cook with them. I had one client who put a few drops of bergamot oil on her feet every day and within only a few days her strong cravings for salt completely went away! *Therapeutic grade* essential oils must be purchased through independent distributors. My favorite are those made by Young Living Essential Oils (see *Resources*). The essential oils available at health food stores are primarily *perfume grade* and not recommended. Whatever form of herbs you choose to use, experiment with small doses of one at a time to see what works best or consult with a knowledgeable herbalist. If you are taking medications, be sure to check for any adverse herbal/drug interactions before you begin.

Homeopathic remedies can also assist in clearing food cravings and addictions. You can do some research and experiment with this approach on your own as well. However, because it is such a specialized modality, it is wise to consult with a qualified homeopath for help if you can. Taking essential fatty acid supplements may be indicated if you are craving fatty foods. Refer back to *Chapter 7 ~ The Basics* for more on this topic. As for taking vitamin supplements to help with cravings and associated nutrient deficiencies, although some advocate this approach, I do not. Isolated nutrients are unnatural and can lead to chemical imbalances and other problems. Finally, the general care of your body and mind are critical as well when trying to elude the clutches of cravings and addictions of any kind. Exercise, stress reduction and quality, supportive relationships can all help in this regard.

A helpful tip for overcoming your desire for certain foods in the psychological department is to stop thinking about them. When you find yourself thinking about how a particular food tastes — stop thinking about it! Just don't let your thoughts go there. Some people advocate smelling a forbidden food or having just one little bite and either swallowing it or spitting it out. You can experiment to see if this works for you (I know a couple people who swear by it), but this approach has never worked for me. You wouldn't tell a heroine addict to just shoot up a little bit

Instead of being eaten when we are physically hungry, food is now consumed to satisfy artificial cravings generated by a brain that isn't working right and whose receptor sites beg for synthetic stimulation from chemicals.

We eat, but we're never satisfied.

We're full, but we aren't contented.

Carol Simontacchi
The Crazy Makers

or just smell it, it would be all over. In my experience it is better to just not go there. Thoughts of these foods and cravings for them will go away, but not if you keep indulging in them. So, whether it's on a billboard or T.V. commercial or worse yet, sitting right in front of you, don't let your mind indulge in thoughts of how good whatever it is you're looking at would taste. Instead, train yourself to ignore it. You will naturally begin to take your thoughts away from poor quality addictive foods as your cravings and desire for them subsides. Making a little conscious effort to do so in the beginning will help things along.

Training yourself not to fantasize about foods is a skill well worth learning. But training yourself not to actually consume them is essential. Whether it's stimulants, pseudofoods, or foods to which you are intolerant, if you don't eliminate foods that are offensive to your system from your diet for at least the time it takes to restore strength and balance, you will never eliminate your desire and cravings for them, even if you are doing everything else right. Breaking the addictive cycle by clearing your system of the physical hold that poor quality foods have on you is what is absolutely necessary in order to truly free yourself from them.

cleanse & clear your system

Cleansing is an age-old concept for restoring health, energy, strength, and balance to the body-mind system that we have, unfortunately, lost sight of in our modern, medically-oriented society. But the most important factor associated with cleansing your system in terms of making the transition to a healthier eating lifestyle is that it is a very effective, often necessary tool for breaking the cycle of cravings and addictions to unwanted foods. Cleansing benefits every cell, tissue, organ, and system of the body by releasing stored waste and toxins, giving your bodily functions a rest, and improving digestion, assimilation, and elimination. As a result of cleansing, your body chemistry will inevitably change and you will lose the desire for poor quality addictive foods and stimulants as balance is restored and the cycle of addiction is broken.

To understand the concept of cleansing, think of your kitchen garbage disposal. If you are using it properly, you feed only enough food into it that it can easily grind and process. If, instead, you keep shoving food into it beyond its capacity to process it, what will happen? First it will slow down, then it may get stuck, and finally it will stop working altogether. So, the garbage will just keep piling up. The same thing happens with your digestive and eliminative system. If you keep shoveling food into it beyond its capacity to adequately digest and eliminate it, more than just your digestive system will start slowing down. You'll also have reduced energy, lowered immune function and will eventually develop a host of other maladies as well. This is especially true when you are shoveling in fake food that your system isn't equipped to process in the first place.

Even if you started eating absolutely pristinely today, you still have all the accumulated waste and chemical imbalances from yesterday to deal with. Just changing your diet and lifestyle will rectify much of this, but that will take consistent action over time and can sometimes take longer than most people want to wait; and some of it can only be released or brought into balance through an internal cleansing program designed to do the job. When you are not getting the results you want, as quickly as you want, the probability for being pulled back into old habits and addictions runs high. And this is where cleansing your internal environment can be a life-saver.

There are many different ways to cleanse the body, including herbal formulas, mono-diets, juice fasting, the Master cleanse (water and lemon juice fast), and colon irrigation. Often these different modalities are combined and are either geared to a general cleansing of the system, or to target specific organs or systems of the body such as the colon, liver/gallbladder, or urinary tract. There are also cleansing protocols designed to address specific conditions such as yeast overgrowth (candida) or parasitic infestations. These two particular conditions often show up together and are both major culprits when it comes to food cravings and sensitivities. They essentially cause people to crave the foods that feed them, primarily sugars, dairy products, and refined grains.

Generally speaking, cleansing the body on a regular basis is considered a part of ongoing self-care in the field of natural healthcare. In addition to helping clear food cravings and addictions, cleansing is especially in order for those who have had trouble losing weight or have been experiencing any kind of

I love the fish bowl metaphor: that you are only as healthy as the fluids in which your body cells swim.

In other words if you are sick you don't treat the fish you change the water.

Dr. Robert Youngs
Sick &Tired

chronic health condition, including arthritis, allergies, sinus trouble, or digestive and eliminative problems.

One method of cleansing that has recently been gaining in popularity is colon irrigation, which has been used as a part of healing protocols in cultures throughout the world since ancient times. Modern day colonics are the quickest, least troublesome, most effective method I know of for cleansing and restoring balance to an ailing body-mind. I highly recommend a series of colonics for anyone who is wanting to restore their health and energy. You can eat the best diet in the world and take herbs and supplements from here until the cows come home, but if you don't clear out all the accumulated waste in your system you'll never get on top of the situation. There are certain physical conditions that prevent some people from having them and there are also different colonic systems to choose from, depending on what is comfortable for you. Consult with a qualified colon hydrotherapist to learn more and see if colonics are right for you.

There are many books and resources available on the topic of cleansing. I have two favorites I would like to share. One is a phenomenal website called Curezone (www.curezone.com). It is a non-profit website filled with a variety of comprehensive information on cleansing, including some rather gruesome photographs (nothing like some of those to motivate you!), and active forums where people write in and ask questions and share their experiences. It has been a Godsend for many people with many different kinds of health problems, as you will discover when you read through some of the postings.

The other equally phenomenal resource on the topic of cleansing is a book entitled *The Amazing Liver Cleanse*, by Andreas Moritz. The information in this book, which primarily focuses on adequately cleaning out congestion in the liver/gallbladder, is key to reversing most any health condition. Because of our poor quality modern food culture, liver/gallbladder congestion is a problem for a majority of people, but unfortunately most never realize that this problem is at the root of what ails them. This is a short, easy-to-read book that makes a lot of sense, and is well worth the read no matter what you may or may not have going on in your body. Deeper kinds of cleansing such as the liver flushes described in Andreas Moritz's book, protocols suggested on the Curezone website, or colonics all require more research, a

---

Most people today are so toxic that fasting stirs old toxins up far faster than their already – overloaded elimination organs can handle.

Feeling worse is often the result.

Jon Matsen, N.D.
Eating Alive

commitment, and may also be something you need to experiment with and work up to doing.

The best place for anyone to start when it comes to cleansing is also the best method for identifying and clearing food cravings and sensitivities: a basic elimination diet. An elimination diet is also a wonderful tool to use in combination with many other kinds of cleansing, such as colonics and liver flushes, as it will enhance and accelerate the overall cleansing and healing process. A stand-alone basic elimination diet, however, is your best friend for breaking the cycle of cravings and addictions and identifying those foods to which you may be sensitive.

basic elimination diet

Many holistic healthcare practitioners advocate following an elimination diet in order to give the digestive system a rest, help clear the eliminative tract, provide an opportunity to test for food allergies and sensitivities, and also as a means of breaking the cycle of addiction to certain foods and stimulants. In a nutshell, a basic elimination diet involves eliminating all common food allergens and any other foods that are challenging to digest, or you suspect may be a problem for you. When used as a tool for testing for food intolerances, after an initial 5-7 days on a strict elimination diet, you then reintroduce one suspect food at a time over the course of the following few days or weeks, taking careful note of any reactions to these foods as you add them back into your diet (i.e., heart palpitations, gas, bloating, headache, fatigue, constipation, diarrhea, depression, anxiety, insomnia, etc.).

An elimination diet can be followed for any number of days depending on the results you are trying to achieve. Many people go on an elimination diet for a day or two to help restore balance after holiday partying, for example. Or do it for a week as a part of a regular internal Spring-cleaning. If you are trying to clear cravings, identify food intolerances, or otherwise reverse any kind of chronic condition, however, following an elimination diet for a minimum of 21 days is best.

The concept of an elimination diet is simple and easy, while the actual implementation can be a bit challenging, at least initially. Consequently, it is something you will want to become familiar with and practice before you make a commitment to doing it for the optimal 21 days needed to clear your system and

> But if you aren't digesting and/or absorbing well, you won't be healthy, no matter how healthful your diet.
>
> You will suffer, believe it or not, from malnutrition – or sludge – which interferes with our cells' ability to function optimally and is a sign of the beginnings of illness.
>
> Dr. Mark Hyman & Dr. Mark Liponis

be able to properly test for food allergies and sensitivities. When done correctly, adhering to a basic elimination diet for 21 days or more is a life-changing experience that will alter your relationship with food. Many people who thought they had no sensitivities to foods are amazed to discover that certain foods are, indeed, causing them *dis*-ease of one kind or another. As their system starts to clear out accumulated sludge, they are also amazed at how something seemingly so simple can have such a profound effect on the way they feel both physically and mentally.

In addition to the reduction or elimination of food cravings and nagging symptoms, increased energy and clarity of mind are what people most often report after being on an elimination diet. Nothing speaks louder to you than your own experience. Don't rob yourself of the opportunity to discover just how good you can feel! Follow the steps for a basic elimination diet outlined next to help you through the initial phase of making the transition to an *Eating-for-Health* lifestyle. You'll be glad you did.

basic elimination diet step-by-step

1 ~ *strategize* the process before you begin
...using the outline provided in Chapter 6 ~ Strategize, to set yourself up for success in every area.

Strategizing an elimination diet is paramount for success. Use the process you learned earlier in *Chapter 6 ~ Strategize* to guide you. As mentioned earlier, 21 days is the best, especially if you want to test for food intolerances. You may have to work up to this, however. Start with one or two days (preferably on the weekend) to get a feel for what will be required in terms of food preparation and how your body will respond. Remember that the first days are always the worst, so don't mistakenly think that if you are feeling bad that you will continue to do so for the whole 21 days. On the contrary, after the first 2-5 days most people start feeling better than ever. For many people, following an elimination diet for only 1-2 days is not enough to get over the initial withdrawal phase sometimes experienced, so just know that if you were to keep going, you would feel better in the days to follow. Also

---

Sidebar:

Every single day your body loses hundreds of billions of cells, and every day they are replaced with new ones.

What are these new cells made from?

The food you put into your body...

The food you eat is going to become you.

Quite literally, your very cells will be built from what you eat.

Harvey &
Marilyn Diamond
Fit for Life II

know that some people start feeling better right away and never experience any kind of withdrawal or detoxification symptoms.

As you are strategizing your plan of action, you will want to be sure that you are prepared in every way to ensure your success. It is very important that you think at least a day ahead and always have food ready to take with you if need be. Don't be caught somewhere without any healthy food choices and be forced to go hungry or resort to something you don't want to eat at this time. As part of your preparation, also be sure to clean sweep your kitchen of any foods that you know will be calling your name, especially any extreme foods you know you will crave in the initial stages. It wouldn't be an effective treatment plan to try and rehabilitate an addict with a refrigerator and cupboards filled with their drug of choice.

Another key element to keep in mind as you strategize this particular program has to do with planned indulgences. Although as part of a general *Eating-for-Health lifestyle* it is wise to take a flexible approach to eating and *not* think that you have to be eating 100% perfectly 100% of the time, when you are doing an elimination diet, this is exactly what you will want to do. You will want to follow the diet exactly as described 100% of the time in order to benefit from the experience and results it has to offer. In this case you will *not* schedule in any planned indulgences unless they fall within the confines of the program. (See #5 for suggestions.) Also be aware that this is a *general* elimination diet. It can be modified further to address specific conditions such as candida, arthritis, gluten intolerance, or blood sugar problems.

> If you are what you eat, why would you want to be a Twinkie or a hot dog?
>
> Gary Null

2 ~ do not eat any common food allergens
...or foods to which you suspect you may be sensitive or may have trouble digesting or eliminating.

This is what an elimination diet is all about: going off all common food allergens, which are generally notorious for causing problems, and any other foods that you suspect may specifically be causing you trouble. This would include, but not be limited to:

- wheat
- soy
- yeast
- vinegar
- chocolate

- peanuts
- oranges
- strawberries
- tomatoes
- potatoes

- coffee
- corn
- sugar/concentrated sweeteners
- all **dairy products** - milk, cheese, yogurt, butter, etc.

- shellfish
- eggs

When we live on highly refined junk food that is full of toxins and does not provide our body with the necessary nutrients for optimal health...

when we consume more toxins than our body can neutralize or eliminate,

when we do not get the prerequisite of exercise – then our bodies lose that magical self-regenerating ability.

Patrick Quillin

Refer back to the *Suggested Foods* list in the previous chapter and you will see all of these common food allergens marked by parentheses. You will find other foods in parentheses and may consider eliminating them as well such as berries and cashews, which are sometimes known to cause allergic reactions, or avocados and bananas, which are sometimes difficult for people with a congested liver/gallbladder to digest. If you suspect that you have a problem with gluten, in addition to wheat you may also want to cut out all gluten grains. If you have blood sugar problems or candida, it would be wise to substitute the fruit with 2-3 more servings of non-starchy vegetables.

3 ~ eat at least the following every day

...of only the suggested foods listed in Chapter 8 that are not in parentheses.

As you're reviewing the *Suggested Foods* list notice all the foods that are *not* in parentheses. These are all the wonderful foods you *can* eat. You will want to have at least the following every day:

- 6-8 glasses pure (not tap) water
- 2-3 servings fruit (preferably cooked or raw, not dried)
- 3 servings raw or cooked *non-starchy* vegetables
- 1 serving whole grains or starches
- 1 serving animal protein
- Or if vegetarian – 1 serving beans, lentils, nuts or seeds, or a non-allergenic protein powder such as rice protein (no whey or soy protein powders, until you have tested them)
- At least 1 tbsp and not more than 4 tbsp extra virgin olive oil, coconut oil or unrefined sesame oil.
- Optional: small handful of *raw, unsalted* nuts or seeds once or twice daily (soak overnight to increase digestibility)

Unless you are not that hungry, consume at least the number of servings indicated above and more if you need to. You may eat whatever size portions you desire, but eat them in about these same ratios so as not to upset the overall balance. Don't, for example, eat 4 bananas and 6 cups of rice a day, as a client of mine once did, then wonder why you feel so constipated! If you are really hungry or weak, be sure to include more concentrated foods, such as protein or starches. Because the whole, fresh, natural foods you will be eating are high-octane fuel for the body, you will metabolize, digest, and otherwise burn through them much faster than the foods you normally eat. As a result, many people will be eating more food, more frequently than usual. Be sure to eat more if you are hungry, especially non-starchy vegetables.

4 ~ keep meals and snacks simple
...and avoid processed foods and foods you don't normally eat.

Because so many processed foods contain common food allergens, it is best to not eat processed foods at all during your elimination diet. If you must, be sure to check the label carefully. Eating only whole, fresh, natural foods is the most cleansing and healing to the body, as you have been learning. If you can, take this opportunity to experience their magic first hand.

Also, do not eat a lot of things that you don't normally eat (such as collard greens, beets or beans) as you may have a sensitivity or cleansing reaction to that particular food, making it more challenging to narrow things down when it comes to testing. This may be initially very limiting, but it is only for a short time.

All produce should be fresh and organic whenever possible, which may require more planning, preparation and food shopping than you are used to doing, so plan ahead. Frozen would be the next best choice and good to have on hand for quick smoothies and back up (check the label for additives). Canned foods are processed foods and devoid of vital life force energy and it is best to avoid them altogether. However, you may want to keep a couple of low sodium, additive-free canned soups on hand (*Shelton's* has a good one made with rice and range-free chicken) in case you run into a situation where you have no time to make something fresh and want to maintain your allergen-free regime.

There are also a couple of brands of bread (usually located in the refrigerator or freezer section at the health food store) and crackers that are free of wheat, yeast and vinegar. These are also

That which makes bodies has made a matching system of food to nourish those bodies.

Nothing but the miraculous has ever made either....

Food is a living miracle.

Your body is a living miracle.

Eat at the same level of miracle that you are.

Grace Parusha

good to keep on hand. Spread on a little raw almond butter or virgin coconut oil and you've got a delicious snack. Be sure to check the label for unwanted ingredients and keep these processed foods to a minimum. Overall, you will want to keep your meals and snacks simple. Follow food-combining principles if needed to ensure adequate digestion and elimination. Familiarize yourself with some of the allergen-free recipes, as well as the food shopping and preparations tips in the next section. General suggestions for what to eat include the following:

breakfast: *whole grain hot cereal (rice, oats, quinoa, or millet); chicken, turkey, steak, or eggs (after you have tested for them); raw or steamed fruit; baked yam, salad or bowl of mixed steamed veggies; small handful of nuts.*

lunch/dinner: *whole grains (rice, quinoa, or millet); chicken, turkey, steak, or eggs (after you have tested for them); baked yam or sweet potato; fresh salad or bowl of mixed steamed veggies; lentils, mung beans or other easy to digest legume.*

snacks: *carrot juice; piece of fruit; apple with a little almond butter; a smoothie or green drink; raw veggie sticks and mashed avocado; a handful of nuts; millet/rice bread or wheat-free rye cracker with a little almond butter or virgin coconut oil; cup of herbal tea.*

salad dressings: *squirt of fresh lemon juice with a drizzle of olive oil; fresh garlic and lemon juice with olive oil and tahini; mashed avocado; olive oil and balsamic vinegar (after you have tested for vinegar).*

condiments: *fresh or dried herbs; sea salt; Bragg's Sprinkle seasoning blend; Bragg's Liquid Aminos (if test O.K. for soy).*

beverages: *water; green drink; caffeine-free herbal tea; carrot and other fresh vegetable juices; fresh or bottled fruit juices diluted by half to maintain steady blood sugar levels.*

Wisdom becomes knowledge when it becomes your personal experience.

Yogi Bhajan

Changing your ideas of what is normal to eat for breakfast or have as a snack is helpful for expanding the possibilities of what to eat. As long as you don't have any trouble digesting bananas, *The Frozen Banana Cream Treat* and the *No-Bake Apple Crisp* (see *Recipes*) are great for planned indulgences. Those around you who are not following the elimination diet will enjoy these treats as well. Preparing food the night before or in the morning for the whole day is also helpful.

5 ~ test for food allergies and intolerances
...by introducing them one at a time, starting on day 6.
If you choose to follow the program to the letter, throughout the program any food that is not included on the previous list should not be eaten. If you choose to test for food allergies and intolerances, all foods, including all stimulants and common food allergens, should be eliminated until you have tested them for sensitivity. Depending on the outcome of your test for any particular food, you will then either add it back into your diet or continue to eliminate it for the duration of your program and beyond, if you choose.

> The body intuitively knows exactly what foods are truly best for it.
>
> We simply must learn to be better listeners.
>
> Mark Percival

The following overall plan for testing for food allergies, sensitivities, and intolerances should make this point clear:

- Entire 21 days – *adhere to suggested foods list, eliminating all processed and packaged foods.*

- First 5 days of program – *eliminate all common food allergens listed earlier, and any other suspect foods you want to test.*

- Day 6 – *begin food allergen/sensitivity testing and continue throughout program.*

As for the food testing specifically, it is wise to test for the foods you eat most frequently and those that you most suspect are a problem for you. As indicated you will stay off all common food allergens and other foods you want to test for the first five days. It is very important that you do not consume even a trace amount of the foods that you want to test for, as this can skew your results. On the sixth day, you will introduce one food back into your diet, such as wheat, for example. Have at least 2-3 generous servings, and then take note of any reactions or changes in the way you feel. Some people will notice symptoms immediately, such as headache, bloating, gastrointestinal distress, fatigue, depression, irritability, etc., while others may not notice anything until the next day, such as constipation, puffiness or bags under the eyes, trouble sleeping, etc. And some will not notice anything at all.

Sometimes things get worse before they get better.

This is surprising to many people and often causes confusion.

This period of intense cleaning is called a "healing crisis."

It is referred to as a "crisis" because it involves somewhat unpleasant symptoms...

It is regarded as "healing" because that is what is happening – the body is experiencing an accelerated period of cleansing and healing.

Dr. Bruce Fife

In many cases, not noticing anything at all is an indication that the food you tested is not a problem for you, but not always. It is important to understand that while it is often the case that someone is able to ferret out a specific food that is causing certain problems, like Marissa who was able to make a direct link between her depression and diet soda, this is sometimes not the case.

Sometimes people's systems are so weakened and backed up from years of poor eating habits that they have to clear their system to a great degree before they can get a clear understanding of what specific foods are causing them problems. In which case, not noticing anything after testing a food may also indicate that you need to do some additional cleansing and stay off the suspect food for a longer period of time in order to clear your system. Then re-introduce the food in two or three weeks, for example, and see how your body reacts. Feeling better when not eating a particular food is also a testament to the possible effects it may be having. Pay more attention to your body's signals, use your intuition, and experiment to know what's best for you.

After you have tested for a particular food, if you *did not* have a reaction and are confident that it is not a problem for you, you may now include it as part of your overall elimination diet for the remainder of your program. You may then go on to test another food the next day, and proceed testing for foods in this same manner for the duration of the 21 days, introducing them one at a time. If you *do* have a reaction to the food you tested, continue to exclude this food for the remainder of your program. Also wait a day before you test for the next food to allow your system to clear from the reaction.

Some people are able to successfully clear food intolerances, or at least greatly reduce their reactions to them, by eliminating any offensive foods for three months or longer while at the same time cleansing, nourishing, and strengthening their body and immune systems with natural, nutrient-rich foods, herbs, and whole food supplements. In general, as we discussed earlier, it is best to limit all common food allergens in your diet, especially wheat, dairy and soy, only having them on a rotational basis about every 4-5 days. You will especially want to do this for any foods you have eliminated for an extended period of time, to avoid increasing or resumption of symptoms. Common food allergens trigger the body. If you don't eat them for an extended period time the body can heal. Much like a wound, if you keep scraping it, it will never heal. If you leave it alone, however, it can repair itself.

6 ~ what to expect as you proceed

…can vary from person to person and may include feeling worse before you feel better.

What you can ultimately expect from following a basic elimination diet is to feel better, for many people better than ever. Some may feel worse before they feel better, however, as their body withdraws from stimulants and foods to which they may be sensitive, and otherwise clears itself of accumulated toxins and waste stored in organs and tissues, and adjusts its functions in search of a balanced state of well-being.

The only way around is through.

Robert Frost

As the body is going through all this initial readjusting, cleansing, and healing, some people experience symptoms that range from mild to severe. Some of the most common include *headache, fatigue, nausea, vomiting, diarrhea, constipation, skin eruptions, muscle aches and pains, loss of appetite, fever, coughing, runny nose, itchy or twitchy eyes, depression, and mood swings.* But any symptom can be associated with this detoxification process, often referred to as a "healing crisis." Most people only experience 2-3 of these symptoms anywhere from a couple of days up to a week. Of course, everyone is different and how your body responds will depend on many variables, such as age, weight, current state of health, genetics, diet and lifestyle factors. In general, those who are in poor health with the worst diets usually experience the most severe symptoms. Don't let these symptoms confuse you. A healing crisis is a normal reaction to an elimination diet or any kind of cleansing.

If you have not already weaned yourself off stimulants such as sugars and caffeine, or common food allergens such as wheat and dairy products, following this basic elimination diet is a great way to get the job done all at once. Just be sure to strategize before you begin to increase your chances of successfully following through with what it will take to get yourself to the other side.

In addition to the aforementioned symptoms, you may also experience strong cravings during the first few days. Remember that these cravings will go away if you push through to the other side of the process, which usually only takes a few days. The symptoms they create, however, such as fatigue, excess weight, digestive problems, etc., will last *forever* as long as you keep indulging in the foods that are causing them! Keeping this in mind as you are experiencing the cravings will help you through. In addition, once most people make it to the other side, they are strongly motivated to stay there, for the simple reason they don't ever want to have to go through those withdrawal symptoms again!

If you feel up to it, gentle exercise, such as walking, yoga, Tai Chi, or stretching will also help you through. Now is not the time to start training for a marathon, go mountain climbing, or attend social gatherings, however. In fact, at least for the first few days of an elimination diet, rest and quiet meditative time to yourself is what's most in order. Given all the factors to consider, as mentioned earlier, it may be wise to work up to a full elimination diet. Modifying the program to some degree can be a great place to begin.

> The only time you don't fail is the last time you try anything – and it works.
>
> William Strong

7 ~ consider modifying the program
...for practice or to best suit your needs at this time.

Everyone is encouraged to participate at a level that they can realistically accomplish. Be honest with yourself and set yourself up to succeed. Before you embark on a basic elimination diet, really think about the time you have available, financial considerations (buying all fresh, natural foods in big quantities may be more pricey than what you may normally be eating), upcoming social events, etc. If you think that the program as outlined above may be a stretch, then think about what would be more manageable for you to do to start. Here are some examples:

- Eliminate common food allergens for 2-3 days a week.
- Eliminate all stimulants, especially those that you struggle with (i.e., coffee, sugar, etc.)
- Eliminate one or more foods to which you suspect you have a problem (wheat, dairy, soy, etc.)

- Follow the guidelines above for 1-2 meals a day.

- Eliminate all processed, packaged foods.

Keep in mind, however, that making slow changes can sometimes be traumatic. Each time you put an addictive food into your body, you are perpetuating an existing chemical imbalance or setting a new one in motion. As a result, your body craves more of that addictive substance, which can lead to a yo-yo effect, going back and forth but never breaking free. This can cause people to become discouraged because they are trying to make improvements, but are not experiencing the desired results. In fact, sometimes they end up feeling even worse. In which case, just going for an all out 21-day basic elimination diet can be the solution.

8 ~ to end your program
...be sure to review, revise and recommit to what you'll do next.

Although you may have the desire to go out and scarf down a double cheese pizza and guzzle a few sodas or beers at the end of a 21-day basic elimination diet, doing so would not be the wisest thing to do. Instead, follow strategizing step #10: *review, revise, and recommit, bringing closure to this phase and devising the next.* The next phase you choose is up to you. As mentioned before, many people are inspired by the way they feel and have no desire to go through withdrawal from bad food symptoms again, which makes them want to continue at least some of what they have been doing. Don't just let things fizzle, however. Be sure to make a clear commitment for a specified amount of time for what you will do next, until the desired changes have been integrated as lifestyle habits.

Be persistent and consistent. Remember that it takes practice before you learn to play the piano and a few tries before most people are able to quit smoking. Apply what you have learned here over and over, if you need to. That's what all the people I know who have been successful at integrating a healthier eating lifestyle have done. The next section is filled with practical tips, tidbits, and recipes that will help you do just that.

As for cleansing, it is something you will want to do regularly. It's like your closet or your garage. Stuff is always

As the positive effects of whole food nutrition, greater energy, and a clearer mind come to you; project your thoughts ahead to the months and years ahead and the ever-increasing benefits you will be experiencing.

This is not a program with a beginning and an end. It is a launching pad for a new life.

The Brain Garden
Food First Program

coming in and you have to clear it out one way or another. For this reason, it is wise to do an elimination diet or some other form of cleansing or combination periodically. Doing a cleanse at the beginning of each season, or one or two days a month, for example, is a long time tradition for many. Health is like a bank account. You can't continue to draw on it without making deposits. Going on an elimination diet or other kind of cleansing protocol is the equivalent of making a sizeable deposit. And the more you cleanse regularly, the less problems you will encounter. More and more, what you can look forward to is a clearer, stronger, revitalized body and mind!

basic elimination diet ~ quick reference

1 ~ *strategize* the process before you begin
...using the outline provided in Chapter 6 ~Strategize, to set yourself up for success in every area.

2 ~ do not eat any common food allergens
...or foods to which you suspect you may be sensitive or may have trouble digesting or eliminating.

3 ~ eat at least the following every day
...of only the suggested foods listed in Chapter 8 that are not in parentheses.

4 ~ keep meals and snacks simple
...and avoid processed foods and foods you don't normally eat.

5 ~ test for food allergies and intolerances
...by introducing them one at a time, starting on day 6.

6 ~ what to expect as you proceed
...can vary from person to person and may included feeling worse before you feel better.

7 ~ consider modifying your program
...for practice and to best suit your needs at this time.

8 ~ to end your program
...be sure to review, revise and recommit to what you'll do next.

Section Four

recipes & more

Delicious Dishes & Time-Saving Tips for Meal Planning
& Food Preparation

Having been raised in the suburban Midwest in the 60's and 70's, I grew up on primarily packaged and processed foods. My mother had 4 children at a young age. Her extended family lived hundreds of miles away. She had no assistance raising her lively brood, except for my father, who was exhausted himself from a demanding job that also entailed a long commute. As a result, for the sake of convenience and because my mother wasn't fond of cooking, we lived primarily on foods that came out of bags, boxes, and cans. On the rare occasions we had fresh foods, it seemed so foreign to our taste buds that we usually turned up our noses. (Except for the fresh corn on the cob we got from the produce stand at the edge of town every summer. Everyone enjoyed that.)

When I went off to live on my own during college I ate pretty much as I had eaten during my childhood, with the addition of much more junk and fast foods which had only been allowed on occasion while living at home. It wasn't until I joined the Peace Corps after college that I began to learn a whole new approach to food and its preparation. In Morocco, where I was stationed, there are no fast-food restaurants, packaged foods or frozen entrees, let alone a microwave to pop them in. Anything canned is questionable and in short supply. The restaurants that do exist are unwelcome places for women, and sometimes officially off limits to them in this Muslim country. Fortunately, I was blessed with two vital resources for learning how to prepare and cook a variety of foods from scratch using locally available foods, or I probably would have starved.

One of them was my roommate, Sunita, who was a fellow Peace Corps volunteer. Although she had grown up in New Jersey, she was born in India and her mother, who had been raised in the old country, taught her how to cook traditional Indian food that would knock your socks off. My other saving grace was our landlord's family. Soon dubbed "my Moroccan family," mama and her three teenaged daughters generously provided me with many a lesson and culinary delight.

Although I loved to indulge in all the exquisite cuisine that was showered upon me, I found it equally as satisfying to learn about the individual ingredients and how it was all prepared. Being a suburban girl from the Midwest, it was fascinating to watch these women as they chopped and kneaded and combined a plethora of fruits, vegetables, grains, meats, legumes, herbs and spices, many of which I had never seen before, into the savory dishes for which both Morocco and India are known. It was an empowering and exotic cultural experience that tantalized all my senses.

After this enriching experience I never viewed food the same again. In fact, I realized that my perception of food had been up until then, very limited. For the most part I was ignorant of the cornucopia of foods that are available, let alone how to prepare them. I remember feeling self-conscious when Sunita, mama or one of her daughters would drop their jaw, aghast at my ignorance of food and its preparation. And a little embarrassed when they would snicker at my awkward attempts to learn new skills, such as finely chopping parsley or kneading bread dough, which for them had become second nature.

That's why when a client or participant in one of my healthy eating programs sheepishly confesses that they don't know what a zucchini looks like or how to cook grains, for example, I can more than empathize. Cooking and food preparation has become a lost art in most American homes. Entrenched in pre-packaged, processed foods, we have become so disconnected from our food source that as a culture we are largely ignorant when it comes to the food we eat, which is having widespread repercussions, as we have seen.

The staggering rates of overweight and obese people in this country prompted former President Bill Clinton to establish The National Nutrition Summit just before he left office, for the purpose of studying why people eat what they do, even when they know it is not healthy. Allocating a few million dollars to uncover the answer to this question wasn't necessary, however. The answer is simple. The current *Standard American Diet* is tremendously influenced by the modern food industry and its intensive advertising and marketing endeavors. In addition, because most people today have very little to do with the source of their food other than to pluck it from the grocery store shelf, they truly don't know enough basic information about whole foods and how to prepare them. Most people in this country are literally unequipped to make healthy changes in their diets.

Health advocates can recommend eating whole grains and avoiding processed foods all they want, but if people don't know what a whole grain is or how to cook it, it's pretty unlikely they're going to eat it. The same is true of processed foods. If people aren't clear about what constitutes a processed food or what they can eat in place of it, it's unlikely they're going to avoid processed foods as recommended.

In working with a multitude of clients and participants in my healthy eating programs, I have gained keen insight into what many average Americans know and don't know when it comes to food. In the beginning I took for granted that people understood the difference between a refined sugar and a natural sweetener, what constituted a processed food, a whole grain, or how to cook a pot of rice. My clients and students quickly taught me that I needed to start with the basics, as most of them had received little to no training in the kitchen. Fully empathizing with their position, I was happy to do so, gratefully remembering those who did the same for me when I was first learning.

At the beginning of a healthy eating program a woman once asked if a bagel or bread, for example, would be considered a whole grain or a processed food. She self-consciously prefaced her question by saying, "I know this is probably a stupid question, but...," while taking a couple of side glances to see how the others were reacting to her "stupid" question. The others did not think it was stupid at all. They anxiously awaited my answer, as most of them indicated they were not sure themselves. They were relieved that somebody had asked it.

Much like I felt during my days in Morocco and when I first began to learn about real foods, there is a sense of guilt and embarrassment on the part of many people regarding their lack of knowledge and confusion about nutrition and food preparation. As I did that evening in response to this woman's question, I want to ease any such feelings that you may have in this same regard, and assure you that if you are feeling this way you are not alone. On the contrary, you've got a lot of company. I want to further assure you that there *really is* no such thing as a *stupid* question. In fact, it is questions such as these that have motivated me to write this book and also helped formulate the guidelines for *Eating for Health* in order that they may be of the most service to the greatest number of people. In that same vein, I now present this final section loaded with recipes and practical tips for food preparation and meal planning. It is designed to increase your practical know-how and your confidence, so you can get on the road to a healthier eating lifestyle and enjoy the journey.

Chapter Ten

be prepared

Tips for Food Shopping, Preparation, Meal Planning & Eating Out

When it comes to making *Eating for Health* a routine reality, *be prepared* is the motto. And that's just what this chapter will help you do. Filled with easy-to-follow instructions for menu-planning, natural foods shopping and preparation, and practical ideas for keeping healthier choices available, this chapter will make eating wholesome foods as convenient as a fast food pick-up at a drive-thru window. In addition, it will provide you with strategies for restaurant dining, party-going, and social gatherings. All of this, coupled with the simple, delicious recipes that follow, will help you transform a natural foods lifestyle, which may have seemed like a galactic-sized feat in the past, into a feat of earthly proportions that is easy, enjoyable, and satisfying. We begin this transformation in the most critical, albeit often most abused and neglected, room of every earthling's abode: the kitchen.

kitchen set up & equipment
In order to successfully integrate consuming an abundance of natural foods as a lifestyle habit and enjoy doing it, it is imperative to create a user-friendly kitchen. Doing so will greatly increase the likelihood of this sacred room being used more frequently for its intended purpose — the proper care and fueling of our human vehicles with nutritious foods. Performing a clean sweep of all pseudofoods is the perfect time to take inventory of what needs to be done. Whether you decide to make a clean sweep or not, there are three main elements of every kitchen that you will want to have in order.

First, you will want to be sure that all areas of the kitchen are well organized and free of clutter as much as possible. Throw out expired foods and kitchen gadgets that are broken or never get used. Organize what remains with like items in accordance with their frequency of use. For example, place frequently used items close to the area in which they will be used and can be easily accessed, such as spices and hot mitts near the stove. Stow away fine China, the turkey roaster, and other *in*frequently used items in the more difficult to access places of the pantry, cupboards or even in a closet or storage place outside the kitchen. Place only those items you use regularly on the counter to free-up adequate space for unencumbered food preparation.

Next, you will want to be sure you have all the necessary kitchenware and equipment. A good set of pots and pans, including a vegetable steamer, a set of sharp knives, a cutting board and lots of hard plastic, or better yet, glass containers with lids for food storage and convenient take-along, are all essential. There are many other items, such as a food processor, blender, grinder, juicer, rice cooker, crock-pot, vacuum sealer, and salad spinner that are also very helpful. Don't buy or keep things around that you don't need or will never use, however, as they will only end up contributing to the clutter you are trying to reduce. Which equipment gets used will be different for everyone. Some people couldn't live without their food processor, while I personally would be lost without my juicer and vacuum sealer.

But the only thing that will keep you from preparing homemade, nutritious foods more than a disorganized, ill-equipped kitchen is a kitchen that is lacking a supply of whole, fresh, natural ingredients to prepare. This is the final all-important element of a user-friendly kitchen oriented toward healthy eating. It must be regularly and adequately stocked with nutrient-rich, natural foods, which usually takes a little forethought.

shopping tips

Making a shopping list before you head to the store is always a good idea, and an absolute necessity when you are first starting to make major changes in your diet. A well-executed shopping list is not only a valuable time-saver and stress-reducer, but will also keep your food choices on the right track. Create a general list of staple goods that you'll want to keep on hand, but won't need to buy every week, such as baking supplies and condiments. Check this list and make note of anything you need on a weekly basis. You will also want to keep a list of things you buy every week, such as produce, eggs, and bread. Finally, you will want to include items that you don't buy regularly, but may need for special meals you are planning for that particular week. As for the actual shopping, the more routines you can establish, the better.

Try to limit your trips to the store to 1-2 times per week, and establish specific days for food shopping, such as Monday for your major food shopping and Wednesday for fresh meats and a few extraneous items. Also, frequent the same stores as much as possible. Knowing where things are will save you time and abate frustration. Following the same route each time you shop will similarly expedite the process, and can also jog your memory for any items you may have forgotten to include on your shopping list.

When checking labels on natural brand processed foods, remember that items are listed in descending order of ingredient concentrations. Also be mindful that hydrogenated oils, refined sweeteners, and ten syllable words you can't pronounce are all best left on the store shelf, even if you found them at the health food store. Unfortunately, an increasing number of *un*natural food items have made their way into what used to be authentic natural foods stores. While scrutinizing labels may be necessary when first transitioning to new, healthier brands, sticking with those you like and have become familiar with will help minimize time spent on this task in the future. Similarly, planning meals in advance will save you precious time, and also make coming up with your weekly shopping list a breeze.

menu planning

Establishing a general plan for each day of the week makes overall menu planning quick and easy. For example, a general weekly plan for dinner might look something like this:

- Monday – fish
- Tuesday – chicken
- Wednesday – pasta
- Thursday – beans and rice
- Friday – natural brand frozen pizza or other entrée
- Saturday – eat out
- Sunday – special dinner

With a general notion of what's for dinner for a particular night of the week, you can easily plug in different dishes from week to week to create variety. Having halibut one week and salmon the next on Monday night, fish night, for instance. Set up your plan to suit your schedule and your lifestyle. When trying a new recipe, be sure to include all the ingredients on your upcoming weekly shopping list.

As for specifics, *Chapter 7 ~ The Basics* provides detailed descriptions of what to eat and how much depending on your individual needs. Following is a brief review to keep in mind when thinking about overall menu planning:

general daily menu plan:
- 0-3 servings protein
- 2-4 servings fruit
- 3-7 servings non-starchy vegetables
- 1-3 servings starchy foods, such as yams, sweet potatoes, whole grains, whole grain bread, or whole grain pasta
- 1-3 tablespoons extra virgin olive oil, coconut oil, unrefined sesame oil, flaxseed oil, ground seeds, or an essential fatty acid supplement
- optional: small handful of raw, unsalted nuts or seeds (not more than ¼ cup)

In terms of more specific menu planning, flip through the recipes in the next chapter to help you brainstorm, and then formulate a plan that's right for you. Lunch and dinner ideas come easily for most people, while breakfast and snack ideas seem to pose the biggest challenge as people request help with them the most. Following are a list of ideas for each that will help. Items in italics indicate recipes included in the next chapter:

breakfast ideas
- *Green Drink, Smoothie,* fresh carrot or vegetable juice combination, alone or followed by any of the following.
- *Carrot-Apple Salad, Creamy Fruit salad,* or *Coco-nutty Fruit Salad.*
- *Raisins & Spice Hot Cereal, Quinoa-Millet,* oatmeal, or other whole grain cereal with raw, unsalted nuts, seeds, or raisins.
- Poached eggs, omelet, *or Scrambled Eggs Ranchero* with steamed veggies and sprouted Ezekial bread toast.
- *Breakfast Burrito* on sprouted grain or spelt tortilla with fresh green salad.
- Organic, nitrate-free turkey, chicken or beef sausages.
- If you can handle a little dairy, *Dr. Budwig Cottage Cheese Dish.*

snack ideas
- Snack bars made with all whole, fresh, natural ingredients (not the overly-processed, overly-sweetened variety!) such as *Govinda* bars or *Rama* bars, made from nuts, seeds, grains, honey, and dried fruit.
- Sliced apple with a tablespoon raw almond butter.

- Baby carrots, celery sticks, cucumber slices and natural brand bottled ranch dressing (*Annie's Cowgirl Ranch* is a good one), *Lemon-Tahini Dressing,* mashed avocado or guacamole for dipping.
- Handful of trail mix – raw, unsalted, and unsweetened, such as pumpkin seeds, sunflower seeds, almonds, walnuts, raisins, and date pieces.
- A few pieces of unsulphured dried fruit, such as dates, figs, apples, or apricots.
- Fresh carrot or other vegetable juices.
- Fruit juice, diluted with water by half to lower glycemic index.
- *Wasa* wheat-free rye crackers, or brown rice crackers, with almond butter, organic cheese, or virgin coconut oil and all-fruit preserves.
- For those working on balancing their blood sugar – hard boiled egg, chicken strips, a couple slices of organic, nitrate-free turkey or beef.
- A *Green Drink* or *Smoothie.*
- *Wheat-Free Blueberry Muffin* spread with butter or ghee – be sure to bake extra muffins and freeze.
- Bowl of unsweetened, additive-free apple sauce, or apple sauce blend, such as apple/apricot or apple/cherry.
- Air-popped popcorn drizzled with melted virgin coconut oil mixed with a little flax oil (remember not to heat flax oil) sprinkled with sea salt.
- A cup of flavorful tea, such as apple/cinnamon, chamomile, or a rich spice tea with a little oat milk and Stevia, maple syrup, or agave for sweetener.
- *Almond-Date No-Bake Apple Crisp* or *Frozen Banana Cream Treat.*

These suggestions should help you in planning ahead and keeping snacks and meals simple, which is the key to healthy eating on a regular basis. If you need more help and have long wished that someone else could plan everything out for you, including a categorized shopping list, your wish has come true. There is a fabulous service called *Menu-Mailer* now available online at a very reasonable cost. Visit their website for a free sample of a week's worth of menu plans and coordinating shopping list at www.menumailer.net. If you decide to subscribe to this service, a menu plan will be e-mailed to you directly each week. Because brand names are not listed, make sure to use only ingredients at *Level I* of *Eating for Health*. In other words, use only natural, additive-free brands, and organic produce and animal protein whenever possible.

Even the best-laid plans can fall apart, however. And it is for this reason that you will want to keep easy-to-prepare food around as back up for those times when you just can't bring yourself to cook up those vegetables, or roast that chicken, or whatever plans you may have had.

maximize availability of healthy foods

It's times when we are the most hurried, stressed or hungry that lead us, usually against our better judgment, to resort to what are sometimes the worst possible food choices we can make. And we don't have to look too far to find them. There exist today many more opportunities to eat poor quality food than ever before. To counter this situation, in order to eat well regularly, it is imperative to create as many opportunities to eat high quality foods as much as possible, whether at home or out in the world. Always have quick and easy-to-prepare foods of a healthier variety on hand that can be made up when there is no time to make something, or take along with you whenever you are headed out the door such as additive-free natural brand frozen and canned foods.

Although I don't generally recommend these kinds of foods because they are devoid of the vital life force and enzymes that give food its magical quality, if it comes down to a last minute choice between a natural brand frozen dinner or can of soup and a stop at the fast-food drive-through, or ordering a pizza covered with plastic cheese, there is no doubt that the first choice would be your best. It is for this very last minute situation that we all face from time to time that I think it is smart to keep a few cans of canned soup and frozen dinners on hand, especially if you have children or are very busy, or on an elimination diet. Knowing that you have a quick can of soup you can heat up (or better yet, have the kids heat up for you!) in a matter of minutes can save you from having many a bad food day. This is much better for your self-esteem, your spirits, and your body-mind system than resorting to something that doesn't belong in your body.

There are now a variety of both canned and bottled all natural soups to choose from on the market today, as well as an increasing variety of savory, additive-free frozen dinners and pizzas made with real, organic cheese. Make sure the products you choose are not the MSG, chemical-laden, sodium-saturated pseudofood variety, however. Check labels carefully, even on the brands made available in the health food stores. Unfortunately, there are a few brands that have made there way into the health foods stores that contain autolyzed yeast extract, which is a source of MSG.

Make up a fresh salad or side of fresh steamed vegetables, and you've got a quick and delicious meal that isn't half bad. *Thai Kitchen* also makes a great rice noodle soup that comes in little packets. Throw in some chopped carrots and zucchini to the boiling water and a tablespoon of virgin coconut oil and you have a satisfying gluten-free meal. Add a raw egg at the end and allow the heat of the water and noodles to cook it for added protein and satiation.

Also be sure to take advantage of the many pre-washed bagged salads, herbs, baby carrots and other chopped raw, veggies now available at grocery stores. Once again, check labels to be sure nothing has been added as a preservative, which is sometimes the case. Similarly, you will want to keep plenty of raw fruit around for a sweet and easy snack. These ready-to-eat raw foods are the healthiest fast foods out there.

When you do head out the door, be sure to pack it in! It's a junk food jungle out there and you can never be sure if whole, fresh, natural foods will be available when going to work, school or social outings unless you bring it yourself. Do so whenever possible and you will feel better all the way around. Because vending machines, convenience food stores and eating out can be very costly, you'll save money too!

One of the smartest things you can do is to bring a bag of the aforementioned grab-n-go foods with you at the beginning of the week and keep it in the refrigerator at work or school, if possible, for quick snacks and lunches all week. Because you don't want to be eating processed foods every day, however, you can pack up leftovers from dinner the night before in plastic or glass serving-sized containers to take along too.

Which leads us to the absolute number one guideline when it comes to making healthier foods available on a regular basis: *whenever you are cooking or otherwise preparing food, always make enough to put leftovers in serving-sized, sealable containers for the following day.* Yes of course, the optimum way to go both aesthetically and health-wise would be to make foods fresh just before you eat them, and if you can do it, by all means do so. But for most of us, it just isn't possible, and leftovers from your wholesome meal the night before are much better than many other choices you could make.

fast-food health food

Keeping packaged, ready-to-eat store bought produce on hand, and planning leftovers for future meals are both a tremendous help in maintaining an *Eating-for-Health* lifestyle. In addition, preparing whole, fresh, natural foods in advance for use in a variety of meals and recipes will turn health food into fast food and further increase the likelihood that you will make healthier food choices regularly. If all the work is left until mealtime when you are frequently tired and hungry, chances are any major food preparation is not going to happen. If, on the other hand, you have done most of the work in advance, and it's just a matter of pulling things out of the fridge and heating them up or tossing them in a salad or quick recipe, chances are you will take the last little bit of effort it will take to throw together a delicious, healthful meal. Start with vegetables, the foods we are supposed to be eating the most, but are unfortunately eaten the least.

preparing vegetables in advance

Because fresh produce begins to lose its nutrients and start the oxidative process as soon as it is cut, it is best to chop vegetables right before cooking or eating them. That is the ideal scenario and if you have the time to do it, great. However, for most people this is not always practical and is one of the reasons why people don't eat enough vegetables. The mere thought of having to do all that preparation before each meal can be overwhelming.

For this reason, the best way to ensure that you are eating vegetables on a regular basis is to have them available and ready to throw in the steamer or add to your chosen recipe at any given time. This can easily be achieved by blocking out a 1-2 hour chunk of time once or twice a week in order to wash and chop vegetables, which can then be stored in the refrigerator for quick and easy access. Adopting this process as a lifestyle habit may take some time, but it is one of the best things you can do for your health. Involving children, spouses, roommates or other household members can lessen the burden on any one person and make it an enjoyable family time together.

There were many years when there was rarely a day that I had a vegetable. Today there isn't a day that goes by that I don't have a vegetable, and more often than not, have three or four or five! This is how it's supposed to be, and can happen for you too, by simply following the *Preparing Vegetables in Advance* process outlined next. The first couple of times you shop and chop vegetables as described will take a little longer, but as you get more familiar with this process it will go much quicker, so persevere. Just follow these three simple steps to always have an abundance of fresh vegetables on hand that are chopped and ready to go:

1 ~ shop

- To ensure freshness, plan to shop for produce the day of, or the day before you plan to chop and store it, whenever possible.
- Shop for produce that is locally grown, in-season, and organic whenever possible.
- Choose vegetables that are dark in color, firm to the touch and have no bruises or bad spots.
- For steaming, roasting, or grilling, choose zucchini, yellow squash, broccoli, cauliflower, bell peppers (red, yellow or green), onions, bok choy, celery, carrots, Portobello mushrooms, green beans, Brussels sprouts, etc.
- You can also steam green leafy veggies, such as Swiss chard, bok choy leaves, kale, collard greens, mustard greens, and beet greens.

(You will definitely want to steam the actual beets as well, but they are too messy to chop and store in advance.)

- For salads, choose lettuce, spinach, fresh herbs, cucumbers, tomatoes, radishes, etc.
- Store all produce in the refrigerator until ready to wash and chop if you are doing so the next day.

2 ~ wash & chop

- Fill sink about a third of the way up with water. Add produce wash as recommended on the bottle if using a commercial brand, or one of the homemade versions provided, to help dissolve any oil-based chemical sprays or waxes to which the produce may have been subjected.
- Place as many vegetables in water as possible and allow to soak for about 20 minutes. (You can also wash produce individually by spraying each piece, but this is more time consuming.) Scrub off any remaining dirt, rinse by running under clean water and place washed produce in colander or clean dish rack.
- Towel dry vegetables before chopping to preserve freshness when stored. To dry leafy vegetables, use a salad spinner or lie flat in single layers on dish towels and blot carefully with another clean towel.
- Using a small serrated paring knife or other knife that feels comfortable for you, cut off any bad spots.
- When chopping the firmer vegetables to be used for steaming, roasting or grilling, chop vegetables that steam quickly, such as zucchini, into larger chunks, and vegetables that take longer to cook, such as broccoli or cauliflower, into small to medium-sized chunks.
- For salad and leafy greens – chop off the ends, separate, chop the stems into bite-sized pieces and tear the leaves with your fingers into manageable-sized pieces.
- Chop cucumbers, tomatoes, radishes and other veggies for salads into bite-sized bits.
- It's also a good idea to chop some of the veggies, such as carrots and celery, into strips for dipping. And also to grate 3-4 cups of carrots (a food processor makes this task fast and easy!) to make *Carrot-Apple Salad* or toss together with green salads.

3 ~ store

- Throw together all the firmer, chopped vegetables for steaming, grilling, or roasting in 1 or 2 large hard plastic or glass containers.
- Place salad and leafy greens in separate containers, preferably large zip-lock plastic bags or large hard plastic or glass containers.
- Place watery and other vegetables to be used in salads in separate containers, such as cucumbers, tomatoes, radishes, celery, etc. It's also a good idea to put chopped onions in a separate container as well, so as not to overpower the taste of the other vegetables.
- Produce will keep approximately 3-5 days chopped and stored in this manner depending on the type of produce, and how fresh it was when you bought it.
- You can double, and sometimes even triple, this storage time by vacuum sealing your chopped veggies in glass (Mason jars), or the hard plastic containers designed for your particular vacuum-sealer. For this reason, a vacuum sealer is a must have in my book. It can save you so much time and money!

That's it. Follow these three easy steps — shop, wash & chop, and store — and you have a week's worth of fresh veggies (and possibly more if you use a vacuum sealer) at your fingertips. You can throw raw veggies together for quick, colorful salads, and grab a handful or two of the mixed veggies as needed for cooking. Have these mixed veggies over rice or pasta with marinara sauce and a little grated cheese or sprinkle of parmesan; add them to burritos, tacos, scrambled eggs, stir fry, lasagna or other casseroles, wraps or pita sandwiches. You can now easily meet your daily quota by throwing veggies in everything you can think of! And at the end of the week, or when your once vibrant veggies first start to look a little sad, throw all the appropriate leftover veggies in a large pot with some broth and seasonings to make a delicious vegetable soup.

While you are in the kitchen washing and chopping your vegetables is also the perfect time to put on a big pot of rice or other whole grains to cook. Make enough to last for a few days and store in convenient-sized containers, preferably vacuum sealing, if possible, for maximum storage time. You can take these fast-food whole grains along for lunches, pull them out for quick dinners, or heat up with a few raisins and walnuts for hot cereal for breakfast in the morning. Another easy thing to do that will maximize this time in the kitchen is to bake a few potatoes, yams, or sweet potatoes that can be reheated for lunches or dinners later.

I also know that it's popular with a lot of people to make food in advance and then freeze it. Unfortunately, I can't help much with this endeavor because

I'm not a big fan of freezing. Whenever I do freeze foods, with the exception of muffins or lasagna, I end up throwing them out more than I eat them. If freezing homemade, healthier foods works for you, however, by all means do it. Once again, it's a much better choice than a lot of others you could make.

Employing this method of preparing vegetables and other foods in advance will increase your likelihood of eating more nutritious foods regularly at least ten-fold. There will also undoubtedly be times when you will venture out into the world to dine, however, and tips for coping with these scenarios are next.

---

homemade produce wash

Add about 10 drops grapefruit seed extract to every 2 quarts pure water, when soaking produce in sink. Or, mix 10-20 drops with water in spray bottle to wash individual pieces of fresh produce.

OR...

Mix 2-3 ounces Dr. Bronner's natural all-purpose Almond Soap with 10 ounces purified water in spray bottle. Spritz on produce directly and rinse off, or add to water in sink for squeaky clean fruits and veggies.

---

tips for eating out & social gatherings

It's the frequency with which you eat out or attend food-related social gatherings that will determine how selective you need to be at any given outing. If you eat out virtually every day of the week, for example, you are going to have to be as prudent as possible, as much as possible, when making food selections. If you only go out to eat once a month, however, you can probably get away with eating whatever you like, if you are truly and consistently eating really well at home. Since eating outside the home a few times a month or even a few times a week is more likely the case for most people, however, arming yourself with the following tips will help keep your intentions for good eating and good health on track.

For personal gatherings with family and friends, if you feel comfortable, you can let your host or hostess know in advance that you are following a special diet. If they are people close enough to you and it feels comfortable, you may like to share more details and even make special requests. You could also suggest bringing a dish to share, that you know you'll be able to eat, so as not to have to trouble them with your particular needs. Any time there is a potluck, you can bring a dish or two of your liking, as well, and just eat that when you get there without having to make any fanfare about your dietary preferences.

Another wise strategy to employ, whether you are planning to eat at a restaurant or attend a social gathering, is to eat before you go. This is especially helpful for situations in which you will have no control over what will be served, and know there will be little, if any, real food available. If you eat before you go, you can just have a few nibbles when you get there without causing a lot of damage, or you can just socialize and not eat at all. Either way, plan in advance how you will deal with the situation and you will greatly increase your chances of controlling it, rather than having it control you. Upcoming parties or special events are a great time to plan an indulgence you can look forward to, and keep yourself on track up until then. Just be sure the frequency with which you do so doesn't get out of hand.

When it comes to restaurant dining, you often have more control over your food choices. You can patronize those establishments that serve only whole, fresh, natural foods as much as possible, for example. Fortunately, at least in the more populated areas of the country, they seem to be popping up more and more. And, whether you are in a healthy restaurant or not, you can always choose what to order and how much to eat once it arrives.

Make the best menu choices possible and special requests if needed, to increase the nourishing nature of your meals. For instance, order salads with dressing on the side, steamed vegetables instead of French fries, or a cup of fresh fruit instead of a sugary muffin or toast. Unless you are dining at a restaurant that serves nouveau cuisine (you know, the ones that bring you a little drop of food in the middle of a very large plate with an artful drizzle of colorful something or rather across the top), most restaurants today serve *way* more than what any one human should be eating in one sitting (which is actually a good reason to go for the nouveau cuisine!) Keeping this in mind and heading this problem off at the pass is the best way to ensure you don't eat too much.

For starters, you can ask that the breadbasket or chips and salsa *not* be brought to the table as soon as you arrive. If it's too late for that, and you find a basket wafting its warm, delightful contents right in front of you and aren't willing to give them up completely, consider designating a reasonable portion that you will eat by taking it out of the basket and placing it on your serving plate. This will keep you from mindlessly eating straight from the basket until, in all likelihood, whatever was in it is all gone. Other tips for avoiding eating too much include ordering an appetizer as a meal; portioning off your plate when it arrives; sharing a dish with a dining companion; asking that your plate be removed as soon as you are satisfied; or requesting that only half your order be brought to the table and have the rest doggie bagged for take home.

Don't be afraid to assert yourself at restaurants. Remember that you are paying them to serve you. Don't confuse assertive with aggressive, however. Be pleasant. You don't want any unwanted substances to find their way into your dish in the kitchen as hidden revenge.

If you're trying to avoid MSG, stay away from soups, dressings, and sauces. You can try asking the waiter, but they usually don't have a clue. Because MSG can be hidden under many different names, even if they do check the label or ask the chef, they often still can't give you an accurate answer. On more than one occasion at Asian restaurants, I have told the waitperson that I am highly allergic to MSG and they, subsequently, directed me to dishes they swore did not contain it. A splitting migraine and a slew of other uncomfortable symptoms sometime later, told me otherwise. After learning the hard way on too many occasions, I will now only go to Asian restaurants that have a sign in their window that states unequivocally that they do not use MSG. Fortunately, once again there are a growing number of such health-minded restaurants.

All of this talk about avoiding this, and switching this for that, reminds me of another very wise, all-important guideline for eating out: *on occasion, just go out and eat whatever you want, however much you want!* Seriously. You don't want to completely take the fun out of dining out. And since it's probably going to happen anyway, you might as well give yourself permission rather than beating yourself up about it later. Please note, however, that I said *on occasion*, which should further be qualified as a *rare* occasion. Refer back to the definition of *rare* provided in the description of *Eating-for-Health Guideline #2* to be sure you are correctly interpreting this recommendation :-)

This unbridled occasion aside, unless you are going to a whole foods restaurant and eating the freshest, most nutritious foods possible, in the best combinations, and most appropriate portions for you, limit the amount of time you eat out as much as possible. The inclination to eat low quality foods, and more of them, is just too great when you're eating out. Preparing wholesome foods at home, where you have total control over all ingredients, is always your best bet from a health and well-being standpoint.

"we want recipes!"

...is the loudest cry I hear from people after digesting all the information you have just been fed. So, I'm guessing that recipes are what you're clamoring for right about now as well. Clamor no more! A series of menu planner cookbooks devoted to *Eating for Health* are on their way (or may already be available, depending on when you picked up this book.) In the mean, time, the next chapter serves up a smorgasbord of recipes that are more than enough to get you started, recipes that prove eating healthy foods can be both fun and satisfying. And when you incorporate the strategies for preparing foods in advance that you just learned, preparing them can be quick and easy, too!

Chapter Eleven

recipes

Healthy Dishes That Are Also *Dee*-licious!

When I first started cooking I was more like Gallagher than the Galloping Gourmet in the kitchen. Even today, I want to eat healthy but don't want to spend a lot of time in the kitchen. Like most, I'm really busy and have other places I'd rather be, unlike two Italian women who once came to a cooking class I taught. They had grown up on homemade marinara sauce recipes that had been passed down and perfected for generations, and gasped when I pulled out a jar of commercial brand pasta sauce (all natural, of course) and suggested that people use it to make recipes such as lasagna, or to drizzle over steamed vegetables to entice kids to eat them. They called it "ketchup" and said they wouldn't be caught dead having it around, let alone eating it.

This led to an interesting conversation about priority expenditure of time. These same women who admitted they were willing to spend hours in the kitchen creating pots of savory sauces and Italian pastries to dazzle friends, family and their refined taste buds, had complained earlier that they didn't have time to chop fresh vegetables. They were both humbled by the realization that it wasn't that they didn't have time, they just weren't making vegetables a priority. Since they both wanted to lose weight and increase their energy, they vowed to free up more of their kitchen time for the all-important, yet often ignored, food group of vegetables.

This chapter is filled with recipes, hot tips and interesting tidbits, all designed to help you make healthier foods a priority. Remember that these recipes are meant for busy people who want to eat healthy on a daily basis, not aspiring gourmet chefs who spend a lot of time in the kitchen. That doesn't mean that taste is compromised, however, as these recipes are quite delicious. But they do take the quickest route in order to help you make *Eating for Health* an enjoyable, routine reality.

main dishes

tomato-zucchini pasta

3-4 cups cooked *Vita Spelt* rotini pasta
1 large yellow onion, chopped
2-4 cloves garlic, pressed
6-8 Roma tomatoes, peeled and diced OR 1 can peeled, diced tomatoes
1 medium green zucchini
1 medium yellow squash
1-2 tbsps. finely chopped fresh basil or 2 tsp. dried
2 tsps. dried oregano OR 1-2 tbsps. Italian herbal blend
Bragg's Liquid Aminos
1-2 tbsp. olive oil
¼ cup grated parmesan cheese (optional)
¼ cup pine nuts (optional)

Cover bottom of large skillet with olive oil. Briefly sauté onions, garlic and spices on medium heat. Add tomatoes and zucchini. Squirt with Bragg's to taste and cover. Simmer on low heat until zucchini is soft. Serve in large shallow bowls spread over cooked pasta. Top with grated parmesan cheese and pine nuts (optional).

tips & tidbits

- *Spelt pasta has a kind of nutty flavor and is a great alternative for many of those with sensitivities to wheat. For those who can't tolerate gluten, try quinoa or rice pasta.*

- *Tomato-Zucchini sauce also goes well served over rice or Quinoa-Millet.*

- *For added protein, sauté chicken strips with onions, garlic and spices until browned before adding tomatoes and zucchini*

vegetable lasagna

16 oz. organic low fat ricotta cheese
1 large egg
2-3 cups shredded organic mozzarella cheese
26 oz. jar marinara sauce of your choice (or homemade)
12 spelt, whole wheat or spinach lasagna noodles, cooked
3-4 medium carrots, grated
1 medium zucchini chopped into ½ inch chunks
1 large Portobello mushroom, chopped

Pour pasta sauce into 2 quart pan. Add grated carrots, mushrooms and zucchini chunks. Mix thoroughly in large saucepan or mixing bowl. Beat egg and combine thoroughly with ricotta cheese in a bowl. Spread small amount of sauce (leaving out zucchini chunks if possible) on bottom of 9½ x 14" baking dish. Layer noodles, pasta sauce, ricotta cheese, and shredded mozzarella, in that order. Continue layering until all ingredients are used.

Bake at 350° for 45-60 minutes. Let sit for 5 minutes, then serve.

tips & tidbits

- *Cut leftovers into square sections and freeze in covered plastic containers.*

- *In place of grated carrots, substitute 1 box frozen chopped spinach, or one bunch fresh spinach, chopped.*

- *Use soy or almond cheese products in place of dairy products for those who are sensitive to dairy, but do O.K. with soy.*

- *Add fresh onions, broccoli, bell peppers, black olive slices, etc. to create a veggie extravaganza.*

- *For a gluten-free version, replace noodles with ¼" slices of eggplant. Some people are very sensitive to eggplant, however, and may experience extreme gas and bloating. If this is you (and you'll know if it is!), use large zucchini or yellow squash in place of eggplant or go with the noodles.*

garlic roasted chicken

1 medium roasting chicken
juice of 1 lemon
4-6 cloves fresh garlic, crushed
Braggs Liquid Aminos
1-2 tbsp. dried parsley
1-2 tsp. paprika
½ tsp. dried basil
½ tsp. dried thyme
OR
Spike salt-free seasoning, in place of dried herbs

Rinse chicken and place in roasting pan. Mix lemon juice and garlic together in measuring cup and pour over chicken. Squirt with Bragg's to taste. Sprinkle with dried herbs or sprinkle generously with Spike and cover. Bake at 400° for 45-60 minutes. Baste chicken with garlic juice at bottom of pan every 10 minutes if desired. Carve while hot and serve immediately.

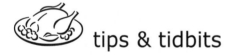 tips & tidbits

- *Garlic is a powerful immune booster, antioxidant and is also known to reduce cholesterol levels and lower blood pressure – and it tastes great too! Add it to almost any dish and reap its many benefits.*

- *When cooking with garlic, rinse hands with lemon juice to eliminate any lingering garlic odor.*

- *If you prefer a little salt, try sprinkling with a bit of* Herbamare *or* Tocomare *seasoning salt by* Bioforce *(available at health food stores).*

tangy lemon-rosemary chicken

4 boneless, skinless chicken breasts cut into chunks
1 large red onion, chopped
3-6 cloves of fresh garlic, sliced or pressed
2-4 tbsps. extra virgin olive oil
1-2 tbsp. minced fresh or dried rosemary
1 fresh lemon
½ tsp. sea salt

Place chicken breasts in large re-sealable plastic bag. Cut lemon in half and squeeze its juice into bag. Cut the peels into wedges and add them to the bag along with remaining ingredients. Seal the bag and let marinate for at least 2 hours or overnight. Place contents of bag in baking dish and bake at 350° for 15-20 minutes. Turn chicken and return to oven for another 15-20, or until chicken is done. Serve with vegetables or over rice with fresh salad.

baked or grilled salmon (or other fish)

large piece of fresh salmon fillet or steak
juice of 1 lemon
Bragg's Liquid Aminos
Spike salt-free seasoning
dash of cayenne pepper
fresh chopped parsley

Place salmon in baking dish. Pour lemon juice over salmon and squirt with Bragg's to taste. Sprinkle generously with Spike and a dash of cayenne pepper. Bake covered at 350 degrees for 20-30 minutes. Or grill steaks on one side for 10-12 minutes and 5 minutes on the other. Grill fillets for 4-6 minutes on one side and 5 minutes on the other. Serve immediately with lemon wedges and fresh chopped parsley.

 # tips & tidbits

- *Rosemary is a wonderful aromatic herb with a variety of medicinal qualities, including being an aid to digestion.*

- *Fish is a great source of protein and is very rich in omega-3 fatty acids that are so important to the body, especially the heart.*

turkey loaf

2 pounds ground turkey
¾ cup dried bread crumbs or rolled oats
1 – 8 oz. can tomato sauce
½ cup zucchini, grated large
½ cup carrot, grated large
½ bell pepper, finely chopped
1 small yellow onion, finely chopped
2 eggs, lightly beaten
2-3 cloves fresh garlic, pressed
2 tsp. dried parsley
2 tsp. dried rosemary
1 tsp. dried sage
2 tsp. Spike Seasoning
sea salt and black pepper to taste
½ cup chopped walnuts or walnut pieces

Mix all ingredients thoroughly in large bowl. Press into a loaf pan. Bake at 350°for 50-60 minutes. Serve hot with ketchup, salsa, or cranberry sauce.

 tips & tidbits

- *Leftover slices of Turkey Loaf make a great afternoon snack, especially for those who have low blood sugar and are trying to stay away from sweets.*

- *Other ideas for leftovers include making a sandwich out of slices, or cutting into bite-sized pieces to add to a salad.*

chicken strips

1 pkg. boneless/skinless chicken breasts cut into strips
Tamari sauce or Bragg's Liquid Aminos
Spike salt-free seasoning

Rinse cut chicken strips in cold water and place in frying pan. Sprinkle Tamari or Bragg's Liquid Aminos and Spike to taste. Cook over medium-high heat turning constantly with spatula until lightly browned all over. Remove from heat immediately. Make enough to refrigerate for snacks and bag lunches.

sunny eggs

4 large eggs
Bragg's Liquid Aminos
Spike salt-free seasoning

Separate eggs (crack egg shells and allow whites to fall out), saving only the yolks in a small bowl. Whisk together adding a squirt of Bragg's Liquid Aminos and a sprinkle or two of Spike. Cook in non-stick or cast iron frying pan, stirring constantly with spatula until gooey. Do not overcook. Serve immediately.

 # tips & tidbits

- *Both these dishes are a great accompaniment to a large bowl of freshly steamed vegetables or fresh green salad.*

- *Add fresh garlic and onions to enhance flavor. Sauté slightly before adding chicken or eggs.*

- *Some people believe that eating only egg whites is healthier, while others believe that the whites contain all the refuse of the egg and should never be eaten. I think the truth is probably in the middle, which means the whole egg is fine just the way Mother Nature made it. However, Sunny Eggs (yolks only, or more yolks than whites) are so creamy and delicious they make a great occasional treat, especially for those who are avoiding cheese. The first time I made them for my honey he thought they had cheese in them!*

scrambled eggs ranchero

5-6 large eggs
1-2 tbsp. extra virgin olive oil or coconut oil
2-3 cloves fresh garlic, pressed
¼ cup diced green pepper
¼ cup diced yellow onion
¼ cup organic chedder or goat cheese
1-2 tbsp. salsa of choice
1 tbsp. low fat organic sour cream (optional)

Sauté oil, garlic, green peppers, and onions in large skillet over medium heat until onions are clear. Scramble eggs in mixing bowl, then pour into pan and cook on medium heat pushing with spatula constantly until firm but gooey. Turn off heat and add cheese, mixing in until melted. Garnish with salsa and sour cream (optional) and serve immediately.

breakfast burritos

Scrambled Eggs Ranchero
2 sprouted grain or spelt tortillas
1-2 tbsp. salsa
1 tbsp. low fat organic sour cream (optional)

Cook up a batch of Scrambled Eggs Ranchero. Heat tortillas in skillet. Place ½ the egg mixture in center of each tortilla. Top with salsa and sour cream (optional). Fold in sides and roll tortilla. Enjoy for breakfast or any time.

 tips & tidbits

- *Pineapple contains the digestive enzyme bromelain, which makes pineapple salsa a wise choice when making Mexican dishes, which typically violates food combining principles, and are therefore difficult to digest.*

- *Some people do better having protein in the morning (especially people who are hypoglycemic). These two dishes are a tasty choice. Served with a fresh green salad, they are also excellent for lunch or dinner.*

avocado, tomato, sprout sandwich

Food for Life sprouted grain bread
1 ripe avocado
1 ripe tomato
fresh sprouts
Annie's Naturals Cowgirl Ranch Dressing

Arrange ½" slices of avocado on slice of bread. Place ½" slices of tomato and a handful of sprouts on top of avocado. Cover with dressing to taste and top with another slice of bread. Cut in half and serve immediately. Substitute cucumber slices for avocado if you have trouble with fats.

mixed veggie pita sandwich

whole wheat or spelt pita pockets
½-1 cup diced tomatoes
½-1 cup carrot/celery salad (diced carrots and celery)
½ cup diced cucumbers
½ cup diced onions
½ cup diced green, yellow or red peppers
½ cup finely chopped broccoli
fresh sprouts
½ cup Lemon/Tahini Dressing
OR
½ cup *Annie's Naturals* dressing of your choice

Toss together diced vegetables and dressing in large mixing bowl. Cut pita in half. Scoop vegetable mixture into pita pocket, top with sprouts and serve immediately.

tips & tidbits

- *These raw vegetable sandwiches are refreshing on a hot summer day. They're also fun and easy when serving a small group of people. Let everyone assemble their own by placing ingredients in separate decorative bowls in center of table with a couple choices of dressing to choose from, and a pitcher of Tangy Lemonade.*

- *To prevent sogginess when brown bagging, place ingredients in separate containers and assemble at time of consumption.*

oriental ginger soba noodles

1 pkg. buckwheat soba noodles
tamari sauce or Bragg's Liquid Aminos
¼- ½" slice of fresh ginger, grated
½ cup yellow pepper diced
½ cup red pepper diced
1 yellow zucchini cut into ¾" spears
1 green zucchini cut into ¾" spears
2 stalks bok choy cut ¾" chunks
OR
2-3 cups already chopped, mixed veggies for steaming
1-2 tbsp. coconut oil

Chop vegetables, if needed, while bringing a large pot of water to a boil. Follow directions on package for cooking noodles. While noodles are cooking, sauté coconut oil, ginger and vegetables in large skillet with enough water to cover bottom of pan. Squirt with Bragg's or tamari sauce, cover and let steam for about 5 minutes. Strain noodles when cooked, toss with vegetables in skillet. Then cover and steam for another 2-3 minutes. Serve immediately.

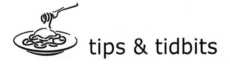 tips & tidbits

- *Buckwheat soba noodles are a hearty substitute for refined white pasta. Most buckwheat soba noodles contain wheat. However, there are soba noodles made only from buckwheat, which is a better choice. Check the ingredients label on the back of the package.*

- *Bok choy is a great vegetable to incorporate into your diet if you haven't done so already. It looks like celery only thicker, and it's white instead of green. A delicious addition to soups, steamed vegetables , and other dishes, boy choy has a mild, sweet taste that many children prefer over the slightly bitter taste of celery.*

spicy goat cheese quiche

1 - 9" whole wheat or spelt flour pie crust
1 cup grated goat cheese (hard goat cheese)
½ yellow onion, chopped
1-2 cloves fresh garlic, crushed
1 small chili pepper finely chopped (optional)
1 tsp. chili powder
pinch of cayenne
1 tbsp. extra virgin olive oil
½ cup broccoli chopped into ½" chunks
½ cup chopped red or green pepper
½ tomato sliced (optional)

Custard:
4 eggs
1 cup plain oat milk
3 tbsp. whole gain spelt flour

Sauté onion, garlic, chili pepper, chili powder and cayenne in small amount of olive oil on low heat, stirring constantly until onions soften. Cover bottom of piecrust with grated goat cheese. Add chopped broccoli, peppers, tomato slices and sautéed onions. Beat together eggs, oat milk and flour. Pour over ingredients in piecrust.

Bake at 375° for 40-45 minutes or until firm in the middle when jiggled.

 ## tips & tidbits

- *Make this delicious quiche for dinner and have leftovers for breakfast or lunch.*

- *To make baking pies and quiche a snap, try ready-to-bake frozen or packaged whole wheat piecrusts with no additives, available at health food stores. Wheat-free versions are sometimes available as well.*

- *Instead of goat cheese, substitute organic cheddar, Monterey jack cheese or dairy-alternative cheese.*

- *For variety, substitute veggies with chopped spinach and mushrooms, and experiment with different herbs and spices.*

mung beans & rice

1½ quarts pure water
1 cup mung beans
1 cup white basmati rice
1 cup chopped carrots
1 cup chopped zucchini
1 cup chopped celery
½ cup ghee or coconut oil
1 large yellow onion, chopped
1 inch piece fresh ginger, finely grated
3-4 cloves fresh garlic, finely grated
1 tbsp. dried basil
1-2 tsp. turmeric
½ tsp. black pepper
1-2 tsp. garam masala (Indian spice blend)
½ tsp. cayenne
½ tsp. sea salt
Bragg's to taste

Rinse mung beans and rice in cold water. Place in a medium to large pot with 1½ quarts water and salt, and bring to a boil. Reduce heat to a simmer. Chop vegetables and add to pot. In separate skillet, sauté onions, garlic, ginger and spices until browned or onions are clear. Stir constantly and add a little water if needed to avoid scorching. Add this mixture to the cooking pot of vegetables, beans, and rice. Add Bragg's to taste and simmer on low to medium heat until beans and vegetables are soft, approximately 40 minutes. Serve hot with a fresh salad.

tips & tidbits

- *This staple dish from the Ayurvedic tradition is like the vegetarian version of a hearty stew - rich, thick and satisfying. It's filling, yet very easy to digest. Best eaten plain health-wise, and really delicious with a little grated cheese melted over the top and a few non-GMO corn chips for a little treat.*

- *A soupier version of this dish, called Kicheree, is the Indian version of chicken soup because it is served to those who are sick or in recovery.*

mexican rice & veggies

½ cup cooked basmati rice (brown or white)
1-2 tbsp. non-fat, spicy refried beans
sprinkle of lemon juice or 1 tsp. apple cider vinegar
drizzle of olive oil (1-2 tsp.)
1-2 tsp. ground flax meal (opt)
1 cup steamed or raw veggies of choice
Bragg's and Spike to taste

Combine rice, refried beans, lemon juice or apple cider vinegar and olive oil in serving bowl and mix well. Mix in veggies and eat warm or cold.

 tips & tidbits

- *This staple dish is a great way to make use of leftover rice and makes one meal-sized serving. Double, triple or quadruple the recipe to increase servings. Don't worry so much about getting the exact amounts. Just make a reasonable estimate, throw it in a bowl, and mix it up.*

- *Refried beans and leftover rice in any combination with a side of mashed avocado, guacamole, vegetables or salad is a quick, easy meal to whip up any time. Add a sprinkling of grated cheese and some non-GMO corn chips for a special treat.*

grain dishes

tips for cooking whole grains

The general protocol for cooking perfect grains every time is as follows:

- *place grain in sieve, remove any rocks or debris, and rinse in cold water*
- *combine grain with water and pinch of salt in appropriate-sized stainless steel or enameled pot*
- *bring grain and water to a boil uncovered*
- *reduce heat to low, stir, cover*
- *cook without stirring until all water is absorbed (time will depend on grain)*

The ratio of one part grain to two parts water works well for many grains, and is a good rule of thumb to use if you have forgotten the specifics for the grain you are cooking. Some grains require a little less water, while others require a little more. Because cooking time and water ratio vary depending on the variety of grain, it is best to write down instructions when buying grains from the bulk bins, or simply follow the instructions given if packaged. Below is a chart that is helpful as well.

per cup	cups water	cooking time
Amaranth	1 ¼	20 min.
Barley	2 ½ - 3	40-60 min.
Buckwheat	2	12 min.
Basmati Rice	1 ¾	15-20 min.
Millet	2 – 2 ½	20-30 min.
Oats (whole)	2	45 min.
Quinoa	2	15-25 min.
Rice (short grain brown)	1 ½ - 2	40 min.
Rice (long grain)	2 – 2 ¼	45-60 min.
Teff	1 ½	20 min.

tips & tidbits

- *When cooking grains, be sure to keep heat on low to reduce risk of scorching or sticking to the bottom of the pan. To loosen grain that has stuck to the bottom, remove pan from heat leaving the cover on for a couple of minutes. Then stir loosened grain up from the bottom. (Works only if grain hasn't been scorched.)*

- *For a nutty flavor, grains may be toasted alone or with a small amount of ghee or oil before adding water. Spices, fresh ginger or garlic are also a delightful addition.*

- *Substitute half or all of the water with chicken or vegetable broth for added flavor. For hot breakfast grains cook with oat milk or apple juice.*

brown basmati rice pilaf

½ cup chopped onions
1-2 tbsp. ghee or olive oil
1 clove garlic, crushed
½ tsp. ground cinnamon (or 1-2" cinnamon stick)
1 cup brown basmati rice, rinsed
3 cups chicken or vegetable broth
¼ tsp. sea salt (optional)
2 tbsp. raisins or currants
2 tbsp. chopped walnuts, almonds or pecans

Sauté onions in ghee or olive oil until soft. Add garlic and sauté briefly. Stir in rice and raisins or currants until combined. Add broth and cinnamon. Bring to a boil, then reduce heat to low and simmer covered until water is absorbed (approximately 45-50 minutes). Remove from heat and let sit for 5 minutes. Fluff with a fork, garnish with nuts and serve immediately.

tips & tidbits

- *As mentioned earlier, brown rice should be avoided if you have any kind of digestive or eliminative difficulties, as it is often difficult to digest. White basmati rice would be preferable in this case. Although it is slightly processed, it is much easier on the digestive system. Make sure it is basmati rice and not regular white or instant rice.*

- *Although rice is a non-gluten grain and may be a welcome change to many wheat-logged digestive systems, for some it may be slightly constipating. In which case, Quinoa-Millet would be a better choice for a staple grain dish.*

lemon basmati rice

1 cup white basmati rice, rinsed
1 fresh lemon
2¼ cups water
1 tsp. turmeric
2 tbsp. light olive oil or ghee
2 tbsp. parsley flakes
¼ tsp. saffron (optional)
½ tsp. sea salt (optional

Juice lemon and set aside. Finely chop one half of the lemon rind. Briefly sauté lemon rind, turmeric, and saffron in light olive oil or ghee, stirring constantly. Stir in rice until coated. Add water and 1 tbsp. parsley flakes and salt. Bring to a boil. Reduce heat and simmer covered until all water is absorbed, approximately 15 minutes. Remove from heat and let sit for 5 minutes. Fluff with a fork, garnish with remaining parsley and serve immediately.

 tips & tidbits

- *Turmeric is a colorful, flavorful herb that has many medicinal qualities. It is especially beneficial to the female reproductive system. In ayurvedic medicine it used abundantly when nursing post-partum women back to health. It is also known to prevent diabetes and cancer, as well as providing relief from arthritis and skin ailments.*

- *Be careful when handling turmeric – it will permanently stain virtually everything! Wash the stain immediately and put it out in the sun.*

- *Store lemon juice in glass jar in refrigerator and use for master cleanse drink the next morning.*

quinoa-millet

½ cup quinoa
½ cup millet
3 cups water

Rinse quinoa and millet with cold water in strainer. Place in 1 quart pan with water and bring to boil uncovered. Reduce heat to low simmer and cover. Cook until all water is absorbed and grains are light and fluffy (approx. 20 minutes). Serve with a dab of butter and Bragg's Aminos to accompany steamed veggies. For breakfast, serve with a dab of butter and teaspoon of maple syrup or honey. (When cooking specifically for breakfast, try substituting half the water with plain rice milk or apple juice to make it sweet and creamy).

multi-grain medley

Combine two or three grains of your choice to create a medley of textures and flavors. Grains that have similar cooking times and require similar amounts of water make this quite easy. When combining grains that have different cooking times, start with the slower cooking grains and add faster cooking grains in at the appropriate time. (See the chart at the beginning of this chapter.) Cook with broth and/or spices of your choice to enhance flavor.

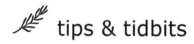 **tips & tidbits**

- *Quinoa-Millet is a staple dish that is so versatile (have it for breakfast, lunch or dinner!), quick and easy to make, nutritious and gluten-free..*

- *Quinoa is higher in calcium than milk and higher in protein than any other grain. This wonder grain is believed by some researchers to come closer in providing all the essential nutrients than any other food. It's also easy to digest!*

- *Millet is cleansing and nourishing to the digestive tract and the preferred grain for those with blood sugar imbalances. It is rich in iron, phosphorous, B vitamins and contains the most complete protein of all the grains.*

raisins & spice hot cereal

1cup *Bob's Red Mill 8-Grain Wheat-less* or *Gluten-Free* cereal
1½ cups pure water
1½ cups pure apple juice
1 bag *India Spice Tea*, by *Yogi Tea's*
handful of raisins
handful of raw seeds (pumpkin or sunflower)
handful of raw nuts (walnuts, sliced almonds, etc.)
2 tsps. ground flax meal
1 tbsp. flax oil or coconut oil

Place water and apple juice in sauce pan with tea bag and bring to a boil. Remove tea bag, add cereal and stir. Reduce heat to low, stirring almost constantly so cereal doesn't lump together. Simmer covered for 8-10 minutes. Stir a couple of times while cooking. Remove from heat when done and let sit covered for 3-5 minutes.

Serve in bowl-sized portions. While still hot, stir in raisins, raw seeds or nuts, flax meal and oil to suit individual tastes.

 tips & tidbits

- *This recipe makes about 4-5 servings. It's great for feeding an entire family or having leftovers to reheat for a couple of mornings.*

- *If cereal lumps together or sticks to the bottom while cooking, remove from heat with cover in place and let sit for 2-3 minutes. Stir out lumps and anything stuck to the bottom and resume cooking on lowest heat.*

quinoa-vegetable pilaf salad

6 cups cooked quinoa
¼ cup coconut oil
½ cup grated carrots
½ cup yellow or green onion, finely chopped
½ green bell pepper, diced
½ yellow or red bell pepper, diced
3 cloves fresh garlic, pressed
½ tsp. dried oregano
½ tsp. dried parsley
1-2 tsp. Spike
½ tsp sea salt
¼ tsp black pepper
1 cup sliced almonds or pine nuts

In large saucepan, sauté oil, garlic, spices, and vegetables until softened. Place cooked quinoa in large serving bowl. Add vegetable mixture and toss with quinoa and almonds.

Serve hot or cold.

 tips & tidbits

- *Quinoa is quick and easy to prepare. Follow the instructions given in the chart at the beginning of this section for cooking the quinoa.*

- *Quinoa is gluten-free and easy to digest – a perfect grain for anyone with digestive or eliminative problems.*

- *For breakfast, cook up a pot of quinoa with half water and half apple juice. Remove from heat and add ½-1 cup dried fruit, chopped, such as dried cherries or cranberries, dates, or raisins, and a handful of sliced almonds for a light, yet tasty and satisfying meal.*

salads & dressings

veggie-pasta salad

1-8 oz. box brown *Vita Spelt* rotini, cooked and cooled
1-8 oz. light *Vita Spelt* rotini, cooked and cooled
1 cup cucumbers, chopped
1 cup fresh tomatoes, chopped
1 cup carrots, chopped
1 cup zucchini, chopped
½ cup green bell pepper, chopped
½ cup yellow or red bell pepper, chopped
1 bunch green onions, chopped fine
½ cup black olives, sliced
¾ cup parmesan cheese, grated
Italian or vinaigrette dressing of your choice, to taste

Toss cold pasta with chopped vegetables and dressing in large bowl. Serve chilled.

This recipe makes a large batch that is perfect for carting along to a potluck or having leftovers for lunches. Adjust the types of vegetables to suit your taste.

tips & tidbits

- *Using your favorite bottle Italian or vinaigrette dressing is the quickest, surest way to go. Drizzling with your favorite olive oil and balsamic vinegar and adding some Bragg's and Spike to taste, can also be quite tasty.*

- *This is a great dish for summer outings and also for taking along on trips. Store in cooler and eat at your leisure.*

- *It usually lasts about 3 days before the vegetables starting wilting. Vacuum-sealing in a large plastic container or glass Mason jars will extend its life up to a week.*

carrot-apple salad

1 medium apple cored and chopped into ½" chunks
2 carrots, shredded
¼ cup sliced almonds, raw Chinese pumpkin seeds,
chopped walnuts or pecans
¼ - ½ cup raisins or currants

Chop carrots in food processor (or use hand grater). Combine with other ingredients. Cover with 2-3 oz. of *Almond-Tahini Dressing* just before eating. Deeelicious!

almond-tahini dressing

½-1 tbsp. raw almond butter
½-1 tbsp. raw tahini (sesame seed butter)
6 oz. pure apple juice

Combine all ingredients in 8 oz. glass jar with lid. Cover tightly and shake vigorously until mixed thoroughly. Mixing is easier when ingredients are at room temperature. Keep refrigerated. Use within 3-4 days.

tips & tidbits

- *Carrot-Apple Salad is a favorite recipe I learned from Grace Parusha (formerly Grace Cropley) a master at whole foods preparation. This and other fabulous recipes are featured in her book,* The Five Essential Laws of Eating. *See* Resources *for ordering information.*

- *Both carrots and apples are very cleansing to the body, especially the liver. This is a really healthful treat to add to your regular diet. Go easy on it to start, however, especially if your system is not used to raw foods.*

- *I save the 8-ounce jars from almond butter and tahini for mixing* Almond-Tahini *and other dressings. Use the 16 ounce jars for larger batches, but remember dressing only lasts 3-4 days (a week or more if vacuum-sealed in glass Mason jar).*

carrot-celery salad

4-5 cups shredded carrots
2-3 cups chopped celery stalks

Mix celery and carrots together. Top with *Almond-Tahini* or *Lemon-Tahini Dressing* and serve immediately. Or store in refrigerator in covered container and add dressing at time of serving.

lemon-tahini dressing

2 tbsp. raw tahini (sesame butter)
juice of 1 lemon (or 1 oz. Santa Cruz Organic Lemon Juice)
1 tbsp. brown rice vinegar
2 tbsp. extra virgin olive oil of your choice
1 tbsp. Braggs Liquid Aminos
1-2 cloves garlic crushed

Combine all ingredients in empty 6-8 oz. jar with lid. Shake vigorously. Use within 3 days. For lighter dressing omit tahini.

 tips & tidbits

- *Carrot-Celery Salad is a good staple to keep in the refrigerator to eat on its own (add avocado slices for extra oomph!) or add to other dishes, such* Mixed Veggie Pita Sandwiches *or salads.*

- *Juice fresh celery for a natural sedative that soothes the nervous system after a stressful day. It's very bitter tasting however, so it is best mixed with other juices, such as carrot and beet, to make it more palatable.*

creamy fruit salad

2 red or gala apples chopped into medium chunks
2 oranges or tangerines sectioned and cut into chunks
2 bananas sliced ½" thick
1 pint fresh strawberries halved
1 cup blueberries or grapes
½ cup walnut pieces or slivered almonds
½ cup raw sunflower or Chinese pumpkin seeds

Toss all ingredients in large serving bowl. Mix in *Yogurt Dressing* and chill covered in refrigerator until ready to serve.

yogurt dressing

6 oz. organic plain yogurt
¼ cup fresh orange or apple juice
¼ tsp. ground cinnamon

Mix ingredients thoroughly. Use within 3-4 days.

OR…
Make things really easy and toss fruit with a few spoons full of yogurt that is already flavored and/or has fruit added. Be sure to check label for those that are sweetened with natural sweeteners such as honey or fruit juice concentrate. Avoid those sweetened with refined sugars or artificial sweeteners.

 tips & tidbits

- Creamy Fruit Salad *and the upcoming* Waldorf Salad *are two refreshing salads that are perfect for a picnic or brunch on a hot summer day – or anytime.*

- *Yogurt contains friendly bacteria that is beneficial to the colon – unless you are sensitive to dairy. If this is the case, substitute coconut milk for the yogurt.*

- *For those who are allergic to oranges, substitute orange juice with grapefruit or pineapple juice. Or try apple juice with a small squirt of fresh lemon juice.*

coco-nutty fruit salad

½-1 apple or pear, chopped into bite-sized bits
1 medium banana, sliced
small handful walnut pieces or sliced almonds
2 tbsp. coconut milk
sprinkle of cinnamon
grated fresh ginger to taste (opt)

Combine ingredients in bowl. Best when served immediately. Serves 1-2.

Options: Double or triple recipe, add berries, cherries, grapes, or orange slices.

dr. budwig cottage cheese dish

½-1 cup organic low fat cottage cheese
2-4 tbsp. ground flax meal
2-4 tbsp. flax oil
½ cup fruit, such as sliced banana or blueberries
pinch of cayenne

Mix by hand in bowl or blender. Great for breakfast or snack.

This is the basic recipe for the healing diet of Dr. Johanna Budwig, a German biochemist. It is a therapeutic recipe that helps in the treatment and prevention of many ailments, including cancer and liver/gallbladder conditions.

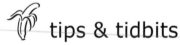 tips & tidbits

- Coco-nutty Fruit Salad *is my favorite breakfast and I have yet to find anyone who doesn't like it, including kids. Adding fresh ginger will increase its digestibility.*

- *Although the* Dr. Budwig Cottage Cheese Dish *is known for its therapeutic qualities, those who are intolerant of dairy may still have a problem with the cottage cheese. Give it a try and see if it agrees with your system.*

waldorf salad

3 large apples cut into chunks
2 stalks celery chopped
1 tangerine sectioned (or 1 small orange)
1 large carrot shredded into large pieces
¼ cup raisins
½ cup walnut pieces or almond slices

Toss all ingredients in large serving bowl. Mix in Yogurt Dressing and chill covered in refrigerator until ready to serve.

moroccan tomato-cucumber salad

3-4 fresh medium tomatoes
1 medium cucumber
1 small red onion
1 bunch cilantro or flat parsley
1 oz. olive oil or flax oil
juice of 1 lemon (or 1 oz. Santa Cruz Organic lemon juice)

Slice and gut tomatoes. Chop gutted tomatoes, cucumber, onions and parsley very fine. Toss together with oil and lemon juice. Sprinkle with garlic powder for extra zest.

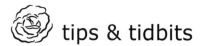 # tips & tidbits

- *Add torn romaine leaves for a delicious variation to the* Waldorf Salad.

- Tomato-Cucumber Salad *is a very popular dish in Morocco that is usually served with fresh baked bread for dipping. Instead of bread, use celery sticks or cucumber slices to scoop up salad. Also delicious when eaten by itself with a fork.*

- *Raw onions are cleansing and help to build the immune system. However, for those with sensitive digestive systems they may cause gas and bloating (not to mention questionable breath!) and are better left alone until the digestive system is stronger.*

soups & sides

potato-onion soup

6-8 small red or yellow potatoes, scrubbed
3 large yellow onions, chopped
olive oil
2" piece of fresh ginger, crushed
5-6 cloves garlic, crushed
¼-½ tsp. crushed red chiles
½ tsp. cayenne
1 tsp. black pepper
1½ tsp. turmeric
Bragg's Liquid Aminos to taste

Cut potatoes into medium chunks. In large soup kettle, briefly sauté onions and all spices in small amount of olive oil and water. Add potatoes and cover with purified water to about 1" over top of potatoes. Cover and simmer on low heat until potatoes are soft. Serve hot, adding Bragg's to taste.

tips & tidbits

- *Onions, garlic and ginger are a classic healthful combination. They cleanse and purify the body, act as a natural antibiotic and boost the immune system, to name just a few of their many beneficial properties. Go easy on the onions and garlic to start as they may cause gas.*

- *This is a favorite soup of the American Sikhs. They have it every day for breakfast (yes, breakfast!) during their bi-annual weeklong yoga retreats. It is designed to be very spicy to increase its cleansing and purifying properties (if you are not used to hot spicy foods, reduce cayenne, garlic and ginger). You don't have to have it for breakfast, but I assure you, it is a warm and wonderful way to start the day.*

ginger vegetable soup

1 large onion, chopped
3-4 cloves garlic crushed
2" piece of fresh ginger, grated
1-2 dashes of cayenne
2 tsp. Salt-Free Spike
1 yellow zucchini
1 green zucchini
1 large carrot
½ cup green beans
½ cup peas
½ cup corn
Bragg's Liquid Aminos or Quick Sip to taste

Chop all vegetables into bite-sized chunks. In large soup pot, sauté onions, garlic, cayenne and spike in small amount of olive oil and water. Add all vegetables and enough purified water to clear top of vegetables by 1 inch. Add squirt or two of Quick Sip or Bragg's (you can always add more at time of serving). Cover and simmer on low heat until vegetables soften. Serve immediately.

tips & tidbits

- *It is so important for your overall health to keep the bowels moving efficiently and regularly. This soup is a great helper for those prone to constipation. Eat it for lunch and dinner for a day or two and it will help get things moving again.*

- *If you are just getting started in the cooking-from-scratch department and not accustomed to chopping a lot of vegetables, you may want to try frozen bags of mixed vegetables (they have mixes with carrots, peas, green beans and corn). Not the best choice, but certainly better than canned soup or some other choices. Zucchini is not available frozen and only takes a minute to chop up, so at least you can have that fresh.*

mama rosa's escarole, bean soup

1 bunch escarole (may substitute with spinach)
1 small onion, chopped fine
1 stalk celery, chopped
1 medium carrot, chopped
1 clove garlic, crushed
1 tsp. parsley flakes
½ tsp. black pepper
1 tsp. dried oregano
1 tsp. dried basil
8 oz. tomato sauce
16 oz. cannellini beans (soaked or canned)
olive oil

Rinse escarole and tear into bite sized pieces. Set aside. In large skillet, sauté onion, celery, carrot and garlic in small amount of olive oil and water. Add tomato sauce and all other seasonings. Simmer on low heat for about 5 minutes. Add 8 oz. purified water and escarole. Simmer for 10 more minutes. Add cannelloni beans and simmer another 10-20 minutes. Serve hot. Add Bragg's to taste, if desired.

(If escarole and cannellini beans are unavailable, substitute spinach and great northern white beans, respectively.)

✿ tips & tidbits

- *Mama Rosa was my former husband's mother. A true Italian New Yorker, she grew scores of tomatoes every summer and spent hours in the kitchen making up large batches of homemade tomato sauce from a family recipe that had been passed down for generations. And that was the just the beginning of her culinary extravaganza! Hats off to Mama Rosa, her Escarole & Beans are magnifico!*

- *Although scrumptious by itself, this dish is traditionally served with fresh Italian bread for dipping and scooping. Fresh whole grain bread or sprouted grain bread would be a better choice (and even tastier, in my opinion) - also quite nice over a bed of rice.*

tara's green beans almondine

1 lb. fresh green beans
3-4 cloves garlic thinly sliced
olive oil
1 large yellow onion sliced thin
1 large red pepper sliced lengthwise
Bragg's Liquid Aminos to taste
1 tsp. Tocomere seasoning
OR
1-2 dashes of cayenne
½ cup whole raw almonds

Wash beans and snap off ends. Cover bottom of large skillet with small amount of olive oil and water. Place beans in skillet, squirt with Bragg's, cover and steam on low/medium heat for about 15 minutes. Mix in onions, garlic, peppers and Tocomere. Squirt with a little more Bragg's and continue to simmer on low heat for another 15 minutes or until beans are soft. Turn with a spatula periodically. Add almonds last, allowing to steam 2-3 minutes (do not overcook or they will get soggy).

 tips & tidbits

- *This is a yummy dish my childhood friend Tara made for me one lazy summer evening. It is a wonderful complement to almost any meat or fish dish. Also great on top of rice or all by itself.*

- *Green beans are very alkaline and therefore very beneficial to today's highly stressed, over-acidic body systems.*

- *Use roasted almonds instead of raw for a special treat. Slivered or sliced almonds work well too.*

carrot-beet casserole treat

6 medium beets
6 medium carrots
1 large yellow onion, chopped
2 cloves fresh garlic, crushed
¼ tsp. black pepper
olive oil
Bragg's Liquid Aminos to taste
½ cup sliced almonds (optional)
½ cup grated Monterey Jack cheese (optional)

Scrub beets and carrots. Steam beets first for about 10 minutes. In skillet, briefly sauté onions, garlic, and black pepper in small amount of olive oil and Bragg's. Remove from heat and set aside. Add carrots to steaming beets and steam for another 10 minutes or so, or until both are softened. Rinse in cold water and scrape off skins. Coarsely grate beets and carrots separately by hand or in food processor. Place in casserole dish and toss with sautéed onions and almond slices. Top with cheese, if desired. Bake or broil at 350° for 5-10 minutes or until cheese melts. Serve hot.

 tips & tidbits

- *This is one of my favorite dishes. I call it casserole treat because it is so rich that it is more than just a side dish. Try it over a bed of basmati rice and a fresh green salad for a light meal.*

- *With its combination of carrots and beets (not to mention the onions and garlic - here they are again!) this dish is not only delicious, but it also packs a powerful punch in cleansing and healing the body. For that reason, it is best to eat only small portions to start and see how your body does with it.*

macaroni & cheese

8 oz. *Vita Spelt* rotini pasta
2½ cups mild cheddar or Monterey Jack cheese, grated
1½ cups oat or cow's milk
2 tbsp. butter
2 tbsp. corn starch
½ medium onion, minced
¼ tsp. Westbrae Dijon Mustard
½ tsp. Herbamere
½ tsp. Spike Salt-Free Seasoning
¼ tsp. black pepper
Bragg Liquid Aminos to taste

Follow package instructions for cooking pasta. While pasta is cooking, melt butter in skillet on low heat. Add cornstarch and whisk for 3 minutes. Then slowly whisk in milk. Add onion, mustard and other seasonings. Simmer on low heat for approximately 15 minutes, stirring frequently. Add cheese to sauce and stir until melted. Drain pasta when cooked and place in greased casserole dish. Mix in cheese sauce and bake at 350° for 30 minutes. Let sit for 5 minutes and then serve.

tips & tidbits

- *Eating for health doesn't mean you have to miss out on some of your old favorites. If you've been feeling that way, this hearty dish will fill that void. Be sure to eat plenty of steamed vegetables or a large green salad with this Mac & Cheese to offset all the cheese and grains.*

- *Some people do O.K. with cheese, but have difficulty with cow's milk. Use the kind of milk that works best for your body.*

- *For a lighter version, substitute cheese with 1 cup low fat cottage cheese and 8 oz. low fat cream cheese.*

baked butternut squash

Cut squash in half lengthwise and lay upside down in shallow baking dish with 1" of water. Bake at 400° for 45-60 minutes. Scoop out squash and serve hot. Add a bit of butter and a splash of Bragg's, if desired.

baked yams or sweet potatoes

yams or sweet potatoes

Scrub yams or sweet potatoes and poke with a fork in a few places. Place in shallow baking dish (do not set on rack, they usually ooze syrup) and bake at 400° for 45-60 minutes. Serve with melted butter and a squirt of Bragg's or sprinkle of cinnamon.

baked yam or potato home fries

yams, or russet potatoes
light olive oil
sea salt, Tocomere or Herbamere

Scrub yams or potatoes and cut into lengthwise strips about ¾" wide. Grease cookie sheet generously with olive oil. Place fries on cookie sheet, rubbing each in the olive oil on both sides. Sprinkle with sea salt or seasoning. Bake at 375° for 10-20 minutes. Turn fries and bake for another 10-20 minutes, or until done.

 tips & tidbits

- *Butternut squash is truly one of nature's delicacies. It's so simple and easy to make, you'll want to make it a regular part of your diet if you haven't already.*

- *Yams are a deeper orange color on the inside as well as out. Sweet potatoes look like faded yams on the outside and are a paler yellow or flesh color on the inside. I prefer yams myself. They are Mother Nature's candy.*

- *These Baked Yam or Potato Home Fries will hit the spot when you get a hankering for their unhealthy counterpart, French fries – and you can actually feel good about eating them!*

steamed veggies & leafy greens

Your choice of the following vegetables, washed and chopped as described in previous chapter:

Green & yellow zucchini, broccoli, bell peppers (red, yellow or green), onions, bok choy, celery, Portobello mushrooms, green beans, brussel sprouts, etc.

Your choice of the following leafy greens:

Swiss chard, bok choy leaves, kale, collard. mustard, or beet greens

Cover bottom of steamer pan with ½ - ¾ inch of water. Place chopped vegetables in basket of steamer and steam for approximately 5 minutes. Place leafy greens on top of steaming vegetables and steam until limp (about 2 minutes). Do not over cook. Serve with dab of butter and squirt of Bragg's Liquid Aminos or tamari sauce. Or serve on bed of pasta or rice and cover with marinara sauce.

grilled veggies

Marinate chopped, mixed veggies for steaming at least 2 hours, and preferably overnight in your favorite vinaigrette dressing or a combination of olive oil, balsamic vinegar and spices to taste. Slide on skewers or place in grilling pan. Grill over medium heat until vegetables soften.

tips & tidbits

- *A mixture of veggies should be eaten every daily by anyone wanting to restore or maintain their health. Your taste buds may argue at first, but just keep eating them and soon they will be in agreement, as well.*

- *If green leafy vegetables are new to you, experimenting is the best place to start. They are one of the most nutrient-dense foods available and wise to eat them regularly. For example, kale is rich in calcium, iron, potassium, Vitamin A and one cup provides more Vitamin C than an orange! If eating greens regularly just isn't going to happen at your house, which is often the case, at least be sure to take green food supplements regularly, as discussed earlier.*

ratatouille

1 eggplant cut into ¾" cubes
1 zucchini cut into ¾"cubes
1 ½ cups chopped broccoli
1 green pepper cut into ½" pieces
1 yellow, orange or red pepper cut into ½" pieces
2-3 fresh Roma tomatoes, cubed (optional)
1 medium yellow onion sliced
1 jar natural marinara sauce
1-3 cloves freshly pressed garlic
¼ cup fresh basil, chopped fine
2-3 sprigs fresh thyme

Steam eggplant, zucchini and peppers for 6-8 minutes. Remove from heat and place in large casserole dish with all other ingredients. Mix well. Bake at 350° 15-20 minutes until vegetables are tender. Serve hot or cold.

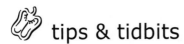 tips & tidbits

- *Ratatouille is a wonderful dish that is satisfying when eaten all by itself. It is also great with chicken, fish or served over a bed of your favorite rice or whole grain dish such as quinoa/millet for a vegetarian meal.*

- *For a special treat (or to entice finicky children to eat it!) grate a little cheese over the top while hot, allowing it to melt slightly.*

- *Many people are sensitive to eggplant causing gas, bloating and other uncomfortable symptoms after eating it. If this is the case, substitute the eggplant with 2 medium yellow squash and/or increase the amount of zucchini and broccoli.*

sweets & treats

blueberry muffins

2 cups spelt flour
½-2/3 cup rapadura sugar
4 tsp. aluminum-free baking powder
½ tsp salt
2 large eggs, lightly beaten
¼ cup softened butter or coconut oil
1 tsp. vanilla
¾ cup oat milk or apple juice
1 ½ cups frozen or fresh blueberries

In large mixing bowl, whisk together eggs, butter or coconut oil, and vanilla. Add oat milk or apple juice and set aside. Combine dry ingredients in separate bowl, then add to wet mixture in mixing bowl. Mix thoroughly. Fold in blueberries. Fill greased muffin tins half full and bake at 400° for 12 minutes, or until tops are slightly browned. Makes about 12 large muffins.

 tips & tidbits

- *This is a basic muffin recipe that can be used to make a variety of muffins. For example, substitute the blueberries with raspberries or mixed berries, or a ¾ cup raisins and ¾ cup walnut pieces.*

- *Spread with butter, ghee or coconut oil for a delicious addition to breakfast or stand alone snack.*

- *These muffins freeze well, so be sure to make extra to freeze for later – if you can keep them around that long!*

carob chip cookies

¼ cup almond butter
¼ cup tahini (sesame butter)
1/8 cup coconut oil
½ cup brown rice syrup
½ tsp. liquid Stevia
1 tsp. pure vanilla extract
¼ cup plain oat milk
1 egg
1½ cups whole grain spelt flour
½ cup rolled oats
¼ tsp. sea salt
¼ tsp. baking soda
½ cup unsweetened carob chips
½ cup walnuts (optional)

Cream together almond butter, tahini and all other liquid ingredients. Stir sea salt and baking soda into flour. Add flour mixture and oats to liquid ingredients. Mix thoroughly, and then add carob chips and walnuts. Drop on greased cookie sheet and press down with fork.

Bake at 375° for 12-15 minutes.

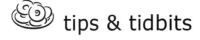 tips & tidbits

- *I highly recommend using insulated cookie sheets for baking. They are great stress reducers. Cookies come out perfect every time - no burning or sticking!*

- *Substitute carob chips with raisins for a healthier version. Or substitute carob chips with naturally sweetened chocolate chips for a more decadent version!*

peanut butter cookies

½ cup natural peanut butter
3 tbsp. coconut oil
1/3 cup brown rice syrup
½ tsp. liquid Stevia
1 tsp. pure vanilla
1 egg
¾ cup whole grain spelt flour
¼ cup amaranth flour
¼ tsp. baking soda
¼ tsp. sea salt (optional)

Cream together peanut butter and all liquid ingredients. In separate bowl, mix together flours, baking soda and salt. Combine with liquid ingredients and mix thoroughly. Drop on greased baking sheet and press down with fork.

Bake at 375° for 12-15 minutes.

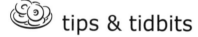 **tips & tidbits**

- *Use honey instead of brown rice syrup for a slightly sweeter version.*

- *For those avoiding peanuts or with a more delicate digestive system, try using raw almond butter in place of the peanut butter.*

- *Natural peanut butter doesn't contain additives (or sugar) and therefore separates, with the oil floating to the top of the jar. Be sure to mix thoroughly before adding to recipes.*

- *Amaranth is a non-gluten grain that is very nutritious. It contains more protein and calcium than milk. Unfortunately it is also underutilized in our culture. Adding amaranth flour to baked goods is one way of reaping some of the benefits of this uncommon grain. It adds a slightly nutty flavor to recipes, as well.*

kelly's carrot cake

1½ cups finely grated carrots, packed (3-4 large carrots)
1 egg
¼ cup organic butter, melted
1 cup plain oat milk
½ cup brown rice syrup
½ tsp. liquid Stevia
1 tsp. vanilla extract
1½ cups whole grain spelt flour
1 tsp. ground cinnamon
¼ tsp. ground nutmeg
¼ tsp. ground allspice
½ tsp. sea salt (optional)
1½ tsp. baking powder

Combine all liquid ingredients. Stir in grated carrots (best if grated very fine using food processor). In separate bowl, stir together all dry ingredients. Add to carrot mixture, mixing in gently and only until thoroughly mixed. Do not beat. Pour into greased 9x9" square baking pan.

Bake at 350° for 45-50 minutes or until knife inserted comes out clean. Allow to cool. Top with cream cheese frosting or spread square pieces with butter or ghee.

 tips & tidbits

- *This moist and delicious cake is rich in carrots that are so beneficial to the body. Add 1 cup raisins and 1 cup walnuts to give it more texture and interest.*

- *Or, add 1 cup fresh pineapple chunks (or 8 oz. can crushed pineapple, drained) to liven things up. It will also make it a little easier to digest, as pineapple is rich in bromelain, a powerful digestive enzyme.*

- *To decorate, ice cake with cream cheese frosting. Then place fresh flowers and leaves around the bottom border and a couple in the center of the cake. Be sure to put flowers on just before serving to prevent wilting.*

cream cheese frosting

4 oz. organic cream cheese, softened
¼ cup organic butter, softened
2 tbsp. honey
¼ tsp. vanilla

Set butter and cream cheese out to soften. Whip cream cheese with butter. Add other ingredients and whip until smooth.

(Do not substitute maple syrup for honey in this recipe. It is too thin and makes frosting runny.)

 ## tips & tidbits

- *Double the* Carrot Cake *and* Cream Cheese Frosting *recipes to make a 9" layer cake, perfect for any special occasion. With electric mixer, beat in a few pineapple chunks or 2-3 pitted dates with small amount of cream cheese frosting to spread between the layers.*

- *To make natural food coloring for borders or writing with icing, boil beets (for red) in small amount of water and add to a portion of icing. For yellow, add small amount of powdered turmeric straight from the bottle. Be careful not to add too much or it will alter the taste.*

almond-date no-bake apple crisp

¾ cup whole raw almonds
8-10 medium, pitted dates
4 red or gala apples - cored
2 tbsp. freshly squeezed lemon juice
4 tbsp. apple juice
½ tsp. ground cinnamon

Grind almonds and dates together in food processor. Press mixture firmly and evenly into bottom of 9 x 9" baking dish. (May mix in a little raw almond butter to help hold together.) Puree 1½ apples in blender with 1 tbsp. lemon juice and cinnamon, adding apple juice as necessary, until mixture is about the consistency of thick apple butter. Dice remaining apples into ¼" chunks by hand or in food processor. Sprinkle with remaining lemon juice. In mixing bowl, mix together diced apples and apple puree. Scoop into baking dish and smooth evenly over the almond/date crust. Serve immediately by cutting into squares or cover and refrigerate until a little firmer. Don't put off having some if you have others in the household, however, because it will disappear fast!

 tips & tidbits

- *This is a great treat that contains all raw foods and no concentrated sweeteners. Eating raw foods ensures you are getting the most nutrients and enzymes from your food.*

- *An apple-coring tool is a must in every health-oriented kitchen. Available in stores that sell cooking utensils, they look like a serrated knife, only curved to cut around the core of the apple and easily pull it out.*

- *Another sweet treat idea comes from my days in Morocco where I spent many a teatime peeling apart sweet, gooey dates and replacing the pit with an almond. Try it. It's a quick and easy natural foods snack that is not only fun, but one of nature's true delicacies – and kids love it!*

big bud's pumpkin pie

1 - 9" whole grain piecrust
1¾-cup fresh pumpkin (or 1 –15 oz canned pumpkin)
2 eggs, beaten
1/2-cup honey or maple syrup
1 tsp. ground cinnamon
1 tsp. ground ginger
¼ tsp ground nutmeg
1-cup vanilla oat milk

Mix all ingredients and pour into piecrust. Bake at 350° for 45-55 minutes or until knife inserted comes out clean. Allow to cool. Serve with spoonful of whipped cream sweetened with honey or maple syrup, if desired.

 tips & tidbits

- *This is a delightful alternative to traditional pumpkin pie recipes, which usually include large amounts of refined sugar and sweetened condensed milk.*

- *We have served this pie many times to guests who rave about it. Only after the first few bites do we let them know that it is sugar free. Just that term seems to sometimes turn people off. Probably because people's first association is to the many commercial products labeled sugar free that contain harmful strange-tasting chemicals.*

- *Pumpkin is rich in vitamin A and helps to regulate blood sugar. It is also very cleansing to the liver and digestive system.*

frozen banana cream treat (dairy-free)

2-3 ripe bananas (peels should be turning brown)
splash of oat milk
splash of maple syrup or honey (optional)

Slice bananas into ¼ inch slices and place flat in square container with lid or on a plate and cover tightly with plastic wrap. Place in freezer until frozen. Remove from freezer and allow to soften just slightly. Blend in food processor or blender with a splash of oat milk and a splash of maple syrup or honey. Top with nuts of your choice and a sprinkle of cinnamon. Yummy!

frozen fruit ice cream

1 part coconut milk or plain, organic yogurt
1 ½ - 2 parts frozen mixed berries or cherries
small squirt of honey to taste (optional)

Blend in food processor and serve immediately.

 tips & tidbits

- *Bananas start to turn brown about 10 days after placing in the freezer, so make the* Frozen Banana Cream Treat *within a few days of freezing the banana slices.*

- *This is a great recipe to teach kids how to make for themselves. It's so easy to make and they love it!*

- *I had a friend once who asked me to stop telling her kids that we were going to make banana ice cream. She was afraid they were going to be disappointed with whatever natural recipe I was gearing up to introduce to them. She apologized later when they started begging for it, just like they would ice cream!*

beverages

green drink

4-6 oz. pure apple or pear juice
12-16 oz. purified water
1-2 tsp. green food powder
2 tsp. non-allergenic protein powder of choice (optional)

Combine ingredients in quart jar or plastic container. Shake or stir frequently.

tangy lemonade

1 cup fresh lemon juice (approx. 8-10 medium lemons)
OR 1 cup Santa Cruz 100% lemon juice (not from concentrate)
4 cups purified water
20-25 drops liquid Stevia
¼ cup + 1 tbsp. pure maple syrup
¼ cup pure cranberry juice (optional, for pink lemonade)

Mix liquids together in pitcher or 1-2 quart glass jar. Add thin lemon slices as garnishment. This is a tangy lemonade that can withstand a little dilution from added ice on a hot summer's day. Makes 1 quart.

citrus apple soda

1 part pure apple juice
½ part pure orange or grapefruit juice
½ part carbonated mineral water

Mix together liquids just before serving to maintain fizz. This is a refreshing drink that is a great substitute for commercial sodas. Contains no concentrated sweeteners or other additives. Leave out the carbonated mineral water for a tasty juice combo.

If the fizz is what excites you about soda, this is a delicious alternative you'll love. This is the basic recipe for starters, but don't feel you have to stick to it. Children especially love to experiment to find their own favorite ratio of the ingredients.

essential three smoothie

1 cup fresh or frozen fruit of your choice
1 ripe banana
¾-1 cup purified water
½ cup pure apple or pear juice
handful each of raw sunflower & pumpkin seeds
¼ cup coconut milk
1 tbsp. coconut or flaxseed oil
1 tsp. green food powder of your choice
1-2 heaping tsps. non-allergenic protein powder
¼" thick slice of fresh ginger

Combine ingredients in blender and blend until smooth and creamy. Add water
if needed for a thinner consistency.

high energy smoothie

12 oz. pure apple juice
18 oz. purified water
2 ½ cups frozen fruits (peaches, grapes, melons, cherries, blueberries)
1-2 tsps. wheat grass powder
½-1 tsp. barley grass powder
1-2 tsps. flax oil or extra virgin olive oil
2 heaping tsps. non-allergenic protein/fiber powder

Mix all ingredients in blender and serve.

 tips & tidbits

- *Smoothies are a great way to start the day in the warmer months. I do not
  recommend consuming them later in the day however, as most people have been
  eating solid food, and throwing in a smoothie on top of it all usually makes for
  digestive disturbances.*

- *Experiment with different fruits according to your own tastes and food tolerances.*

- *Commercial smoothies often contain common allergens, such as strawberries, orange
  juice, bananas and milk products), essentially negating the otherwise healthful
  benefits for those who have food sensitivities.*

creamy ginger smoothie (dairy-free)

1 sliced apple
6 oz. oat or almond milk
2 oz. purified water
2 heaping tsps. non-allergenic protein powder
¼-½" thick slice of fresh ginger
sprinkle of cinnamon

First, grind up ginger with apple juice in blender. Add remaining ingredients. Blend just slightly for a chunky smoothie that's fun to eat or, if you prefer, blend until mixture becomes a traditional smooth consistency.

delicious date shake

2-3 pitted dates
4 oz. oat or almond milk
3 frozen bananas
1 tsp. pure vanilla extract
½ tsp. liquid Stevia OR honey to taste
sprinkle of cinnamon

First, grind up dates with milk in blender. Add remaining ingredients. Blend until smooth, scraping sides as necessary. Serve immediately. Better than the malt shop!

 # tips & tidbits

- Creamy Ginger Smoothie *is not the ideal food combination and for that reason may not be a prime choice for those with sensitive digestive systems. Works fine for many, so try it and see.*

- *This* Date Shake *is a wise choice for those who are transitioning off dairy and sugar. Certainly not something you'd want to indulge in every day, but for a once in awhile delectable treat, it is a much better choice than what the corner fast-food restaurant has to offer.*

- *Add a little honey in place of the Stevia if you do O.K. in the blood sugar department. Top off with peanuts or sliced almonds for added texture.*

fresh juices

Fresh juices are packed with nutrients and very beneficial to the body. For optimal digestive action, "chew" fresh juices, letting them remain in the mouth a short time to allow them to mix with saliva. It is also best to drink juices on an empty stomach, as they move through your system quickly. Go easy if you are not accustomed to raw foods or fresh juices, as they can have a heavy detoxifying effect and can also cause gas and bloating initially (especially if you drink them too fast). Once your digestive tract has strengthened and acclimated to this nourishing nectar, you can increase the quantity you consume.

You can purchase very inexpensive juicers today. They are great for getting started if you have never juiced before. Sometimes they leave the juice a little pulpy (pouring through a strainer helps) and aren't quite as durable as some of the more expensive ones (I burned out the motor on my first inexpensive model!) I recommend either the *Juiceman II* or *Juiceman Jr.* They are both reasonably priced, make pulp-free juice, and are relatively easy to clean.

Individual and combination juices have been used for years to rejuvenate ailing bodies. Drinking only fresh juices for 1-2 days periodically (also known as a juice fast) is also a great way to cleanse and rejuvenate your system. Once every season is a good place to start. It allows your digestive organs to rest and clears the body of toxins and unwanted debris that could be making your system sluggish. People report increased energy and clarity of mind after juice fasting.

Drinking only watermelon and watermelon juice for a day or two is a regular cleanse I do every summer. It is very cleansing and beneficial to the liver, kidneys, and colon. Watermelon juice is also incredibly delicious if you have never tried it. Following are a couple of my favorite fresh juice combinations. For more help, there are entire books that contain only juice recipes, or experiment on your own.

tips & tidbits

- *Both fruit and vegetable juices are concentrated and often very sweet. For that reason, it is wise to dilute fruit juices by half and vegetable juices by one quarter. This is easier on your blood sugar and a little easier on the digestive system as well.*

- *It is best to drink fresh juices within a few minutes after juicing to obtain the most nutrients. Fresh juice is still better than fresh store bought or bottled juice. So, if you don't have time to juice every day, make enough to last a couple days and store remainder in glass jars in the refrigerator. Vacuum seal for added freshness.*

carrot-apple-ginger juice

2-3 large carrots
2-3 large apples
¼-½" thick slice of fresh ginger

Run ingredients through juicer. Serve immediately.

This is a great formula for fighting off colds (much better than orange juice, which can be very mucous producing). Ginger is a real immune booster and is also beneficial to the digestive tract. Make this juice as hot as you like by adding more ginger or tone it down by adding less.

carrot-celery-cucumber juice

1 large or 2 small carrots
2 stalks celery
1 medium cucumber

Wash vegetables. Peel cucumber if it had wax on it. Cut off celery leaves for less bitter tasting juice. Run vegetables through juicer. Serve immediately.

Especially good for the skin, liver/gallbladder and for relaxing (celery juice is a natural sedative), this juice combination is more of a healthful, medicinal juice. Taste is not it's forte, but you sure do look and feel good if you drink it regularly.

 # tips & tidbits

- *If you want to find out how efficient your digestive system is at moving things through, drink a small amount of beet juice (best if mixed with carrot or apple juice) and count the number of hours it takes before your stools appear reddish. Beet juice is also a powerful liver cleanser.*

- *Add a small bunch of fresh parsley to any juice as a powerful blood purifier. Also very beneficial to those with gallbladder problems. Start with a small amount as it is very potent. If you do O.K., add more the next time you juice.*

teas & coffee substitutes

Although coffee has become a staple in the average American diet, as the second guideline indicates I recommend eliminating coffee and it's constituent caffeine from your diet, or having it only on occasion in reasonable amounts. Caffeine is a stimulant that taxes your adrenal glands, upsetting your energy levels and the overall biochemical balance of your body, and has been linked to a variety of detrimental health conditions (including high blood pressure, nervousness, fibroids, PMS, menopausal complaints, depression, etc.).

There are a variety of teas and roasted grain beverages that serve as tasty substitutes for coffee. You may even find that you like one of them even better than that old cup of java (which in my opinion leaves something to be desired in the taste department anyway). Following are some favorites:

- **India Spice Tea, Cocoa Spice Tea, & Green Tea Kombucha**
  all by the Yogi Tea Company

I love all the teas by this company, but these 3 are my favorites. The Yogi Tea Company also offers quite an array of medicinal teas, high quality teas that are worth exploring.

- **Bengal Spice & Roastaroma**
  by Celestial Seasonings

These two caffeine-free teas are both very flavorful and satisfying. The *Celestial Seasonings* boxes they come in are beautiful and offer inspiring thoughts as well.

- **Kukicha (twig tea)**
  by Eden Foods, Inc.

This Japanese favorite contains a bit of caffeine and is therefore a good stepping-stone for those who experience harsh withdrawal symptoms, such as headaches, when going off coffee. It is also available in a caffeine-free version. It is best simmered for up to 20 minutes to bring out its full flavor. When steeped it tends to be a little weak.

- **Kaffree Roma**
  by Worthington Foods

An instant, caffeine-free roasted grain beverage made with malt barley and chicory, this is about as close as you can get to coffee when it comes to taste. In fact, when I served it to some unsuspecting habitual coffee drinkers, they thought it was instant coffee!

- Cafix
  by InternNatural Foods

Cafix is very similar to *Kaffree Roma*, but with added rye and beetroots.   This drink has the added benefit of the cleansing and detoxifying power of the beetroots. So go easy to start. For some people it may be *very* cleansing (if you know what I mean!).

- Teeccino
  by Teeccino Caffé, Inc

Teeccino is a blend of herbs, grains, fruits and nuts that are roasted, ground and brewed just like coffee. Dark, rich, and full-bodied, Teeccino brings you all the satisfaction of a robust brew with no caffeine reaction.

quick & easy herbal iced tea

For a delightful and easy to make cold tea, place 3-4 bags of your favorite fruit tea , such as blackberry, peach, strawberry/kiwi, etc., in a quart jar of purified water. Let steep in refrigerator and within a few hours you have a refreshing fruit tea. Add a tad of Stevia or natural sweetener, although it tastes wonderful all by itself.

fresh ginger tea

2-3 - ¼" slices fresh ginger
2-3 cups purified water

Combine ingredients bring to a boil and simmer for 20-30 minutes. Serve hot.

 # tips & tidbits

- *There's nothing like a hot drink to soothe one's spirits at almost anytime. However, the choices that have become the social norm (coffee or caffeinated tea) are not soothing to the body – quite the opposite. Why not make this practice truly comforting, by drinking quality herbal teas that are healing and nourishing to the body.*

- *Add rice, oat or almond milk instead of cream or cow's milk to teas and coffee substitutes. To sweeten, add a small amount of Stevia, maple syrup, agave, or honey instead of refined sugar. Or drink plain and enjoy the natural taste*

The End

A *drop of juice slid down the palm of my hand. I caught it with my tongue before it got away, spit a couple of seeds into the sink and ravenously went for the next juicy bite. It was then, when I sunk my teeth into the sweet flesh of the fruit, that it dawned on me. I had been eating watermelon with reckless abandon almost every morning for the last two weeks since I had started writing this book. The irony of this brought a smile to my face.*

I remembered that day so long ago, when I had regretfully declined the offer of fresh cut watermelon, which brought that fateful question, heavy with despair, to my lips. It was a pivotal day in my life, I now thought. Surely the day this book was unknowingly conceived. I marveled at how my life had changed since then. With each passing year since, my health had progressively improved. Eating watermelon had now become part of my regular summer routine, a recently adopted routine that revolved around working on my book.

Before indulging in watermelon, I'd jog around the lake enjoying the restored strength of my body and the inspiration of the Rocky Mountains that loomed to the West. I'd think about my book, what I wanted to say, and exactly how I might say it. I'd think about the people who would read this book and my wishes for how it would serve them. I wished for it to be a friend and a coach. To stand by the reader's side, tell them what they needed to know, walk with them through the process, pick them up when they fell, move them closer to their goal. It was what I yearned for as I struggled through my own transition to health and to a better way of eating, never realizing until now, that I was creating it all along.

My thoughts drifted back to that day in the magical mountains of New Mexico. As I recalled the sickness and despair that had consumed me, I was struck by the revelation of that prophesied answer to my fateful question so long ago and how it had indeed come true. Everything suddenly became clear to me and I now knew exactly why it had all happened. I had learned. I was well again, better than ever, and I was now teaching and helping others to be well, too.

My eyes teared with reverence as I lifted my gaze out the window and up to the sky where the heavens reside. Time stopped for just a moment. A moment that filled me with humbled gratitude and a deep knowing of something much greater than us at play. And with that came the biggest and final wish for all readers — that they too, would have such a moment.

Resources

recommended websites

- www.foodfitnessbyphone.com & www.wellnesscoaching.com
  Kelly Hayford's websites, healthy eating programs, free e-zine, information

- www.cspinet.org
  Center for Science in the Public Interest website

- www.nosmsg.com, www.msgmyth.com &
  http://www.ideatown.com/ntxa/index.html
  Lots of valuable information on MSG

- www.truthinlabeling.org
  Food labeling issues and more information on MSG and

- www.organicconsumers.com
  Information on organic foods and the biotech industry (GMO's)

- www.foodyoucaneat.com
  Fabulous site for those with food allergies or avoiding allergenic foods

- www.feingold.org
  Proven dietary techniques for better behavior, learning and health

- www.safe-food.org
  Mother's for Natural Law

- www.menumailer.net
  Menu planning service, e-mailed weekly

- www.foodnews.org
  Best & worst produce choices for pesticides

- www.themeatrix.com & www.eatwellguide.org
  Factory farming issues, locate sustainably raised meats & dairy in your area

- www.curezone.com
  Lots of information on cleansing, connect with others in active forums

- www.coopdirectory.org
  Online directory of food co-ops throughout the country

- www.soyonlineservice.co.nz/ & www.wholesoystory.com
  Soy Online Service, uncovering the truth about soy

- www.citizens.org
  Website for Citizens for Health, *a natural health consumer advocacy organization*

- www.thefutureoffood.com
  Fabulous documentary on the topic of genetically modified organisms

- www.supersizeme.com
  Official site for the documentary Super Size Me *& associated info.*

recommended products

- www.juiceplus.com
  Provides nutrition from 17 different fruits, vegetables, and grains in convenient and inexpensive capsule form

- www.youngliving.com
  Source for Berry Young Juice *& therapeutic grade essential oils*

- www.nutriplexformulas.com
  Dr. Vic Shayne's fabulous professional line of whole food supplements

- www.simplycoconut.com
  Order high-quality organic coconut oil, products, recipes, etc.

- www.tahitiannoni.com
  The original, high-quality Tahitian Noni juice

- www.lifeforce-intl.com
  Source for Body Balance *whole food supplement*

recommended books

- *Eating Alive: Prevention Thru Good Digestion*, by Jonn Matsen, N.D.
- *Food is Your Best Medicine*, by Dr. Henry Bieler
- *Sugar Blues*, William Dufty
- *Lick the Sugar Habit*, by Nancy Appleton
- *Caffeine Blues*, by Stephen Cherniske

- *Nutrition and Physical Degeneration*, by Dr. Weston Price
- *The New Whole Foods Encyclopedia*, by Rebecca Wood
- *The False Fat Diet*, by Dr. Elson Haas
- *How to Eat Away Arthritis*, by Lauri Aesoph, N.D.
- *Preventing & Reversing Arthritis Naturally,* by Raquel Martin
- *Healthy Healing,* by Linda Rector Page
- *Fast Food Nation*, by Eric Schlosser
- *Food Politics* and *Food Safety*, both by Marion Nestle
- *Politically Incorrect Nutrition*, by Michael Barbee
- *The Crazy Makers*, by Carol Simontacchi
- *The Wheatgrass Book*, by Ann Wigmore
- *Fit for Life*, by Harvey & Marilyn Diamond
- *The Healing Miracles of Coconut Oil*, by Bruce Fife
- *Excitotoxins*, by Russell Blaylock
- *Battling the MSG Myth,* by Debby Anglesey
- *In Bad Taste: The MSG Syndrome,* by George R. Schwartz, M.D.
- *Eat, Drink & Be Healthy*, by Dr. Walter Willett
- *Our Stolen Future*, by Theo Colburn
- *Hormone Deception: How Everyday Foods and Products Are Disrupting Your Hormones*, by D. Lindsey Berkson
- *Mother Prevent Your Daughters From Getting Breast Cancer,* by Sherrill Sellman
- *Food Fight*, by Kelly Brownell
- *The Mind-Body Makeover Project*, by Michael Gerrish
- *Dr. Abravanel's Body Type Diet*, by Dr. Elliot Abravanel
- *The Five Essential Laws of Eating*, by Grace Purusha (formerly Grace Cropley, available at www. radiantaliveness.com or 808-875-6123)
- *The Whole Soy Story: The Dark Side of America's Favorite Health Food,* by Kaayla T. Daniel, MS, CCN
- *Wheat-Free Recipes & Menus*, by Carol Fenster, Ph.D.
- *The Diet Cure*, by Julia Ross
- *Eat Here: Reclaiming Homegrown Pleasures in a Global Supermarket,* by Brian Halweil
- Books by Dr. Bernard Jensen and books by Gary Null

References 📁

ABC News Special Report: How to Get Fat Without Even Trying, host Peter Jennings, (December 8, 2003), ABC News Productions.

All-You-Can-Eat Economy is Making the World Sick, (Worldwatch Institute News Release, May 24, 2001) – retrieved July, 2001, from http://www.worldwatch.org/alerts/010524.html

Ballentine, Dr. Rudolph, *Diet & Nutrition: A Holistic Approach,* (Honesdale: Himalayan International Institute, 1978.)

Brownell, Kelly D., *Food Fight: The Inside Story of the Food Industy, America's Obesity Crisis, and What We Can Do About It,* (New York: McGraw-Hill, 2004.)

Center for Science in the Public Interest (CSPI), *Diet, ADHD & Behavior: A Quarter Century Review,* (CSPI Pamphlet, 1999) - retrieved January, 2004, from http://www.cspinet.org/new/adhd_resch_bk02.pdf

------ *Food Additives: The Chemical Cuisine,* retrieved August, 2003, from http://www.cspinet.org/reports/chemcuis.htm

------ *A Parent's Guide to Diet, ADHD & Behavior,* (CSPI Pamphlet, 1999) - retrieved January, 2004, from http://www.cspinet.org/new/adhd_bklt.pdf

------ *Studies Show that Diet May Trigger Adverse Behavior in Children: HHS urged to Recommend Dietary Changes as Initial Treatment.* (October 25, 1999) - retrieved November, 2003, from http://www.cspinet.org/new/adhdpr.html

------ *Sugar Intake Hit All-time High in 1999: Government Urged to Recommend Sugar Limits,* (May 18, 2000) – retrieved February, 2004, from http://www.cspinet.org/new/sugar_limit.html

Cherniske, Stephen, *Caffeine Blues: Wake Up to the Hidden Dangers of America's #1 Drug,* (New York: Warner Books, 1998.)

Chronic Disease Overview: Costs of Chronic Disease, National Center for Chronic Disease Prevention and Health Promotion. Retrieved July, 2004 from http//www.cdc.gov/nccdphp/overview.htm

Diamond, Harvey and Marilyn, *Fit for Life II: Living Health,* (New York: Warner Books, 1987.)

Do Artificial Sweeteners Help You Lose Weight? (Nutrition Action Health Letter. Vol. 14, No. 4, May, 1987.)

Food Allergy & Intolerance Facts, retrieved February, 2004, from http://www.savorypalate.com/food_facts.htm

Ford-Martin, Paula. *The Growing Problem of Obesity and Its Impact on Our Kids.* Retrieved July, 2003, from http://diabetes.about.com/library/weekly/aa021901a.htm

Finucan, Brandon & Charlotte Gerson, *Soy: Too Good to be True,* (Gerson Institute Newsletter, Volume 14, #3) – retrieved January, 2004, from http://www.mercola.com/2000/feb/13/more_on_soy.htm

Gardner, Gary and Brian Halwell, *Hunger, Escaping Excess*, (World Watch, July/August, 2000.)

Harvard Center for Cancer Prevention: Cancer Fact Sheet, (April, 2002) - retrieved March, 2004, from http://www.hsph.harvard.edu/cancer/press/archives/cancer_fact.pdf

Jacobson, Michael F., *Liquid Candy How Soft Drinks are Harming Americans' Health*, retrieved December, 2004, from http://www.cspinet.org/sodapop/liquid_candy.htm

Liptak, Adam, *Saving Seeds Subjects Farmers to Suits Over Patent*, (New York Times, November 2, 2003) - retrieved January, 2004, from http://www.organicconsumers.org/ge/tupelo110503.cfm

Liebman, Bonnie, *The Gathering Storm: The Pre-Diabetes Epidemic*, (Nutrition Action Health Letter. Vol. 31, No. 5, June 2004.)

Mercola, Dr. Joseph, *The Potential Dangers of Sucralose*, retrieved February, 2004, from http://www.mercola.com/2000/dec/3/sucralose_dangers.htm

------ *Each Daily Soda Increases Obesity Risk 60%*, (February 28, 2001) – retrieved from http://www.mercola.com/2001/feb/28/obesity_soft_drinks.htm

Myth: Artificial Sweeteners Promote Weight Loss, (University of California, Berkeley Wellness Letter. Vol. 2, Issue 12, Sept. 1986.)

Nestle, Marion, *Food Politics: How the Food Industry Influences Nutrition and Health,* (Berkeley and Los Angeles: University of California Press, 2002.)

Papazian, Ruth. *Sulfites: Safe for Most, Dangerous for Some,* (FDA Consumer Magazine, December, 1996) – retrieved January 2004, from http://www.fda.gov/fdac/features/096_sulf.html

Pollan, Michael, *Power Steer,* (New York Times Magazine, March 31, 2002) – retrieved January, 2004, from http://www.nelivestockalliance.org/news/nytimes33102b.shtml

Quillin, Patrick, *Beating Cancer with Nutrition: Combining the Best of Science and Nature for Full Spectrum Healing in the 21st Century,* (Tulsa: Nutrition Times Press, 2001.)

Schlosser, Eric, *Fast Food Nation: The Dark Side of the All-American Meal,* (New York: HarperCollins Publishers Inc., 2002.)

Simontacchi, Carol, *The Crazy Makers: How the Food Industry is Destroying Our Brains and Harming Our Children,* (New York: Penguin Putnam, 2000.)

Starfield, B., *Is US Health Really the Best In the World,* (JAMA, July 26, 2000)

Statistical Abstract of the United States, (U.S. Census Bureau, 1999.)

Stauber, John and Sheldon Rampton, *Trust Us We're Experts: How Industry Manipulates Science and Gambles with Your Future,* (New York: Penguin Putnam, 2001.)

U.S. Junk Food Intake Worsening, (Annual Experimental Biology 2002 Conference New Orleans, LA April 22, 2002) – retrieved March 2004, from http://www.mercola.com/2002/may/8/junk_food.htm

Willett, Dr. Walter C., Eat Drink & Be Healthy: The Harvard Medical School Guide to Healthy Eating, (New York: Simon & Schuster, 2001.)

Winter, Ruth, *A Consumer's Dictionary of Food Additives,* (New York: Three Rivers Press, 1999.)

~ Index ~

About the Author

Affectionately dubbed the Erin Brockovich of food by her enthusiasts, Kelly Hayford, C.N.C., is on a mission to help people eat better. She delivers the truth about our popular food culture and the devastation it is causing in bite-sized portions the average person can easily swallow, then dishes out no-nonsense nutritional information and practical solutions, which is what people are really hungry for.

Inspired by the successful navigation of her own healing journey, Kelly Hayford is a nutrition and health coach, author, speaker, and healthy lifestyle educator. She has over 16 years experience in the holistic healthcare field and is certified as a nutritional consultant, herbalist, and coach.

As a recovered junk-food junkie formerly in a state of chronic *dis*-ease, Kelly knows what it takes to get from where you are to where you want to be when it comes to diet and health issues. She is committed to helping others achieve optimal health and well-being so that they too can experience a second chance at life. She does this through her *Food Fitness by Phone* healthy eating teleconference programs, in-person lectures, and workshops. Taking a truly holistic approach to healing, Kelly teaches people how to incorporate a combination of nutrition and lifestyle changes, whole food supplements, and cleansing protocols to reverse *dis*-ease, restore health and energy, and successfully navigate their own healing journey.

In addition to her experience in the holistic healthcare field, Kelly holds a Master's degree from the University of Chicago in Cultural Geography; has served as a Peace Corps volunteer in Morocco (TEFL); and has formal training and experience in elementary education. She also continues advanced study in the areas of body-mind healing, nutrition and natural healthcare.

websites: FoodFitnessByPhone.com, WellnessCoaching.com & IfItsNotFoodDontEatIt.com

e-mail: info@FoodFitnessByPhone.com

snail mail: Kelly Hayford, P.O. Box 17394, Boulder, CO 80308-0394